TEACHING 'PROPER' DRINKING?

DRINKING?

CLUBS AND PUBS IN
INDIGENOUS AUSTRALIA

TEACHING 'PROPER' DRINKING?

CLUBS AND PUBS IN INDIGENOUS AUSTRALIA

Maggie Brady

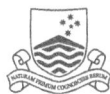

Australian
National
University

PRESS

Centre for Aboriginal Economic Policy Research
College of Arts and Social Sciences
The Australian National University, Canberra

RESEARCH MONOGRAPH NO. 39
2017

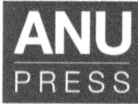

ANU PRESS

Published by ANU Press
The Australian National University
Acton ACT 2601, Australia
Email: anupress@anu.edu.au
This title is also available online at press.anu.edu.au

National Library of Australia Cataloguing-in-Publication entry

Creator: Brady, Maggie, author.

Title: Teaching 'proper' drinking? clubs and pubs in Indigenous Australia / Maggie Brady.

ISBN: 9781760461577 (paperback) 9781760461584 (ebook)

Series: Research monograph (Australian National University. Centre for Aboriginal Economic Policy Research) ; no. 39.

Subjects: Aboriginal Australians--Alcohol use.
Drinking of alcoholic beverages--Australia--attitudes.
Alcohol--Physiological effect.
Alcohol--Social aspects.
Aboriginal Australians--Services for.

Cover design and layout by ANU Press

Cover Image: *Civilisation*, Tommy McRae sketchbook, National Museum of Australia

The writing below the image reads: 'The natives who have been employed at shearing time on some station and have taken out their wages in plenty goodfellow clothes and made themselves along a whitefellow swell. The Australian natives are very fond of copying whitemen's manners in dress when they can manage to do so.'

Contents

List of figures

List of maps

List of tables

List of abbreviations

AA	Alcoholics Anonymous
AAA	Aboriginal Alcoholics Anonymous
AAFR	Alcohol Awareness and Family Recovery
ADC	Aboriginal Development Commission
ATSIC	Aboriginal and Torres Strait Islander Commission
CAA	Council for Aboriginal Affairs
CAAAPU	Central Australian Aboriginal Alcohol Planning Unit
CAAC	Central Australian Aboriginal Congress
CAEPR	Centre for Aboriginal Economic Policy Research
CDC	Commercial Development Corporation
CMS	Church Missionary Society
DAA	Department of Aboriginal Affairs
FASD	Fetal alcohol spectrum disorder
HRSCAA	House of Representatives Standing Committee on Aboriginal Affairs
IBA	Indigenous Business Australia
KALACC	Kimberley Aboriginal Law and Culture Centre
LHA	Laynhapuy Homelands Association Inc.
LWA	Living with Alcohol
MLG	Management Liaison Group
MSC	Missionaries of the Sacred Heart Mission

NPY	Ngaanyatjarra, Pitjantjatjara, Yankunytjatjara
NTER	Northern Territory Emergency Response
ORIC	Office of the Registrar of Indigenous Corporations
PRHA	People's Refreshment Houses Association
RLPC	Renmark Local Progress Committee
SAFA	Student Action for Aborigines
UAM	United Aborigines Mission
UCNA	United Church in North Australia
WAA	Women Against Alcohol
WCTU	Woman's Christian Temperance Union

Preface

Since the repeal of the state liquor regulations in Australia that prevented Aboriginal and Torres Strait Islander peoples from having legal access to alcohol, numerous strategies have attempted to minimise the harms associated with problem drinking. This book tells the story of how governments, their advisers and Indigenous people themselves believed they could minimise such harms by changing the way people drank: how they tried to 'civilise' the drinking act itself. In a sense, this endeavour started in 1789 when Governor Arthur Phillip first taught the captured Aboriginal man Bennelong to raise his wine glass in a toast; however, it was two centuries before the notion found its way into policy in the form of government-endorsed liquor outlets serving Indigenous people in or near remote communities. In the 1970s and 1980s, canteens and clubs were licensed to serve rations of beer in remote Indigenous communities, and government agencies made it possible for Indigenous organisations to purchase public hotels whose sales were affecting their communities. These two approaches to the distribution of alcohol were originally driven by the belief that drinking on regulated premises over which Indigenous people had some control would help to inculcate moderate drinking patterns, and help to prevent damaging binge drinking and sly grog sales. This idea, that people would be able to 'learn to drink' in a conducive setting, forms a narrative thread throughout this book.

Both of these somewhat controversial approaches (having drinking clubs and purchasing hotels) attempted to manage Indigenous drinking by making the sale of alcohol a *social enterprise* that drew in community members as participants, and ostensibly benefited them by allowing them to share in the income generated by alcohol sales. The idea that these outlets could help to cultivate moderate 'civilised' drinking patterns while simultaneously making a profit created a number of moral and social dilemmas and unforeseen outcomes that also form a major theme for the book. Indigenous social clubs and hotels were social enterprises insofar as they were (and are) run (or at least advised) by community-based organisations with participatory governance structures that gave voice to community stakeholders. Perhaps most importantly, as quasi-social enterprises, these projects were intended to benefit their owners by reinvesting profits in charitable or community-led activities. Even if a club or a hotel could not make a profit, the money they spent on wages and other locally sourced production costs would stay in the community.

Some of these ideas about reducing drunkenness by regularising drinking venues, making local citizens shareholders and allocating profits for the betterment of the community had been popular in nineteenth-century Europe. The Swedish 'Gothenburg' system, for example, was a style of alcohol control based on the municipal or community ownership of liquor outlets. Designed to improve standards of behaviour and to civilise uproarious drinking, the Gothenburg system offered an alternative to prohibition by emphasising moderation, and downplayed profiteering by employing 'disinterested' managers who had no pecuniary interest in alcohol sales. As documented in this book, the idea of community ownership of hotels was disseminated from Sweden to Britain and later to Australia where the (non-Indigenous) citizens of several rural South Australian towns purchased their local public hotels as co-operative ventures. I use the principles of the Gothenburg system and its variations as an analytical framework with which to examine the case studies presented in the second part of the book.

This book is based on fieldwork conducted in Indigenous communities and towns in northern and central Australia, visits to community hotels in South Australia and interviews with Indigenous and non-Indigenous protagonists and knowledgeable observers. It also makes use of documentary evidence from reports, archives, local libraries and newspapers. The book contributes to three fields of scholarship: it is a socio-historical study of alcohol; it examines the history of Australian Indigenous policy; and it constitutes a study of social enterprise.

The opening chapter examines the social history of the idea that people can learn to drink in moderation: that drinking, along with other aspects of personal comportment, can be 'civilised'. The work of Norbert Elias sets the scene here. An example from early Australia illustrates the rudimentary attempts made by elites to impart the rules of cultured, moderate comportment around food and drink to the representatives of the invaded Aboriginal groups encountered during the first days of colonisation.

Offering alcohol to Aboriginal people in and around Sydney Cove, and seeing how they responded and how quickly they could learn, was a test of how amenable they might be to 'civilisation' and assimilation. The chapter continues by addressing the more modern formulation of the idea of learning to drink that arose in the 1930s and 1940s following the end of Prohibition in the United States (US) (1920–1933) and restrictive war-time policies in other countries. At this time, with the influence of the temperance movement waning, the public wanted an alternative to abstinence. By the 1960s, behavioural psychologists working in addiction programs began to experiment in teaching alcoholics and others with drinking problems how to control their drinking. I argue that this thinking, together with the idea that drinking was a *learned* behaviour, permeated the Australian policy approaches to Indigenous drinking that accompanied the repeal of alcohol prohibitions.

Since the 1830s in Australia, legislation had created a number of prohibitions attached to the possession and consumption of alcohol by people classified as Aboriginal as well as people of mixed descent, Torres Strait and Pacific Islanders. Following federation, these became state or territory laws that varied by jurisdiction and applied differentially to Indigenous people depending on their perceived degree of assimilation and where they lived. This form of race-based 'prohibition' in Australia thus differed markedly from the National Prohibition Act (the Volstead Act) enacted in the US in 1920, which involved amendments to the Constitution, grew out of local option laws and was the culmination of a politically effective social movement led by the Anti-Saloon League and the Woman's Christian Temperance Union (WCTU). The Volstead Act was repealed in 1933 following the election of Franklin D Roosevelt and the loss of popular support.

In Australia, the 'prohibition' laws affecting Indigenous people were repealed in each state and territory between 1957 and 1972. This was accompanied by the gradual removal of racial discrimination from state laws and the recognition of Indigenous civil rights. However, there were (and are) exceptions. Despite the official end of the prohibition on selling or serving alcohol to Aboriginal people, some publicans continued to refuse them service in a variety of overt or covert ways: in the 1980s, several Aboriginal non-government organisations explicitly requested licensees to desist from selling alcohol to members of their communities; and in the Northern Territory in particular, but in other regions as well, some Aboriginal communities continue to apply their own local 'prohibition' laws and maintain their lands as dry areas by choice.

Chapter 2 traces how the Gothenburg ideas of alcohol control were disseminated to Britain, the US and ultimately to Australia. In the late nineteenth century, local citizens of several towns along the Murray River bought hotels to raise funds for local causes and to diminish sly grog sales. They raised funds through their personal resources or bank loans and 12 premises were purchased in South Australia: nine of the original 12 are still in community hands. In a parallel but separate development that began in the mid-1970s, several Indigenous community associations also bought hotels, usually in an attempt to curtail the troublesome sales practices of their owners. To make the purchases, Aboriginal groups obtained loans or grants from various Aboriginal economic development funds, first established by the Australian Government in 1968. I pay particular attention to the Aboriginal Development Commission (ADC), appointed and funded from 1980 to 1989, and its successor agencies. I present case studies of these enterprises later in the book. Chapter 2 continues by outlining how the investment policies pursued by Indigenous business and development agencies changed over time, forcing some enterprises to concentrate on commercial rather than socially responsible goals; with alcohol as the commodity, this indifference to social objectives sometimes had undesirable outcomes. Reference is also made to kava, a mood-altering substance over which an Aboriginal association held licensing and distribution rights. Like the Gothenburg system, the arrangement created a monopoly, raised revenue that was distributed for community benefit and created an antidote to illegal sales.

At around the time of the first experiments in Aboriginal ownership of hotels, some Australian state and territory governments encouraged remote communities to establish beer canteens and licensed social clubs as a means to communicate moderate and sociable drinking behaviour to Aboriginal people who were adjusting to newly granted drinking rights. Many of these enterprises evolved from the beer rationing systems through which 'native administration' officials had hoped to inculcate moderate drinking patterns. Chapter 3 deals with this episode in policy thinking: it focuses on the influence of government advisers, community superintendents and missionaries that led to the birth of these clubs and the mixed motivations that underpinned their development. Primary among these motivations was the belief that Aboriginal people could 'learn' to drink in more acceptable ways if they were presented with limited amounts of alcohol in pleasant settings—a reprise of earlier ideas about the so-called civilising process of the eighteenth century, about managing the post-Prohibition era of the 1930s in the US and about adopting middle-class norms in the 1950s. In the Australian Indigenous policy context, it was an exercise in assimilation.

The second part of the book (Chapters 4 to 7) presents case studies of community-based clubs and community-owned pubs to illustrate how theories of community and citizen ownership and notions of teaching moderate drinking were put into practice. In Chapter 4, I describe the Murrinh Patha Social Club, one of the earliest of its kind, instigated by Catholic missionaries at what was then known as Port Keats, now Wadeye, in the Northern Territory. The Tyeweretye Club, the topic of Chapter 5, was located in a town (Alice Springs) rather than in a remote community. Instigated by an Aboriginal non-government organisation, the club was designed to provide a convivial and non-racist drinking venue for Aboriginal town dwellers and visitors from outlying communities alike. Both clubs were intended to cultivate moderate drinking styles, but only Tyeweretye achieved this goal, and then only partially. I relate how each of these clubs became the subject of vigorous resistance, primarily from Aboriginal women's groups' campaigns against grog in all its forms, and analyse why neither club survived for much longer than a decade.

Chapter 6, 'Indigenous communities buy hotels', describes the sequence of hotel purchases made by, or on behalf of, Indigenous organisations— an initiative that started in 1975, before the advent of Aboriginal development agencies. Some of these projects, such as the Oasis Hotel at Walgett and the Woden Town Club in Canberra, both funded in the 1980s by the ADC, proved to be disastrous and short lived. By contrast, other premises, such as the Transcontinental Hotel at Oodnadatta and the licensed roadhouse at Mt Ebenezer in the Northern Territory, have lasted for a decade or more. The chapter is primarily made up of observational and interview data from fieldwork visits, but also pieces together the fragmented documentary record on these enterprises. Chapter 7, 'The Indigenous purchase of the Crossing Inn', is a case study of a 'community' hotel in Fitzroy Crossing, one of a suite of enterprises purchased by an Indigenous investment company representing the peoples of the Fitzroy Valley, Western Australia, with funds from the ADC. Despite early hopes that ownership of the hotel would constrain sales and 'civilise' drinking, there were accidental and deliberate deaths, hundreds of injuries and cases of violence against women; there was also an increase in alcohol-related damage to unborn children. By 2007, the situation was so serious that the State Coroner conducted an inquest into 22 deaths in the region (many of which implicated the Crossing Inn): two courageous Aboriginal women sparked a grassroots movement to petition for an end to the inn's takeaway sales; the director of liquor licensing imposed restrictions on sales; and child health experts called for a major study of fetal alcohol spectrum disorders. I analyse how the original ambition for the hotel to be a crucible for moderate drinking was thwarted by the investment policies of the Indigenous business and development agencies that funded the project, as well as by the hotel's own Indigenous controlling body. The concluding chapter reminds the reader of the major themes that make up the book.

A number of questions have pursued me throughout this research. Can people learn to drink differently? Do the social clubs introduced into some remote communities help to cultivate moderate drinking styles, or do they make things worse? Is Indigenous ownership of pubs in small country towns a viable and sustainable strategy to bring about local control over sales? Does such ownership provide the economic and social benefits envisaged by the Indigenous proponents of such enterprises? As well as answering these questions, I want this book to show how a policy of 'self-determination' encouraged a certain type of engagement between Indigenous people and the supply and sale of alcohol.

Acknowledgements

An Australian Research Council QEII Fellowship (DP 0772382) funded this research, which was undertaken at the Centre for Aboriginal Economic Policy Research (CAEPR) at The Australian National University. An ANU Press Publication Subsidy contributed to editing costs. I thank the centre directors, Jon Altman, John Taylor, Matthew Gray and Jerry Schwab, for their support during the project; professional staff, Denise Steele and Tracy Deasey; and my co-investigator, Boyd Hunter, with whom I had many lively discussions about the economics of the Gothenburg system. The project was conducted, with some interruptions, between 2008 and 2014.

Fieldwork for the project took me primarily to Western Australia, South Australia and the Northern Territory, where many people gave generously of their time and ideas. I am grateful for the help I received in and around Fitzroy Crossing from Grant Akesson, Bill Arthur, Emily Carter, Maureen Carter, Patrick Green, June Oscar, Ron Radford, John Rodrigues and Kathryn Thorburn. In South Australia, the managers of several community-owned hotels (as well as local historians) kindly received me and answered questions, including Verity Wyld (Nuriootpa), Robyn Cusick (Loxton), Peter and Carla Magarey (Loxton), Pauline Mitchell (Loxton), Tony Hogan (Streaky Bay) and David Carr (Ceduna). I also appreciate the help provided by Reverend Paul Albrecht, Richard Bradshaw, Margaret Bain, Chris Charles, Andrew Duguid (deceased), Reverend Bill Edwards (deceased), Tom Gara, Pamela Lyon and John Summers.

I would like to thank long-term residents, honorary residents, fieldworkers and colleagues in the Northern Territory for giving me their time with such patience. They include two venerable Territorians who have since died, Reverend Jim Downing and Father John Leary, as well as others who are very much alive: Bob Durnan, Shirley Hendy, Jane Lloyd,

Elizabeth Moore, Anne Mosey, David Nash, Jane Simpson and Gill Shaw. Thanks also to the Northern Land Council staff in Timber Creek, to Kim Barber, Britta Duelke, Jonathan Hunyor of the North Australian Aboriginal Justice Agency and Colin McDonald QC. Bill Ivory and John Taylor were of great help during my visit to Wadeye. In 2013, I spent time at the Centre for Addiction and Mental Health in London, Ontario, Canada, and thank Marg Rylett and Kate Graham for updating me on alcohol-control measures in First Nations communities. I visited the Nk'Mip Spirit Ridge First Nations winery in Osoyoos, British Columbia, with the assistance of Willie Waddell.

A number of people read and checked specific chapters or parts of the text: many thanks for doing so to John Boulton, Xavier Desmarchelier, Mike Dillon, Bill Ivory, Stephen J Kunitz, John Taylor, Michael Thorn and Kaely Woods. My errors are my own. I am immensely grateful to Robin Room whose work has always inspired me and who has been unstinting in his support and interest in these topics. Carol Watson and Peter Murray have long been friends and colleagues, full of wisdom and ideas about all alcohol-related issues, as well as being generous hosts in Alice Springs. I owe a huge debt to Tim Rowse whose detailed reading and numerous perceptive suggestions enabled me to knock the book into much better shape than it would have been otherwise. Thanks to my official readers; to Frances Morphy at CAEPR who has been a patient adviser; and to my friends, Julie, Dave, Nic, Ros, Jacquie, Jake, Pat and Jim, for their support. This book is for Alan, who was here at the start and who would have savoured the finish.

1

Learning to drink: The social history of an idea

The idea that you could teach people to drink sensibly has been around for decades. In the United States, this notion was of particular interest after the end of Prohibition in 1933,[1] prompted by the challenge of encouraging moderation after years of binge drinking, criminal gangs selling illicit grog, adulterated drinks and speakeasies.[2] One who rose to the challenge was American etiquette aficionado Alma Whitaker (1933: 2), who endeavoured to communicate to post-Prohibition drinkers what older, more experienced countries knew about the 'precious creed' of moderation. In her aptly titled book *Bacchus behave! The lost art of polite drinking*, she stressed the need to appreciate the sacred rituals of etiquette to experience the benefits of wines and spirits as social lubricants. In this way, we could *learn* to drink and, 'properly fortified with instructive information, we may yet learn to carry our liquor like gentlemen. It's deucedly messy when we don't' (2). Whitaker declared that the 'right quantity imbibed under the right conditions affords a pleasant stimulation', while people who became drunk revealed all their nastier

---

1 Prohibition (1920–33) was a political failure, but was positive in other ways. There is good evidence that there was less drinking and abuse than before World War I; the cirrhosis mortality rate dropped sharply then plateaued, as did the alcoholism mortality rate. There was a differential affect across social classes and across regions: while the law was flouted in the north and east (and in New Orleans), the working-class people of the south and west were largely dry (Cook 2007: 26).
2 Speakeasy: an illicit drinking venue of the Prohibition years.

inhibitions (4–5).[3] She believed that women had a civilising influence on men and that they would be an important influence in post-Prohibition America. Above all, Whitaker argued that it was deplorable to drink enough to become beyond one's self. To avoid any such loss of composure, her first simple rule of behaviour was never to get drunk. Intoxication has remained morally reprehensible, or at least questionable, in most public discourse throughout the modern period (Room 2005: 149). However, rather than banishing alcohol altogether, societies have held out hope that neophyte drinkers, as well as established drinkers with bad habits, could learn or re-learn 'civilised' moderate drinking. In the 1970s, behavioural research suggested that this would indeed be possible. Many of these ideas permeated Australian governments' thinking about the potential solutions to problem drinking among Indigenous people.

Taming undisciplined consumption

In the tradition of books of manners through the ages, Whitaker (1933) not only advised on personal comportment, but also provided advice on being a good guest, serving the right sort of food and drink for particular occasions and which customs should be frowned upon. By the time she was writing, the cultures of the West had come to despise a lack of self-control and to attribute success and respectability—indeed morality itself—to the power of a disciplined will (Room 1985: 135). However, the qualities of self-constraint and control over one's conduct were not innate: they had to be conditioned in people and *produced* through the internalisation of socially constructed rules of politeness and good manners. Norbert Elias (1982) described how this conditioning—the 'civilising process', as he called it—required the pacification of the individual and the absorption into social norms of notions of bodily propriety, cleanliness and order, so that people came to believe that these represented the features of a good and proper life (Frykman & Löfgren 1987). These notions had their origins in post-medieval European courtly society, during a transformative period that served as a bridge between the Middle Ages and modernity, as observed by Elias (1982) in his analysis of books on manners and the concept of *civilité*.[4] During this period, manners among the elite were softened to

---

3   I am grateful to Robin Room for alerting me to Alma Whitaker's book and to the work of Morris Chafetz and others.
4   *Civilité*: civility, politeness, courtesy.

distinguish them from the coarse manners of peasants. At the same time, outward manifestations of bodily propriety came to be seen as expressions of the inner, whole person. These 'civilised' ways of comporting oneself were elaborated further among the elite in the eighteenth and nineteenth centuries. Eventually, these behaviours became transformed into the dominant, mainstream culture of modern European society. In fact, they became the norms of Western middle-class culture: second nature. Elias (1978) saw civilisation both as a process and a concept. As a concept, it was a self-conscious construct by the 'West' in which European society came to believe itself to be superior to earlier societies, as well as to contemporary but more 'primitive' ones (3–4). In their analysis of the making of the middle-class world view of nineteenth-century Swedes, Jonas Frykman and Orvar Löfgren (1987) went further, suggesting that barbarism was eliminated by using health as ammunition in the civilising process: a civilised person had to be convinced that if he or she transgressed or failed to internalise social norms, then he or she would actually come to physical harm (255). In this way, 'civilised' people who worried about their physical as well as their spiritual health had to watch themselves; they had to be clean, wholesome, of good conduct and exert self-discipline. By contrast, 'uncivilised', unconstrained, rowdy comportment (such as uproarious drinking among peasants) demonstrated a heedlessness of the consequences.

In pre-industrial England, daily drinking was the means by which social relations were both generated and reinforced. Among the labouring classes, there was a mutual obligation to treat others with drinks, as it was through this giving and exchanging of drinks that people established and remade the social ties of obligation and reciprocity. For English villagers, these symbolic values were more important than the possibility of a drunken accident or a bad hangover; not to drink was virtually unheard of, as it would represent a complete withdrawal from socially meaningful existence (Adler 1991: 381, Schivelbusch 1993).[5] These descriptions of the symbolic meanings attached to alcohol in English village society prior to 1830 bear remarkable similarity to the meaning of drinking among many Aboriginal people in Australia today. For Aboriginal people, as for eighteenth-century English villagers, the integrity of social relations rest on claims to rights and the fulfilment of mutual obligations that are

---

5   The same was true of colonial Sydney, according to an account by F Fowler in 1859, in which 'not to drink is considered a crime. *Aut bibat, aut abeat*—which means, in Australia, if you will not "stand" you may walk' (Birch & Macmillan 1962: 156–7).

often prior to other considerations. With the advent of modern industrial society in Europe, there was additional reason to subdue the excesses of the labouring classes, often expressed through unrestrained drinking at carnivals and festivals as well as shared daily drinking. Rural labouring work, such as haymaking and sheep shearing, had been punctuated by four or five meal breaks a day accompanied by pints of strong beer, but this could not occur in a factory, for the timing, location and style of this kind of drinking threatened the orderly development of industrial production. A new industrial workforce had to learn the disciplines of punctuality, routine and perseverance (Adler 1991). It became necessary to quarantine drinking, confining it to acceptable physical and temporal limits, and to create a separate sphere for leisure time. By the late eighteenth century, the eight-hour day was widely adopted in industries in Britain and Australia (Melbourne, in particular, was a focus of eight-hour day activism) and this helped indirectly to create the notion of recreational time and, with it, a burgeoning of alternatives and counterattractions to drinking for members of the public: sport, outdoor activities, dancing and museums.

Modern societies expect that adults will respect the divide between work and leisure: adults are expected to be soberly attentive and conscientious when in charge of small children, when driving, using machinery and at work (Room 2011). Of great assistance in this project was the temperance movement that arose in England and America (and Australia) in the nineteenth century. By preaching discipline, sobriety and self-control, the temperance movement's urgings dovetailed well with the needs of an emergent industrial economy. Indeed, by discouraging workers from spending their wages at the tavern, and by encouraging a middle-class home life and promoting thrift, temperance became a vehicle for the transmission of a middle-class domestic ideology (Adler 1991, Kociumbas 1995, Burnett 1999). Ideas of temperance and moderation helped to create a domestic market for consumer goods; there would, after all, be more cash and leisure time available to devote to buying things. The temperance movement itself was class conscious: wine, for example, (considered a civilised drink consumed by the educated classes) was not often singled out for condemnation, whereas 'spirituous liquors' (preferred by the lower orders) were. Reflecting this inclination, the temperance movement initially called for moderation, thus allowing for the consumption of wine rather than complete abstinence. It was only later in the nineteenth century that temperance advocates rejected social drinking altogether and promoted abstinence from all alcoholic beverages.

For employers, controlling their workers' alcohol consumption and giving support to temperance activities were ways in which they could improve productivity and ensure a healthy industrial labour force. This explains why, in late nineteenth-century England, several villages and 'garden cities' were built by industrialists for their workers. It also explains why these complexes not only provided appropriate accommodation for the workers, but were often designed to be alcohol-free towns, equipped with dry 'temperance' hotels (Howard 1902). The socially reformist businessmen and philanthropists of the time genuinely wanted to improve the living conditions and quality of life of their workers, but they also wanted to secure and protect their labour force from the evils of drink.[6] For example, chocolate maker John Cadbury (2010) was a Quaker and a supporter of the temperance movement who eventually became a total abstainer. To house his chocolate-factory workers, he built the 'model' village of Bournville near Birmingham in the 1890s. As a result of his influence, Bournville remained free from pubs and off-licence sales until recently, although it did have two licensed working men's clubs.[7] In Cheshire, William Lever created a planned village ('Port Sunlight') to accommodate workers at the nearby Lever Brothers Sunlight soap factory. The social reformer Joseph Rowntree, who was a member of another chocolate and confectionary-making family, believed that temperance would improve the lot of the working classes. He later became a supporter of the Swedish Gothenburg system of municipal or community control over alcohol sales as a means of diminishing drunkenness. Like these philanthropic capitalists in Britain, the teetotaller Chaffey brothers in Australia tried to protect their workforce by making their 'irrigation colony' on the border between Victoria and South Australia alcohol free. When this became unworkable because of sly grog sales, Gothenburg-style community-owned hotels were deemed the lesser of two evils and several were opened in South Australia. The idea that a more controlled hotel environment would trammel citizens' excess drinking, thereby helping them to learn to drink in a more civilised manner, flourished. This 'lesser of two evils' thinking also influenced the repeal of prohibition for Indigenous Australians, provoking experiments

---

6   In Austria, supporters of workers' temperance, including 'socialist teetotallers' such as Viktor Adler, were, in effect, trying to 'impose a bourgeois-puritanical model on the working class' largely for political rather than health reasons (Schivelbusch 1993: 166).

7   In September 2015, in a controversial decision, a local shopkeeper was granted the first licence for 120 years to sell takeaway alcohol in Bournville (Finnigan 2015).

in social learning in the form of beer rations in canteens and fostering hopes for controls over sales by having Indigenous people themselves take on ownership of licensed hotels.

The 'civilising' toast

In the earliest days of the colony of New South Wales, only the most cursory attempt was made to mould or curtail the drinking behaviour of Aboriginal people. Indeed, it appears that some early colonists and visitors freely offered alcoholic beverages to Aboriginal people, as they would have to other colonists, probably assuming that Aboriginal people did not need to 'learn' about alcohol. Peter Mancall (1995) suggested that this was the case in North America too: when English explorers encountered Algonquian leaders, they greeted them with wine, meat and bread (43).[8]

Within a few days of arriving at Botany Bay in January 1788, a British second lieutenant on board the First Fleet offered a glass of wine to two spear-bearing Aboriginal men they met on the shore. Philip Gidley King (1980: 34–5) of HMS *Sirius* wrote in his private journal:

> Governor Phillip then went up another branch & I followed the one we were in, & soon perceived that the natives were following us, we soon came to the head of this inlet where we perceived the same party of Indians, wading over, we rowed up to them & many of them came up to the boat, we made them a few more presents, but found it necessY [sic] to put a stop to our generosity as they were increasing fast in numbers & having only a boats crew with me I was apprehensive that they might find means to surprise us as every one of them were armed with lances, & short bludgeons—I gave two of them a glass of Wine which they had no sooner tasted than they spit it out, and we asked them the name of a number of articles.[9]

---

8   Of course, there are numerous historical accounts from Australia and elsewhere of alcohol being forced upon Indigenous people in an uncharitable and prurient manner to deliberately provoke inebriation and spectacle.

9   For an Aboriginal oral history version of this story, see Brady (2008) and Bertie (1924).

King's tone in this description was entirely matter-of-fact: he was simply trying to make contact. He offered wine: they spat it out; he asked for some vocabulary.[10] Similarly, accounts of the first meetings between Tasmanian Aboriginal people and the men of Nicolas Baudin's two ships, the *Geographe* and the *Naturaliste,* suggest that alcohol was offered without ill-intent. The Frenchmen, Baudin (1974: 318) wrote, frequently embraced the 'naturels' and on numerous occasions offered them food and drink (bread, fish, brandy and arrack from Mauritius). They also danced together and the Frenchmen performed tricks, sang and played instruments.[11]

These early Europeans who offered wine or spirits may not have fully realised that the people they encountered in Australia or North America and elsewhere did not have any comparably strong alcoholic drinks of their own. While we now know that Aboriginal people in some regions did make mildly alcoholic fermented drinks, they had no strong alcoholic drinks (e.g. as strong as wine) prior to contact with outsiders (Brady 2008). It is likely that early visitors assumed that some form of liquor did in fact exist, if only because they had experienced such drinks in other locations in the region. Mariners, such as James Cook and Dumont d'Urville, had been offered (and had consumed) the narcotic drink kava, used widely in Melanesia and Polynesia, and may have thought that the native Australians had something similar. In the Malay Archipelago to Australia's north, on the island of Savu and at ports such as Kupang and Batavia, Europeans had drunk locally made palm wine, mild toddies and strong spirits, such as aniseed-flavoured arrack, and they also would have observed local people chewing betel nut and smoking opium.

As the colonisation project proceeded at Port Jackson, there were instances in which Europeans offered alcohol to Aboriginal people as a test of their level of civilisation and as a 'civilising' gesture—an active experiment across cultures in the teaching of manners surrounding food and drink. Alcoholic beverages, particularly wine, were understood to be

---

10   It seems a little surprising to us now that an exploratory party about to land on an alien and potentially threatening shore would even have wine on board, but this was apparently common, especially when water was unpredictable and scarce. In May 1788, George Worgan (1978: 45), also of the *Sirius,* described taking a 'delightful excursion' up the harbour in which his party partook of cold kangaroo pie, plum pudding and a bottle of wine.

11   However, the Tasmanians (and, indeed, Aboriginal people in other parts of Australia) frequently rejected the food and drink offered to them by Europeans; even food that was recognisable to them, such as fish, was treated with suspicion (Plomley 1983). Europeans were disconcerted and puzzled by such refusals.

a natural feature of such an endeavour. From medieval times in Europe, the conditioning of polite behaviours was just one aspect of the overall civilising process designed to improve the peasants and the lower orders, as Elias's (1978, 1982) work demonstrates. In the eighteenth century, it was considered desirable to avoid public displays of passionate anger, hot temper and drunkenness, and women were to be treated with respect and decorum (Gascoigne 2002: 149, Salmond 2003: 393).[12] People had to learn the rules of behaviour expected at the table: for example, how one should sit (with a goblet and a well-cleaned knife on the right, the bread on the left) and how one should lift food to the mouth by means of a fork, rather than fingers (it was considered 'uncivilised' to put food into one's mouth with fingers, even from one's own plate—a rule that had little to do with the danger of illness and more to do with being seen in society with dirty fingers) (Elias 1978: 126). An important part of the spread of courtly manners to the broader populace in the early eighteenth century was drinking to the health of guests:

> It is civil and decent for a prince to drink first to the health of those he is entertaining, and then to offer them the same glass or goblet usually filled with the same wine … nor is it a lack of politeness in them to drink from the same glass, but a mark of candour and friendship. (93)

These manners and rules of comportment communicated distinction, refinement and social civility. It seems to have been relatively common for sea captains, such as Arthur Phillip and James Cook, to selectively invite certain 'natives' or chiefs to dine with them on board their vessels or onshore.[13] In Tonga, a chief joined Cook for a dinner of fish and a glass of wine (Salmond 2003: 217). In Tahiti in 1773, Cook invited local chiefs Tu and To'ofa to take dinner on board his ship. Tu, who had already learned European manners, showed To'ofa how to use a knife and fork, and how to salt his meat and drink wine from a glass (248). Similarly, at Sydney Cove, Governor Phillip invited Aboriginal 'chiefs' to dine with him at his house: Arabanoo was first in December 1788; a year later, Bennelong

---

12   Despite an overall lack of rights for women in Europe, the status of women was considered an indicator of social development; it is significant, then, that diarists of colonial Australia frequently referred to the downtrodden position of Indigenous women (Gascoigne 2002: 149).

13   Although James Cook was brought up as a Quaker, he evidently had no qualms about offering strong alcoholic drinks to the indigenous people he encountered on his travels, including children. In 1773, he gave three glasses of wine to a sulking 14-year-old Maori boy, making him very drunk (Salmond 2003: 187).

and Colbee were invited.[14] By then, the distinction between savagery and civilisation had become entrenched in the thinking of European colonists. In inviting Bennelong and Colbee to dine with them, the English hoped that their 'dinner-table diplomacy' would serve as a civilising influence, facilitating peaceful dealings with the 'natives' (McIntyre 2008: 39.6).

It seems likely that there were mixed motives behind some of these invitations—especially considering that the Aboriginal 'guests' had been taken into the settlement by force. The invitations were intended to facilitate good relations and to demonstrate the superior customs of English society; however, they were also designed to test the alacrity with which Aboriginal people could learn such manners and habits and thus, ultimately, be amenable to assimilation and civilisation. When Aboriginal guests observed and mimicked English manners, it pleased their hosts. Arabanoo, for example, reportedly used his cup and saucer 'well' when taking tea with the governor (Hunter 1968: 132). King was surprised and pleased that Bennelong was so polite, imitating all the actions and gestures of every person in the governor's family, 'bowing, drinking healths, returning thanks, etc. with the most scrupulous attention'; this was considered remarkable, especially given the 'state of nature he has been brought up in' (Hunter 1968: 405). The English dressed him in trousers and a red woollen cloth jacket. An initiated Wanghal man, Bennelong (Woollewarre) not only accepted Phillip's hospitality, he also formed a relationship with the Englishman, sometimes calling him Been-en-aa ('father'), perhaps in an attempt to find a place for Phillip and his officers in the traditional kinship system (Smith 2001). As Isobel McBryde (2000) has pointed out, Governor Phillip and Bennelong needed each other to gain advantage and to ensure the survival of their respective groups, and they manoeuvred around each other to achieve this (254).

Introducing the ritual of raising glasses of wine to drink toasts to health was a key feature of such interchanges and was often mentioned by diarists. Toasting reached a peak of popularity in the late eighteenth and early nineteenth centuries and drinking to the health of the King of England was the most common toast of the time. In Tahiti, for the observation of the Transit of Venus in 1769, Cook and Banks, celebrating the King's

14 On many occasions in the early colony, Aboriginal people refused to consume the food and drink offered to them. Arabanoo initially only drank water and refused bread and salt-meat; later he became an 'avid' drinker of tea. Bennelong's wife, Barangaroo, refused to taste wine (Tench 1996: 96, Hunter 1968, cf. Baudin 1974: 305).

birthday, invited Tupaia, the Polynesian navigator, and others, on board. Tupaia drank all the toasts to 'Kihiargo' (King George) and became enormously drunk (Salmond 2003: 80, cf. MacAndrew & Edgerton 1969: 43).[15] Another Tahitian, Mai, taken back to London on the *Adventure* in 1774, showed his prowess with English customs by learning to ice skate and play chess; he also drank to the health of 'King George!' whenever toasts were proposed (Salmond 2003: 297). At Sydney Cove, wine was offered at Phillip's dinners, but only Bennelong accepted the drink and learned to raise his glass and drink to the King—a process that he called '*daging*'. George Barrington, in his 'impartial and circumstantial narrative' of life at Botany Bay, reported that Bennelong:

> Having observed, when at the governor's house, his majesty's health drank in the first glass after dinner, and had been taught to repeat the word before he drank his own glass, he imagined the liquor was called the king: and when he afterwards came to know that it was wine, yet he would frequently call it king. (Rickard 2001: 92)

Bennelong later realised that wine itself was not really called *daging*, but he continued to make a joke of his mistake and to refer to wine in that way, knowing it would provoke a response (Smith 2001, McIntyre 2008).[16] Bennelong was described at the time by diarists such as Watkin Tench and King as someone who drank socially and who held his liquor well; it was later that he either became or was labelled a 'heavy drinker' (Collins 1971, Kenny 1973, Smith 2001: 44).[17] It is ironic that Bennelong was later stereotyped as the first Aboriginal drunk (*Sydney Gazette* 1813, Kenny 1973): he should be remembered for the much more significant reason of being the first Aboriginal individual to have been taught Europe's most important drinking ritual: the toast (Schivelbusch 1993: 169). Not only is it the oldest European drinking custom (dating to at least the sixth century), bearing magical and cultic associations, but it also communicated aspects of 'civilising' behaviour.[18] Toasting acknowledged

---

15   Although, on this occasion, Tupaia and the other Tahitians did accept wine and become intoxicated, it appears they disliked the experience and their distaste for alcohol lasted several years (MacAndrew & Edgerton 1969).

16   In time, the term '*daging*' (meaning alcohol) was taken up by Aboriginal people across a wide area of New South Wale (Troy 1994: 48).

17   As it turned out, the civilising 'project' around Bennelong was a failure from the British point of view. In David Collins's (1971, vol II: 134) last reference to Bennelong, he reported that by 1798 Bennelong preferred the 'rude and dangerous' society of his own countrymen instead of living 'peaceably and pleasantly' at the governor's residence.

18   For cultural variations in drinking customs and toasting styles, see Douglas (1987). See also Schivelbusch (1993).

and celebrated the sovereign as well as old and new lands and the countries of foreign guests—it remembered absent friends and it honoured, linked and integrated those present. A toast could seal a mutual pact and acknowledge mutual dependence. As Julie McIntyre (2012) points out, while Bennelong must have absorbed the power of meaning contained in the triumphal tone of the toasts, he would not have realised that, by toasting the King, the colonists were also toasting empire and thus the inexorable dispossession of the Indigenous people (42).

Toasting punctuated meals and, because it was (and is) associated with the consumption of food, served to moderate, somewhat, the amount of alcohol consumed; however, it was certainly not always thus. In the early days of the colony of New South Wales, toasting was not inevitably associated with restraint. Every prisoner and all officers and private soldiers at Sydney Cove received a special ration with which to drink toasts to the King's birthday in June 1788, as well as numerous other public toasts. On that occasion, Worgan (1978: 53), a surgeon on the First Fleet, reported that 'Port, Lisbon, Madeira, Teneriff and good old English Porter' went 'merrily round in bumpers'.[19] Fifty years after Bennelong's experience, John Sweatman (1977), a diarist and clerk on HMS *Bramble*, noted that the toasts at formal dinners could be endless. He described one Sydney dinner of 80 people and five kinds of champagne at which an alderman sitting near him became 'very cunnublified' and had to be led away (65). While this kind of determined toasting slowly declined in popularity as the decades passed, diarists and other observers still thought it worth a mention (and clearly found it amusing) on the occasions when they came across an Aboriginal person being taught to toast, or going through the motions of a toast. Tom Petrie (1904), in his reminiscences of life in rural Queensland in the 1840s, described a settler inviting an Aboriginal man called Billy to come and have a glass of grog with him:

> Now Billy, hold the glass so, and say 'Here's good health, gentlemen'. The squatters all stood round, and Billy, who could not say 'health' took the glass, and this was his toast 'Gentlemen, here you go to hell!' Of course, this caused roars of laughter. (276)

---

19   Bumper: a wine glass or other vessel filled to the brim.

In the western district of Victoria, an Aboriginal man, Corwhorong, who was known as Wilmot Abraham, appeared on drunkenness charges more than anyone else in the Warrnambool district. On one occasion, he used his supposedly patriotic toasting as a means of outwitting the magistrate:

> Wilmot informed the bench with an indignant air that it had been the Queen's birthday, and as a loyal person he had been drinking toasts to her health. The presiding magistrate could not withstand his confession of loyalty ... Wilmot escaped with a caution. (Critchett 1998: 41)

In New Zealand, the Maori elite adopted the etiquette of European toasting with great sophistication. Marten Hutt (1999) proposed that the appropriation by Maori of European drinking customs, such as toasting leaders, showed that alcohol was being linked to political allegiances and alliances. At a Maori hui in the 1860s, each chief took turns to propose a toast. As he proposed a toast to the Queen, one asked that she should send 'plenty of powder, plenty of rum, and may both be strong! And may she send and open a public house here' (27).

McIntyre (2008) has argued that teaching Bennelong and his small group of companions to drink wine during dinner in the first years of the colony was part of a considered strategy to persuade Aboriginal people to abandon 'savagery' and to test the potential for them to become 'civilised':

> In terms of the practical scope of the project of 'civilising' the Aborigines by exposing them to 'civilised' British culture, it is significant that only the Aborigines who had particular acquaintance with the Governor and other officials took part in dining rituals at which wine was served. These Indigenous Australians were shaped as an elite, reflecting exclusiveness of the white elite. In assembling this intimate company Phillip and his men developed affection for the Aborigines they knew, but did not attempt to draw any others into the close circle of British authority in the colony. (39.10)

Wine itself was a marker of wealth and political power in late eighteenth-century England, consumed as a traditional part of social gatherings for celebration, bereavement or companionship (39.3). Above all, wine (as opposed to spirits) was considered a civilising drink. In an eighteenth-century form of drug substitution, wine was thought of as an antidote to the consumption of much stronger liquors that were the bane of the colony. Colonists believed that even the cultivation of wine grapes (and the practice of horticulture in general) would promote civility. Indeed, even the Australian countryside itself, encumbered with the 'dreary eucalyptus', could be beautified and tamed by vineyards. In this idealised vision, the bush would eventually give way to the civilising industry of winegrowing that could employ many thousands of workers; the lower classes would be led away from drinking spirituous liquors through viticulture and wine consumption; and, once good quality light wines were freely available, people would surely begin to drink like the peoples of the Mediterranean (McIntyre 2011: 199). Colonists would then be 'merry instead of mad' and 'animated instead of boisterous' (Dingle 1980: 242). As long ago as 1776, Adam Smith, in his Enlightenment text *The Wealth of Nations*, extolled the so-called Mediterranean drinking style, perhaps making him the earliest in a long line of commentators to do so (McIntyre 2011).[20] Smith promulgated the idea that wine had the power to bring about sobriety in itself, declaring that the people of wine countries such as Spain and Italy were the soberest people in Europe. Possibly because he was an economist rather than a sociologist, he attributed the apparent sobriety of Spaniards and Italians to financial rather than social reasons. He believed that the cheapness and easy availability of wine in those countries was responsible for their relatively moderate consumption patterns, rather than the fact that alcohol (in the form of wine) was an accompaniment to food and consumed sociably.

Learning by observation

Far from this idyllic bucolic fantasy of what might have been going on in parts of the Mediterranean, the settlers and convicts of New South Wales drank themselves literally to oblivion in several cases documented by the Lieutenant Governor of the colony, David Collins. In his journals, Collins noted that the superintendent of convicts drank half a gallon of Cape Brandy and died; that a marine died of an inflammatory complaint brought on by heavy drinking; that two women and a child drowned after the women had been drinking; a drummer's wife expired in a fit of intoxication; and that two young men had a drinking competition

---

20   The deregulation of liquor laws in Australian cities in recent years to allow for more small bars (e.g. in Sydney) has often been idealised and promoted as reproducing a 'Mediterranean lifestyle' and a concomitant (supposedly) trouble-free style of drinking. However, the idyllic archetype relates to a few cultures on one side of the Mediterranean, and even these do not escape the casualties of liver cirrhosis (Douglas 1987: 5, Room & Mäkelä 2000: 481, Blocker et al. 2003: 583). In the United Kingdom, a critic of new 24-hour licensing laws that aspired to mimic a European drinking culture, described them as a fantasy based on 'too many Tuscan holidays': longer hours would not mean more sensible drinking, just more drinking (Measham 2006: 259).

with raw spirits and one died on the spot (Collins 1971). From 1793, all convicts working for officers were paid partly in rum and by 1796 illicit distillation was widely practised.[21] By the 1820s, the drinking habits of the inhabitants of New South Wales had:

> Assumed certain distinctive characteristics. They were heavy spirit drinkers. Their average of around four gallons per head was four times greater than that of their countrymen in Britain … some colonists drank [wine] regularly and in significantly larger quantities than the British per capita average of a third of a gallon between 1800 and 1830. Beer however was only consumed in relatively small quantities. (Dingle 1980: 241)

The problem was not only how much people drank, but *how* they drank. By the 1820s, the Rocks district of Sydney had a population of 1,200, one-quarter of which was Irish. Just as it had been in the pre-industrial setting of rural Britain, drinking was communal and collective, and it was very public; brawling and gambling were considered normal behaviours and disputes were settled in public, often in angry and violent confrontations (Karskens 1999: 56). Men from the ships binged on two months wages in two nights ashore at pubs like the Whaler's Arms, named for its clientele; the same pattern was repeated by pastoral workers from the inland.[22] The Austrian naturalist and traveller, Baron Charles von Hugel (1994: 43)), made a number of acerbic comments about Sydney, its criminal population and the drinking habits of the English, when he visited there in 1833:

> The only thing standing between the English and their rapid progress towards world domination is the fascination alcoholic beverages hold for them … A bottle of brandy or a bottle of claret compensate an Englishman for the absence of all other joys of life … But, among the lower orders, brandy [*branntwein*—spirits or brandy] is the supreme and ultimate object in life.

Servants, the Irish and the lower orders in general were said to be particularly prone to a lack of restraint. According to Mrs Charles Meredith of Sydney, one could not leave wine or strong liquor of any kind accessible to one's servants, as they would often be trundled home drunk on a handbarrow

---

21 Distillation became legal in the colony in 1821.
22 In 1958, Jeremy Beckett wrote that the recurrent bouts of wild drinking among Aboriginal men in outback New South Wales recalled the 'benders' of white itinerant labourers: 'It is hard not to believe that the aborigines have modelled themselves on their white brethren' (232).

or 'shouldered like a sack of potatoes' (Meredith 1973: 163, Cunningham 1966: 280). There were undoubtedly less extreme drinkers among the colonists too, but those with more restraint were drinking in private.

As they increasingly ventured into the settlement and came into contact with convicts and settlers, there were plenty of opportunities for Aboriginal people to witness the antics of people who became intoxicated in public. To begin with, supplies of alcohol and food had been precious and expensive and it is unlikely that much of either was freely given to Aboriginal people in or near Sydney Cove. In 1798, Collins observed that Aboriginal people were extremely robust, which he attributed to their 'good habit of body' and the fact that they were free from the use of spirituous liquors and the 'luxuries of the table' (Collins 1971, vol II: 134).[23] However, supplies improved and English, French, Russian and other visiting mariners were soon bartering alcohol for artefacts,[24] which meant that Aboriginal and non-Aboriginal people were mingling. The 'woods' around the settlement were increasingly populated by runaway convicts and vagabonds, and Collins (1971, vol I: 405) noted that several native teenage boys were living among the settlers in different districts. The 1830s marked the heaviest spirits-drinking period in Australian history. By then, Aboriginal people were washing out empty rum casks and drinking the mixture of rum and water, which they called 'bull'; they were also drinking openly from bottles in the streets of Sydney. Scenes of staggering, ragged Aboriginal people were common enough to be depicted by artists of the day such as John Carmichael and Augustus Earle.[25] In the years after the early experiments of teaching Bennelong and his cohort the social ritual of the toast, Aboriginal people were left to themselves to interpret the meaning of alcohol, and what happens after imbibing it. They 'learned' by looking around at the motley collection of Europeans and were often puzzled by what they saw.

---

23   With the *Endeavour* at Cooktown in July 1770, Joseph Banks (1963, vol II: 130) commented similarly that the Aboriginal people they met were 'happy', being unlike Europeans for whom strong liquors and tobacco had degenerated from luxuries into 'necessaries'.

24   In an early case of sly grog selling (in contravention of Governor Macquarie's regulation against supplying natives with alcohol), one Russian navigator negotiated for 'rarities' (three spears, a shield and clubs) with two bottles of rum, 'which showed their passion for drinking. As they would not otherwise have agreed to the barter described, I was obliged to satisfy their desire' (Barratt 1981: 25).

25   Earle's lithograph, *Natives of N.S. Wales as seen in the streets of Sydney* (1830), depicts a partly clothed family group drinking 'bull' outside, apparently excluded from a licensed hotel frequented by Europeans. One woman holds a fish she has caught and another has decorated her hair with clay or gumnuts in the traditional manner; the child is pot-bellied and malnourished (National Library of Australia).

Aboriginal people's exposure to the drinking behaviour of the English came to be seen fatalistically, as an unstoppable process: a mix of passive contamination and active modelling. The first German visitor to South Australia in the 1830s, Dr Hermann Koeler (2006: 76–7), lamented the inevitability of this process, seeing Aboriginal 'alcoholism' developing through a kind of social osmosis:

> Only a few blacks who had been employed as rowers or for other kinds of assistance by the whalers in Encounter Bay, had already become accustomed to drinking, and in time the South Australians will presumably also become friends of spirits just like the Aborigines of New South Wales and on the whole almost all savages who come into constant contact with the English. For no civilized nation is more devoted to alcoholism than 'Albion's proud children', and since the Ethiopian race, to which the South Australians belong … normally only imitate and adopt the vices which they perceive in their white neighbours, even without speaking of other contributing factors, alcoholism will soon begin to effect the physical decline of the Adelaide tribe.

In a similar vein, the *Australian Temperance Magazine* published the opinion that:

> Savages, as the New Hollanders for instance, resist it [alcohol] at first, and only learn its pernicious influence by obeying the imitative principle and partaking of it out of compliment to the European. Indeed, it may be doubted whether the earliest tasters of spirit were pleased with its penetrating odour, its pungent effect upon the palate, and the burning sensation it communicates to the throat and stomach: habit, and habit alone, can make it a pleasant beverage.[26]

The influence of observation, habit and 'custom' on drinking behaviour was repeatedly stressed in early temperance tracts, which showed a surprising awareness of the power of the social environment on everyone, not just Indigenous people. 'From long habit and the power of association, the price of many men in New South Wales is a glass of rum', observed the *Australian Temperance Magazine*, which also noted that it was 'custom—daily custom—[that] brought the two powerful feelings of covetousness and appetite to bear upon grog'.[27]

---

26   *Australian Temperance Magazine* 1837, I(2):17.
27   *Australian Temperance Magazine* 1838, II(2):19.

The practice of observing and imitating white men is described in an oral history account from far north Queensland that reveals how mystified Aboriginal people were by the drinking of whites. The story, translated from the Kuuk Thaayorre language, also described the introduction of alcohol in Cape York:

> Long ago we didn't know the taste of it but saw the whites drinking. None of us here went near it to actually swallow alcoholic drinks though others elsewhere did but we still kept our distance. When we saw stray men drinking here and there and commented 'Oh yes, those men there, what are they gulping? Is it food? I'll first go and have a look to see what they are swallowing!'

> 'Whacko, there it is, finished!' One man was roaming around and the whiteman said, 'come on chaps, there's plenty more of this liquor!' … We were quite oblivious of alcoholic drinks. I was telling you about the whiteman's drinking that he passed on to us. So he kept on drinking and still went back for more! (Foote and Hall 1995: 2)

Learning by observation is still cited by Aboriginal people as the means by which they were (and are) introduced to drinking; however, more recent accounts, such as those below, describe the powers of example and persuasion presented not by Europeans, but by other Aboriginal men. A woman from Yirrkala in northeast Arnhem Land described the visual effect of family members who were able to drink at a mining canteen:

> One thing that I noticed at that time was they'd come home and they'd be drunk, but I remember them being really happy drunk. They used to make jokes, make us laugh … we'd say 'hey, so and so is drunk, quick', and then us kids would all run up to this man and he'd joke and do a lot of funny things that would make us laugh and we thought having *nanitji*[28] to be funny, to make other people laugh, you know to be a good thing for them, we thought, at that time. But of course as the years went by they wanted more and more … Seeing my brothers drinking … follow their footsteps, like watching movies getting ideas … ideas from family and relatives … I seen them and I start following. (Wearne 2001: 47–8)

---

28   This is the term used for alcohol among Yolngu; it is a loan word from the Makassar language.

Pitjantjatjara-speaking men in South Australia made similar comments:

I came from college there and, hey, 'that's how they drinking!' I was watching you know. I was sitting down, you know, just watching them. Men (they passed away now) they told me 'hey, you want to get warm? Try this!' *Uwa*, yes, it was really cold too and I bin try 'em you know. First [time] I got really drunk. Yes, I couldn't walk. I gotta crawl to the camp. I was really headache then. Boss of me then. I was drinking, drinking, drinking. (Young Mr May, in Brady 1995: 130)

When you watch, you follow, you know? When somebody do things, see them and you follow their example. They drink—well, you drink too! You get in there with them, they share you, 'hey, come on, come on here, drink, here!' And you drink. That's it. The grog get hold of you. And you drink, drink, drink. (Keith Peters, in Brady 1995: 137)

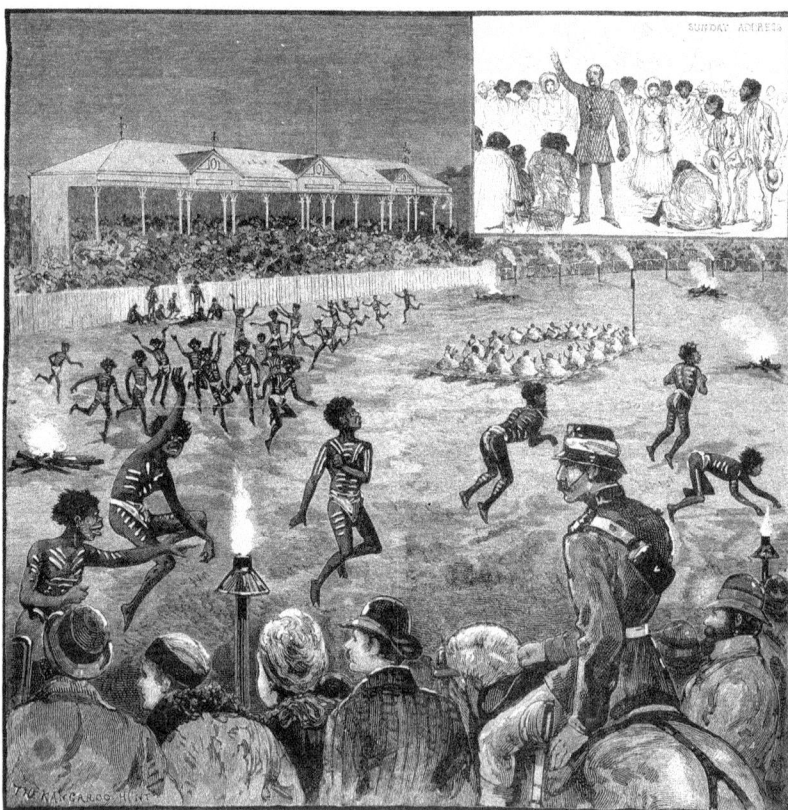

Fig. 1 Aboriginal Corroboree at Adelaide, 1885
Source: Reproduced in *Australasian Sketcher* 29 June 1885, SLV Mp009675

Performing drunkenness

In the very early days of the colony, George Worgan (1978: 18) observed that Aboriginal people were 'expert at the art of Mimickry, both in their Actions and in repeating many of our Phrases … the Sailors teach them to swear'. Russian expeditioners in Sydney observed Aboriginal people quarrelling and wife-beating and noted that 'from the convicts they have acquired the expletives, curses, and oaths of the English rabble' (Barratt 1981: 38). We can conclude from such firsthand accounts that Aboriginal people were keen observers of the behaviour of colonists and settlers— and that they took a great interest in the drunken comportment of these people. They learned the bodily and verbal manifestations of intoxication so well that not only did they know how they were supposed to act when drunk, but they were also able to accurately mimic and re-enact faux intoxication even when they were sober.

The visiting Quaker, temperance campaigner and social reformer, James Backhouse, also observed the 'force of example' set by European drinking and the imitative behaviour that followed. Backhouse (1843) described seeing Aboriginal people soaking empty sugar-bags[29] in buckets of water, avidly drinking the sugary infusion and then, in an apt illustration of drunken comportment as learned behaviour, enacting pseudo-intoxication:

> The Blacks of Sydney reel after drinking the infusion of sugar-bags, and put on the appearance of intoxication so well, that it has generally been supposed, that the liquor really made them drunk. The following circumstances satisfied an acquaintance of ours, that this appearance of intoxication was feigned, and our own observation has confirmed this view. (327)

Backhouse went on to describe an Aboriginal man who, after drinking salty water (with no alcohol content) and having been told it was rum, began to throw his arms about and adopt a staggering gait, declaring that he was 'murry [very] drunk like a gentleman' (327). It is difficult to tell from such descriptions whether the Aboriginal men in question were mocking white men or trying to emulate them. In these instances of pseudo-intoxication, it was clearly more important to appear intoxicated than to actually be drunk. We can only guess at the reasons for this:

---

29 Bags of fine sacking were used to store sugar and the term 'sugar-bag' later became incorporated into Aboriginal English to describe honey, especially honey from the native bee (JM Arthur 1996: 61).

to cause amusement; to earn tips; to advertise the fact that the person is drunk and not responsible for his actions. Drunkenness is usually feigned to take advantage of the excuses that such behaviour can provide, but in these examples, the motive is not so clear. This is because the pretence was taking place at a cultural boundary, as Room (2001) has explained:

> In the context of interaction between people from very different cultures. At such boundaries, the expectations and attributions about drunken behaviour take on an added dimension: each side in the interaction has expectations, whether well-founded or not, about drunken comportment in the alien culture. Further, each side builds up some knowledge of what is expected of them by the other. (196)

Mac Marshall (1981) discussed anthropological field studies of pseudo-intoxication and the ability of people to turn their drunken behaviour on and off in the context of the (supposedly) inevitably disinhibiting effects of ethanol on human beings. If drinkers can demonstrate a full range of culturally appropriate drunken behaviours ('murry drunk like a gentleman') whether drunk or not, then 'sober up' at a moment's notice, he suggests that the disinhibiting effects are called into question.

Aboriginal people's mimicry of drunken comportment found its way into formal performance contexts in dance-music events that were publicly staged to settler audiences. In Adelaide in the mid-nineteenth century, such events evolved into a tradition of regular 'corroborees', as they were called, conducted for tourists in public spaces, such as parks and ovals, and drinking seems to have been a common theme (Parsons 1997). A newspaper story noted that the Aboriginal men of Gawler Town (north of Adelaide):

> Have introduced English dialogue into their corroborees, and the following short one is a great favourite—A native, who staggering drunk, comes into the ring, and addressing himself to another who is supposed to re-present a licensed retailer, says, 'Give me a pint of beer', to which the other replies, 'I shan't—you're drunk already'. A third black then says, with all the intonation of authority, 'Send for policeman' when chorus of voices gives exultingly, and with great vociferation, a sententious 'put him in jail' and, finally, young and old join in applauding the performance.[30]

---

30 *Moreton Bay Courier* 16 January 1847: 4.

In 1860, the citizens of Angaston in the Barossa Valley found a group of Aboriginal people from the Murray River encamped outside the town. The local newspaper noted approvingly that they were 'well clad and well behaved', and that they performed corroborees that included demonstrations of drills and marching. Another part of the performance included the 'imitation (minus the liquor) of a *whitefellows' drinking party*' (emphasis added), in which performers asked each other:

> 'What will you take?' and 'what will you take?' etc. 'I'll take a glass' and 'I'll take a nobbler',[31] concluding all with 'hip, hip, hoorah!'[32]

Later in the nineteenth century, Aboriginal men from the Coorong and the Murray River performed corroborees on the Adelaide Oval. Some of these events were controversial, described by disapproving white observers as being a circus or a sham, inauthentic because of the cross-cultural elements incorporated into the action. One article described such performances derisively as a 'whitey-black corroboree', because of the 'utilisation of appliances of civilisation in the display'.[33] Nevertheless, in May 1885, 20,000 Adelaide citizens turned up to watch a dramatic night-time corroboree lit by coloured lights, flaming torches and fireworks, in which semi-naked Aboriginal performers walked onto the oval singing God Save the Queen. After a kangaroo dance, they performed 'a little satire on civilization' that involved 'liquoring up' and a pantomime on intoxication—falling down, yelling and tumbling about (see Fig. 1). One account interpreted the performance as:

> Affecting to teach the whites the evils of intemperance … there can be little doubt that the second part of the program had both moral significance and a certain amount of irony. Evidently most of the Aborigines performing it belonged to a Blue Ribbon organisation and, having become abstainers, wanted to illustrate the principles they had adopted. (Whimpress, no date: 5)

Drunkenness was performed at temperance meetings as well, usually in the form of cautionary dramas on the evils of drink as a way of promoting sobriety. At the Point McLeay Mission (now Raukkan) in South Australia

---

31 Nobbler: a small drink of beer, spirits or wine; a term first recorded in 1852 (Baker 1978: 228).
32 *South Australian Register* (Adelaide, SA) 26 October 1860: 3.
33 *Australasian Sketcher* 29 June 1885, 13(194): 99. Apart from performances at the Adelaide Oval, there were other public corroborees in Adelaide at this time, including one at the Kensington Oval (*The Observer* 6 June 1885: 30). I am grateful to Tom Gara for drawing my attention to these accounts.

in 1888,[34] Aboriginal members of a temperance group performed a number of recitations, dialogues and action scenes representing the evils resulting from the use of intoxicants for the benefit of visiting members of the Aborigines' Friends' Association (1888: 16).

In 1924, Torres Strait Islander dancers were filmed re-enacting drunkenness. Frank Hurley's film, *Pearls and Savages*, featured them wearing traditional *dhari* headdresses and grass skirts with trousers and rolling around feigning drunkenness while holding cups and bottles. Hurley's inter-title read: 'Dancers with bottles mimic the movement of drunk men'.[35] Anthropologists Ronald and Catherine Berndt (1993) documented a 'modern' ceremony while they were doing fieldwork among the Yaraldi in South Australia in the 1940s. Their informant related how tempers flared easily when people were drinking, and how men simulated drunkenness in the ceremony by stumbling and waving empty bottles and singing songs about quarrels, tempers and how being 'silly' with drink caused them to 'bring out stumbling words' (219).

The content of these public, private or ceremonial performances of intoxication (involving stumbling, falling, waving arms and bottles, quarrelling and fighting) reveal that Aboriginal people not only learned and took on the Europeans' ways of being drunk themselves, but also absorbed European beliefs about what alcohol does to people: that alcohol loosens the inhibitions that constrain and excuse bad behaviour; that it contributes to male bonding and allows for disinhibited sexuality and so on. Aboriginal observers could see that, when drunk, people usually became loud, abusive and feisty, vomited, walked unsteadily, sang and passed out.[36] In a volume of detailed anthropological studies of drinking in Papua New Guinea, Marshall and colleagues (1982) showed how these beliefs and behaviours were taken on, largely unchanged, by Papua New Guineans, becoming merged with their local cultural perceptions of intoxication (cf. MacAndrew & Edgerton 1969).

---

34 The missionary at Point McLeay, George Taplin, was a strict teetotaller. There were regular temperance meetings and Aboriginal people were persuaded to 'sign the pledge'.

35 *Pearls and Savages* (New York, 1924). The introduction to this film sequence shows Mer Island, where it was presumably filmed (National Film and Sound Archive ID 6810-0012).

36 Burbank (1994: 63) described how children in East Arnhem Land (in the late 1980s) associated 'drunk' with aggression while play-acting at drinking 'beer' from an empty lemonade bottle.

Although the Irish and English were the most persistent models for drinking and drunken comportment in Australia, they were not the earliest. In the north of the country, the first drinkers of strong liquors observed by the Yolngu and other coastal peoples were maritime visitors from Southeast Asia. These men (the 'Macassans') were bêche-de-mer fishermen who sailed from Makassar, south Sulawesi, to northern Australian coasts between around 1720 and 1907. They arrived each year in December, usually beaching and setting up camp at the same locations where they processed their catches onshore, and staying for around four months until the monsoon winds turned around. These lengthy and regular stays required the negotiation of friendly relationships with local Aboriginal traditional owners. Along with other desirable items traded or presented to local people (such as cloth, rice, steel axes and tobacco), the Macassans brought a favoured and portable alcoholic drink: the distilled spirit arrack.[37] Among most Aboriginal groups in contact with the Macassans, arrack came to be known by the borrowed term '*nganitji*' (from the Macassan '*anisi*', meaning 'strong drink'), and the term is still in use in Arnhem Land today to describe alcohol in general. We know very little about the social contexts within which *nganitji* was consumed: exactly how much was imported; with whom, exactly, it was shared; what kind of behaviours the visitors might have exhibited; and whether these Southeast Asians consciously 'inducted' Aboriginal people into its use.[38] However, given that a 'drunken Macassan' dance is still regularly performed in northeast Arnhem Land in the *nganitji* sequence of an ancestral song cycle, we do have some indication of its affect (Evans 1992, Brady 2008). In the dance, Aboriginal performers stagger around with empty soft drink bottles, miming the drinking of arrack—much as their counterparts had done on the Adelaide Oval in 1885.

In Australia, as settlement advanced, Aboriginal people soon began to confront contradictory information about how Europeans themselves interpreted alcohol. While most drank heartily, binged frequently (often until unconscious) and offered or forced strong spirits upon Aboriginal

---

37 At home, the Macassans also consumed other fermented drinks, such as toddies and palm wine (*sagueir*); however, these did not travel as well as distilled spirits. Wallace (1989: 224) observed that although the Macassans were 'nominal Mohammedans' they were lax in their religious observances and consumed alcoholic drinks with gusto.

38 Oral histories of the Macassans provide conflicting accounts of their drinking behaviour as well as that of their Aboriginal hosts. Consequently, the historical reality is difficult to distinguish from the now heavily mythologised depictions of these Southeast Asian visitors (Warner 1957, Macknight 1976, Searcy [1909] 1984, Hercus & Sutton 1986, Wallace 1989, Brady 2008: 12–14).

people for amusement or enticement, others—the missionaries of the many Christian denominations, the temperance campaigners, and many ordinary 'upright' citizens—abstained, portrayed drinking alcohol as a sin and attempted to protect Aboriginal people from its worst excesses. As a result, there were numerous mixed messages about alcohol circulating in colonial Australia.

The fantasy of (re)learning how to drink

The historical examples discussed here have demonstrated that, in the early decades of colonisation, Aboriginal people adopted many of the drinking practices of the British, Irish and others, as well as taking on European beliefs about alcohol. Aboriginal people, in a sense, did 'learn' (as neophyte drinkers) from outsiders. However, the only example of a formal induction into one aspect of the practice of drinking alcohol was when Governor Phillip taught Bennelong to raise his glass of wine in a toast in the earliest days of the colony.

Once the period of 'dinner-table diplomacy' with Bennelong and his cohort came to an end, the colonial administration (and those that followed) seemed to abandon any rudimentary notion they might once have had of easing the Indigenous inhabitants into a sociable familiarity with alcohol, and instead resorted to legislation prohibiting its sale or supply to them. For most of the nineteenth and some of the twentieth century, Aboriginal people were banned from drinking in hotels[39]—the traditional focus of Australian drinking. Consequently, they were prevented from mixing with, and adapting to, what would later become an eclectic range of drinkers in relatively controlled licensed environments. They were also prevented from experiencing the changes in drinking behaviour that developed over time. Due to this race-based prohibition policy in Australia (and indeed in other British colonies), Indigenous people missed the opportunity for a long-term familiarisation process: they were denied the opportunity to experience the waves of change in patterns of consumption and attitudes to alcohol that affected the general population over the decades.

---

39   Only Aboriginal people with exemption certificates issued for 'good behaviour' could drink in hotels. In rural New South Wales, Beckett (1958) found that many Aboriginal people who would be eligible for exemption did not bother to apply. They drank fortified wine, rum and methylated spirits and consumed them rapidly: 'Once bought, the bottle is never safe until it is emptied, so … behind a fence, perhaps, or under some hedge, it is gulped down as quickly as possible' (225).

There have been many rises and falls in consumption. The law was effective in keeping people out of hotels, but it did not prevent them from obtaining and drinking alcohol surreptitiously. After conducting anthropological fieldwork in inland New South Wales in the 1950s—a period of mostly illicit consumption of alcohol by Aboriginal people—Jeremy Beckett (1958), commenting on the widespread drinking and drunkenness among Aboriginal men, argued that:

> It is not enough to regard this sort of behaviour as merely a social aberration or a symptom of spiritual emptyness [sic]; among aboriginal men it has become institutionalised; it is a central value in their lives, to which they will adhere in the teeth of strong pressure. (223)

It is both ironic and unfortunate that, by the time Aboriginal prohibition began to be repealed in Australia (i.e. mainly during the 1960s), the influence of the temperance movement was on the wane and consumption in the general Australian population was reaching levels at least as high as those of the gold rush era of the 1850s. The six o'clock swill was one of the vestiges of the temperance movement that had kept closing time to the early evening. Per capita consumption increased by 20 per cent between 1969 and 1975, which was a dramatic shift in drinking practices (Drew 1977: 80). Sales of sweet wine—the drink favoured by Aboriginal drinkers—grew by 40 per cent between 1970 and 1981 and alcohol availability generally increased (Room 1988: 418). In another unhappy coincidence, the era in which Indigenous people were finally able to drink legally also marked the beginning of the decline of the hotel as the prime focus for Australians' drinking. Rather than hotels—places where sociable drinking and some basic rules of comportment could be fostered—this period was characterised by the growth of the bottle shop and the drive-in liquor store, and the increasing popularity of cheaper packaged alcohol that made it easier for drinking to take place in unregulated spaces.[40] The liberalisation of liquor laws in the 1960s meant that bottle shops could now sell single bottles of alcohol for consumption off premises, whereas previously bottle shops had had 'gallon licences' in which the minimum takeaway purchase was 12 large bottles. This marked the real beginning of takeaway alcohol sales. Hard on the heels of changes to bottle shop licences, the alcohol industry introduced innovations such as the beer can

---

40 Another influence on Australian drinking patterns and the decline of the hotel was the advent of random breath testing that commenced in Victoria in 1976 but was not fully operational in all states and territories until the early 1980s. The liberalisation of liquor laws in the 1960s extended opening hours, including Sunday trading for hotels, bowling and golf clubs.

(in 1962), the ring-pull can and, later, rip-top stubbies of beer, which increased sales of this bottle size by 90 per cent (Welborn 1987). In the 1970s, Australia invented the wine cask, a silver wine bladder encased in a cardboard box. Since the wine did not go off, casks became the stock item of the takeaway trade for home or outdoor consumption (Stockwell & Crosbie 2001). For reasons of cheapness and convenience, takeaway cask wine became the drink of choice for Aboriginal drinkers (see Fig. 21).

In the few decades during which Indigenous people were able to, and chose to, drink on licensed premises—that is, the brief period from the end of restrictions until the proliferation of takeaway alcohol—progressive thinkers of the time viewed hotels as settings that facilitated a form of social learning and social contact between the races. The psychologist Norelle Lickiss (1971), whose work is largely forgotten, believed that the public drinking house served a number of functions for Aboriginal people. She nominated its value as a social centre: a communication centre (for people who were often mobile); a place for tension discharge and stress release; and as an agency for integration 'with non-Aborigines in similar socio-economic circumstances' (214). Hotels provided the setting within which Aboriginal people could moderate their consumption of alcohol, 'enjoying the social benefits of drinking without trying to get drunk', according to rural medical practitioner Max Kamien (1975: 295, Lickiss 1971). In the 1950s, before the laws were changed, Aboriginal men protested that if they were allowed into hotels they would drink beer at the normal rate, as whites did. Beckett (1958) thought there was some force to this argument, particularly if those in question were anxious to conform to 'white drinking conventions' (226). However, he found that older, more hardened, drinkers preferred wine and rum, and he heard that when a couple of hotels had briefly opened their doors to Aboriginal people, their drunken and disorderly behaviour had become 'quite intolerable'.

Drinking off premises, relatively unencumbered and unrestrained, is now so entrenched in many regions that drinking on premises in licensed venues is atypical. In 2007, when restrictions were placed on the licence of the Crossing Inn in the largely Aboriginal town of Fitzroy Crossing (Western Australia), drinkers were no longer able to buy full-strength takeaway alcohol from their hotel, and instead were compelled to purchase full-strength drinks for on-premises consumption only. The manager reported that many of his Aboriginal customers had never drunk in bars before and did not know that they were not allowed to become intoxicated in licensed premises. They had no idea of bar rules and became aggressive when refused further service (Henderson-Yates et al. 2008, appendix VIII: 109).

Behavioural studies of drinking

The idea that people could be 'taught' to drink moderately reached its zenith in the 1960s and 1970s. In the post–World War II period, alcohol researchers and psychologists in the United States and the United Kingdom developed a critique of the disease concept of alcoholism that opened the way for a new conceptualisation of drinking problems as being fundamentally behavioural in nature: that drinking to excess was a disorder of behaviour over which control could be exercised (Cook 2007: 37, McCambridge 2011: 567). Once this new science of drinking problems took hold, it made way for a host of different approaches and treatments to be trialled, including social-learning models, brief interventions and controlled drinking. Researchers began to try to understand and inculcate varieties of self-control over alcohol consumption: perhaps people with damaging drinking habits could be (re)taught how to drink after all?

An influential research program in the United States produced dozens of research papers examining different cultural styles of drinking (e.g. Jewish, Italian, Irish, Mormon and Protestant). By examining 'positive' examples of drinking styles (e.g. Jewish and Italian) as well as 'negative' ones (e.g. Irish and Mormon) the purpose of these studies, as directed by the Yale Center of Alcohol Studies, was to design ways to train Protestant Americans to drink more sensibly. This tradition of research was continued by Dr Morris Chafetz who, in 1970, became the influential first director of the United States National Institute on Alcohol Abuse and Alcoholism. Chafetz believed that beverage alcohol should be presented as a normal part of life—the Mediterranean approach—rather than as an alluringly illicit substance, and that this would encourage responsible drinking. In 1971, in a submission to Congress, he observed that in societies with a low incidence of alcoholism, the beverage was sipped slowly, consumed with food and taken in the company of others in relaxing and comfortable circumstances. In these cultures, intoxication was abhorred (Chafetz & Demone 1962, Room 1976, Room & Mäkelä 2000).[41] In an attempt

41   The idea that a society's drinking norms explains, at least in part, its rates of drinking problems is now widely accepted; however, at the time, the adoption of this position was a rare example of the influence of sociological thought on public policy, as Room (1976: 1048) pointed out.

to both mimic and inculcate this integration of drinking into everyday life, Chafetz proposed that schools should teach children how to drink responsibly by providing them with heavily diluted sherry. Believing that alcohol was here to stay, he argued that people must learn to develop a healthy attitude towards it.[42]

In keeping with the hypothesis that even problem drinkers could be taught better habits of drinking, and with clinical psychologists exerting a growing influence on alcoholism treatment research, studies turned to ways of teaching controlled drinking to people who were alcoholics, including those who had been hospitalised. Reports that some diagnosed alcoholics could return successfully to a limited drinking pattern threatened the prevailing dictum that abstinence was the only treatment for such individuals. These findings, which also challenged the disease hypothesis, were vigorously debated, primarily because the 'disease' of alcoholism was thought to be characterised by a loss of control, while the emergent research was showing that, under some circumstances, alcoholics were able to exert control (Thom 1999, Cook 2007, McCambridge 2011). English psychologist Jim Orford recalled angry reactions to his suggestion in the late 1960s that alcoholic drinking was a learned behaviour and that people could perhaps learn to drink less harmfully (Thom 1999: 144).

In the 1960s and 1970s, aversion therapy, including electrical aversion (electric shock administration) and chemical aversion (the use of nausea-inducing drugs), was used within the armamentarium of behavioural approaches to alcoholism (Mills et al. 1971). Less confronting behavioural studies looked at gulping and sipping behaviour and typical intake, and experimented with training in self-regulation, social modelling, supervised drinking and teaching and practising how to drink (Collins & Marlatt 1981, Strickler et al. 1976, 1981). Other studies compared different approaches to drinking, including direct instruction in how to drink moderately, practising target behaviours and requiring subjects to observe a model. Using insights from social-learning theory, these were often referred to as 'learning approaches' to alcohol abuse. While much of the research into learning approaches was based in the United States or United Kingdom, similar studies were undertaken in Australia (Thom 1999: 144). It is intriguing to ponder the extent to which the behavioural research studies prompted by Chafetz and his colleagues in the United

---

42   As an indication of Chafetz's influence, his obituary noted that he changed the view of alcoholism in the United States (*New York Times* 21 October 2011).

States filtered through to influence Australia's 'post-prohibition' era in general, and the post-prohibition era for Indigenous Australians in particular. In 1969, for example, a Sydney-based doctoral student began a project to see whether he could train drinkers to discriminate their own blood alcohol concentrations—that is, to teach people to monitor their own levels of intoxication. He later wrote what was described as a 'watershed' study into trials of controlled drinking (Caddy & Lovibond 1976, cf. McLean 1987, Thom 1999: 145). A British clinical psychologist who later moved to Sydney to become director of Australia's National Drug and Alcohol Research Centre, Nick Heather, was a leading figure in the controlled drinking debate in this country. He argued that problem drinking is better regarded as a learned behavioural disorder than a disease (Heather & Robertson 1989). The behavioural social-learning studies and interventions conducted within and beyond Australia were relevant to helping people diagnosed as dependent on alcohol. They were not necessarily relevant to the task of teaching responsible alcohol consumption to those who had little or no previous exposure to alcohol. Nonetheless, such studies permeated the Aboriginal policy environment and influenced approaches to improving the lives of Aboriginal people.

Unlike the United States, which had a nationwide constitutional ban on alcohol from 1920 to 1933 that prompted individuals such as Alma Whitaker to advocate the importance of learning to drink, Australia never had total prohibition for all its citizens. Only a few regions of Australia, such as the Chaffey brothers' irrigation colony near Renmark, voted under local option laws to be dry. With prohibitions on the consumption and possession of alcohol, the discrete reserves and mission settlements where many Aboriginal and Torres Strait Islander people lived were all 'dry' for most of the nineteenth and part of the twentieth centuries. Recognising the new era of civil rights, and aware that the prohibition era for Aboriginal people was really over, in 1963, Aboriginal activist Kath Walker told the prime minister that Aboriginal people were going to have to 'learn to live with alcohol, the white man's poison' (Bandler 1989: 98). Over the next 10 years, the idea that Aboriginal people should learn to drink responsibly began to take off, as government agencies and their proxies, the missions, started to put the idea into practice. Governments and mission authorities were agreed that once prohibition laws in the states and the Northern Territory were repealed, some protection against the potentially disastrous consequences of the sudden and unrestricted availability of alcohol was going to be necessary for Aboriginal people. The solution appeared to be a graduated approach to availability, combined with some form of instruction or education in 'learning to drink'—ideas that led to many experiments in several remote missions and settlements in which alcohol was made available. Initially, these trials took the form of beer rations being distributed a few times a week, often under the control of an Aboriginal council; some ration systems developed into canteens or clubs with a degree of Aboriginal governance (see Chapter 3). However, other than making alcohol available in small amounts through beer rations or canteens, there were no attempts to implement the social-learning techniques tried elsewhere, such as direct instruction, supervised drinking and learning to self-monitor. Further, at the time of repeal,[43] it seems that there were few, if any, health education programs for Indigenous people focused on the strength, contents and risks of alcohol.

Sociologist of alcohol Robin Room urged caution about optimistic plans for engineering change in drinking habits, and not just in minority or indigenous populations. While moving towards a 'continental' or 'Mediterranean' culture of sociable drinking has long been a dream for English-speaking societies with bingeing problems, such as Australia and Britain, this fantasy has run up against the 'stubborn realities' of cultures that attach value to intoxication.[44] Cultural norms and the interactions of everyday life possess their own dynamics and can generate pressures towards heavy drinking and determined drunkenness (Room & Mäkelä 2000: 476, Measham 2006, Ormerod & Wiltshire 2009). The societies and subcultures in which heavy drinking is normative value this style of drinking positively, ensuring 'that learning to drink heavily will be transmitted from generation to generation' (Kunitz & Levy 2000: 173). Once established, such norms are difficult to shift. As Room (1982: 448) observed, cultural change comes slowly and unpredictably, particularly if someone is trying to engineer it from outside.

---

43 Northern Territory Aboriginal people ceased to be labelled 'wards' in 1964. This change brought restrictions on their civil rights, including the right to possess and consume alcohol, to an end.

44 Continental southern Europe is made up of predominantly wine-consuming countries where wine is usually drunk with meals and usually in moderate amounts, although, as Room and Mäkelä (2000) have cautioned, one should be sceptical about the idealisation of drinking in these countries. Northern European countries, including Scandinavia and the United Kingdom, can be typified as beer- or spirits-drinking societies, as they have different consumption traditions to those further south. Prior to the introduction of the potato, beer was a major source of nourishment for central and northern Europe, with 'beer soup' being consumed for breakfast (Schivelbusch 1993: 22). However, even this north–south distinction is becoming blurred, as wine consumption increases in northern Europe and beer consumption rises in Mediterranean countries (Hupkens et al. 1993).

A seductive—but elusive—goal

The idea that people could be formally taught good habits of drinking, and that these would replace bad habits, has been a recurrent theme over many decades. It is a seductive idea, especially in cultures imbued with a strong belief in human perfectibility, such as American, British and Nordic cultures.[45] However, to say that drinking alcohol is, or can be, learned, perhaps by using the 'instructive information' of which Whitaker wrote in her etiquette manual, or through the use of staged, pretend bars set up in the alcoholics' wards of hospitals,[46] seems to present the idea rather too neatly. It is 'redolent of knowledge gravely imparted and respectfully received', as Justin Willis (2002: 9) rather tartly put it. The process of learning, of course, is far more indirect, chaotic and ad hoc than one might think. Even the social-learning researchers were uncomfortably aware that people are influenced indirectly and contagiously by those around them. They found, for example, that research subjects who were exposed to heavy drinkers drank more than subjects who were exposed to light drinkers (Collins & Marlatt 1981)—that is, that low-risk, normal drinkers, increase their consumption if they drink with 'pretend' heavy drinkers; and that people who drink in groups tend to adjust the pace of their drinking to the fastest drinker among the group (Watson & Sobell 1982, Heath 2000, Ormerod & Wiltshire 2009). Social-learning researchers noted that it was difficult for subjects to maintain moderation after treatment when they were re-exposed to the same environments and the same reinforcing stimuli that had influenced them in the first place (Strickler et al. 1976). These research studies, including ethnographic observational studies, reinforce what common sense tells us about drinking: that people 'learn', or are influenced informally, by how those around them are drinking.

The idea that Indigenous drinking patterns were learned from Europeans on the frontier has been criticised as presenting a static view of Indigenous patterns of behaviour, as if, once adopted, such patterns were incapable of change (Saggers & Gray 1998: 78).[47] There is undoubtedly some truth in this critique. While many other variables influence drinking behaviour,

---

45 Robin Room, pers comm, 6 March 2013.
46 For example, in the 1970s, seven-week training sessions for 'excessive drinkers' were conducted in a simulated bar in the Psychiatry Department of the Baltimore City Hospital (Strickler et al. 1976).
47 Kunitz and Levy (1974), writing of changing ideas about alcohol use among the Navajo in the 1970s, found that they had reconsidered earlier interpretations of heavy drinking and redefined it as deviant.

and while there have been some changes, there has also been considerable persistence in longstanding patterns of consumption that tend towards episodic heavy drinking.[48] Jeffery Stead (1980) argued that the patterns of alcohol use apparent in the late 1970s varied between different Aboriginal groups depending on their historical circumstances, exposure to different policies, contact with Europeans and individual social and cultural organisation. Serving as a reminder of the importance of the setting or context in which alcohol use is learned, Stephen Kunitz and Jerrold Levy's (Kunitz et al. 1971, Kunitz & Levy 1994) groundbreaking long-term research revealed significant differences in drinking patterns and disease outcomes between the neighbouring Navajo and Hopi peoples of Arizona. Both these Native American groups learned alcohol use in the nineteenth century by observing Anglo-American frontiersmen, but their established cultural values influenced their adoption of the colonists' drinking styles. The Navajo drank overtly in flamboyant binges, whereas the few Hopi who drank did so in a covert and clandestine way to avoid being ostracised by other Hopi. The two groups lived close to each other and were socio-economically similar, but their different approaches to drinking alcohol resulted in different patterns of morbidity and mortality. Comparing them demonstrates the significance of different styles of drinking as a determinant of health and illness.

Australian data on Aboriginal drinking styles are not disaggregated by locality. Therefore, a comparative study of Aboriginal Australians is not feasible, but it is plausible to conclude that the effects of alcohol consumption will vary according to learned styles of consumption. Historically, and still today, there are few accounts of sensible alcohol use by Aboriginal people, perhaps because it is not thought worthy of reporting (cf. Broome 2005: 25). Nevertheless, we know that there has been change in the choice of drinks. Devoted Aboriginal drinkers in rural and remote areas have largely moved on from drinking fortified wine (port) from flagons or bottles as they did in the 1960s and 1970s; now they prefer sweet wines such as moselle or 'fruity lexia' drunk from casks, or spirits and pre-mixed drinks in cans. In 2000, Kunitz and Levy (2000: 159) reported that among the Navajo Indians of Arizona and New Mexico there had been a shift from fortified wine to beer. After 30 years of

48 Unfortunately, irregular, episodic heavy drinking is one of the most damaging ways of consuming alcohol: it is associated with coronary heart disease, stroke and diabetes. These diseases are exceptions to the usual dose–response relationship between the volume of alcohol consumption and the burden of disease (Room et al. 2005: 520).

research among the Navajo, they also found signs that, despite consistent peer pressure to drink, drinking behaviour was potentially moderating, as implied by declines in mortality and amounts of alcohol consumed. In 1994, they had noted milder drinking styles among Navajos living permanently off-reservation (Kunitz & Levy 1994). Kunitz and Levy (2000: 159) hypothesised that:

It may be due to increasing exposure to a variety of different, and more moderate, drinking styles, although our data are not really adequate to deal with this issue ... the shift from wine to beer is important as a marker of a profound change in tastes and, we believe, as an indication of the penetration of the Navajo economy and culture by the advertisers' art and the tastes of the larger regional population.

Despite the scepticism expressed by some commentators about the rather too orderly implications of the idea of a formalised process of learning how to drink (and re-learning how to drink differently), the idea persists that people can be taught to drink in a different way. Certainly, Aboriginal people themselves believe that they learned their (mostly bad) habits of drinking by observation—initially by watching Europeans' public drinking behaviour and, later, by seeing and following the behaviour of their own family members. Further, in Australia as elsewhere, Indigenous people still express a wistful desire for someone to 'teach' them how to drink and often lament the fact that Europeans never inducted them into the proper use of alcohol. In 1972, John Lame Deer, a Sioux medicine man, wrote with grim humour:

Those clever white men always try to teach us poor, dumb Indians something new. I sure wish they'd teach us how to drink. When you buy a camera or a tape recorder, it always comes with a little booklet which tells you how to use it, but when they brought us the white man's whisky, they forgot the instruction book. This has caused us no end of trouble. (Lame Deer & Erdoes 1972: 71)

In the 1980s, another Native American account compared 'Indian drinking' to white men's drinking with a similar message:

'See, a white man could sit around, drink with a cup'—he mimed drinking tea, little finger in the air—'go for maybe four to five hours. White man enjoys it and don't get quite as intoxicated. You give a quart to one of our guys, he drinks it up, chugs it down, jus' like he used to when it was illegal. Never learned how to drink'. (Lincoln & Slagle 1987: 26)

Although many white Australians drink to excess,[49] Aboriginal people compare their own drinking unfavourably to the drinking practices of settler Australians, and they express the view that their people should learn to drink like the white man.[50] For example, at Yirrkala in northeast Arnhem Land, soon after the repeal of restrictions on consumption in 1964, Yolngu objected to the licensing of a hotel and bottle shop only a few kilometres from their community. With the failure of their objection, and realising that community members would now go to town to drink, the Yirrkala Village Council said that 'Aborigines should learn to drink, like the wise white citizens drink—not too much'. Council member Roy Marika suggested that Yolngu could have a wet canteen as a way of avoiding trouble, 'spoiling *manikay* [clan songs], hurting women and children, and [training] Yolngu to drink sensibly'.[51]

The idea—the aspiration—that people can set aside habitual drinking customs of excess and learn to 'carry their drink like gentlemen' still has traction 80 years after Whitaker's missive on polite drinking. Politicians still yearn for the 'Mediterranean style' of drinking to become the norm in Australian cities. Aboriginal people in remote communities continue to grapple with the dilemmas of alcohol availability, pressures to revoke restrictions and policy options that allow for limited, controlled access. Faced with seemingly endless uproar around alcohol availability and alcohol-related trouble, Aboriginal community leaders—even those who usually support strict controls and dry communities—sometimes relent and once again invoke the desire that people should learn to do better. In 2014, Noel Pearson was reported as suggesting that:

> If there is a model that can encourage responsible drinking then I think it is worth trialling. The ideal position is that we don't have alcohol in Aboriginal communities because alcohol and the strong kinship don't mix, they drink until there is nothing left. But if Indigenous communities insist that they have the same rights as other Australians to have a drink, then they have to learn to drink responsibly like the Greek people, the Chinese people, the whitefellas. (cited by M McKenna 2014: 5)

---

49   A 2016 poll of Australian attitudes and behaviours around alcohol found that 37 per cent of drinkers (more than 4 million people) drink to get drunk (FARE 2016).

50   See Brady (1995) for further examples of Aboriginal men comparing their drinking to that of white Australians.

51   Notes from Yirrkala Village Council meeting, 14 October 1970, courtesy of Dr Nancy Williams.

2

The Gothenburg system, monopolies and the community good

In late Victorian Britain, social and temperance reformers initiated a lively debate about how to encourage civilised drinking and dissuade intoxication through the dual mechanisms of improving the ambience and the serving practices of the public house: the pub. Community or municipal ownership of licensed hotels was one strategy for doing this, together with 'disinterested'—rather than profit-driven—management. This style of ownership, known colloquially as the Gothenburg system, was put into practice in parts of Britain and in Sweden. In the 1890s, these ideas filtered through to influence developments in Australia, particularly South Australia, where, over several decades, 12 community-owned hotels were established in rural towns as a way of benefiting the community and improving amenities. These hotels (nine of which are still trading under community ownership today), distributed a portion of their profits for the good of the community and the betterment of the town. They also aimed to discourage heavy drinking by providing a family atmosphere with access to food and non-alcoholic beverages.

The Gothenburg system provides a useful analytical lens through which developments in the Indigenous domain in Australia can be considered. Commencing in the 1970s with financial assistance from newly constituted business-oriented government agencies such as the ADC, several Indigenous community-based associations purchased licensed hotels.

They hoped to achieve many of the same aims as their non-Indigenous counterparts: to reform drinking premises, control excess and direct profits to community needs. These ideas influenced the policy climate that allowed licensed social clubs and canteens to be opened in remote Indigenous communities. In the case of the narcotic drug kava, used in some Aboriginal communities in northeast Arnhem Land, regulated access and a monopoly over sales was seen as preferable to prohibition. Nineteenth- and early twentieth-century arguments for and against the principles underlying Gothenburg-style hotels, and the debates between citizens, abolitionists and publicans, provide a foretaste of the political and community agitation that accompanied Indigenous forays into social and commercial liquor enterprises in Australia in the 1980s and 1990s.

The 'Scandinavian plan'

The notion that excessive drinking could be moderated by removing the commercially driven profit motive from alcohol sales and replacing it with a softer, community-benefiting rationale, seems to have originated in Scandinavia in the mid-nineteenth century. The idea gave birth to a liquor-control model that came to be associated with the city of Gothenburg.

Gothenburg was Sweden's second city: a commercial town and seaport that suffered deep poverty and increasing degradation under the 'blight and curse' of the drink traffic (Pitman 1877: 220). Despite being a well-educated town with a system of compulsory education and philanthropic schools for poor children, it had a culture of extreme spree drinking of spirits. Sweden had a strong temperance tradition; however, rather than opting for prohibition, as had other Scandinavian countries, Gothenburg chose to experiment with restrictive alcohol-control measures that had been tried in the smaller town of Falun (Room 1993: 173). The guiding principle of the system was to disconnect the sale of alcohol from the profit motive, thereby reducing the pressured selling that led to excess consumption and intoxication. The system proposed ownership of licensed premises by a semi-private trust that regulated the sale of spirits on philanthropic principles. The shopkeeper selling strong liquor was restricted to taking only 5 per cent profit, with the municipality, county and state dividing any additional profit (Brown 1972, Blocker et al.

2003: 603). Licensed outlets were to be run by 'disinterested' and salaried managers who had no pecuniary interest in pushing sales of alcohol. As one supporter explained:

> The secret of most of the mischief now worked by the [liquor] trade is that the monopoly of the sale of liquor is connected with private interests … The brewer, the distiller, the publican, the shareholder, are all deeply interested in promoting the sale of liquor. (Wilson 1894: 7)

Eliminating the stimulus of personal gain from a legitimate commercial activity was a revolutionary idea. It was based on the belief that the 'drink traffic', as it was called, was so abnormal that it should be treated differently to other kinds of trading activity (Pitman 1877: 223).[1] The system was originally targeted at working-class restaurants in Sweden, but it also provided for municipal ownership of taverns and was later extended to shops providing off-premise sales of spirits. Spirits such as *brännvin*, a type of vodka distilled from potatoes and grains, were the most damaging drinks, while ale and beer were considered barely intoxicating at all. Apart from civilising the drinking act and minimising social disruptions related to drinking, the system aimed to improve standards in licensing, make alcohol subject to local control and cut out any political influence on the trade (Room 1993). The authorities could control the licences and minimise drunkenness while the community shareholders received a return on capital, with any surplus going to the municipal coffers.[2]

In 1865, a charter was granted by the Swedish Government and a *bolag* (company) was formed with the following objectives:

- to reduce the number of public houses
- to improve their condition as to light, ventilation, cleanliness
- to make public houses eating houses where warm, cooked food was available at moderate prices
- to refuse sale of spirits on credit or pledge

---

1   The sentiment that alcohol differs significantly from other consumables and trade items was reiterated 116 years later when a major World Health Organization–sponsored study was given the name *Alcohol: No Ordinary Commodity* (Babor et al. 2003).
2   In Bergen, Norway (where the system started in 1877), the beneficiaries of the company's profits included the orchestra of the Christiana theatre, the Young Men's Association, civic plantings, fountains, the Society for Homeless Youth and the Country Housekeeping Society (Gould 1893: 190).

- to employ as managers respectable persons who should derive no profit from the sale of spirits, but should be entitled to profits from the sale of food and other refreshments, including malt liquors
- to secure strict supervision of all public houses by inspectors of their own, in addition to the police
- to pay to the town treasury all the net profits of sales of spirits. (Pitman 1877: 223)

Similar monopoly companies established in Scandinavia mandated other rules, such as not selling to those intoxicated or underage, and some employed their own police detectives to monitor breaches on premises. Most of these principles are recognisable within modern alcohol-control policies as harm-reduction strategies; indeed, since the nineteenth century, strong evidence has accumulated that government monopolies on the manufacture, supply and sale of alcohol tend to result in reduced harm. Seven countries belonging to the Organisation for Economic Cooperation and Development now permit a state-owned monopoly at some stage in the alcohol production and sale cycle. According to a 2005 review of regulations:

> Unlike private suppliers with a strong profit motive, a state-owned monopoly can pursue other objectives including restricting the volume and availability of what it supplies. Rather than seek to innovate and expand the number of markets, a state-owned liquor monopoly has no incentive to, for example, introduce alcohol milk products or alcohol-caffeine mixes or to advertise heavily. On the contrary, it can price discriminate to suppress demand for most popular items and those appealing to high risk drinkers especially. The benefits to health outcomes from this approach would need to be balanced against the economic loss that will result from monopoly. (Marsden Jacob Associates 2005: 38; cf. Babor et al. 2003)

What became known as the 'Scandinavian plan' was vigorously debated and implemented to varying degrees in the United Kingdom (Wilson 1894, Brown 1972), the United States (Pitman 1877, Gould 1893, Gordon 1911, Room 1993) and Australia (Malins 1899, Butler 1899). The United States Commissioner of Labor was interested enough to send a statistician, ERL Gould, to Scandinavia to investigate and collect data on the system. Gould (1893) subsequently compiled an impressive and positive overview that included data on intoxication, alcohol-related symptoms and deaths and rates of refusals of entry to premises, and reported a notable decline in drunkenness. He concluded:

That the system is perfect no-one will be sanguine enough to maintain; but that it represents the best means which have yet been devised for the control of the liquor traffic where licensing is permitted ... few who ... have studied its operation would be bold enough to deny. (243)[3]

In the United States, United Kingdom and Australia, the Scandinavian plan had two main groups of opponents: brewers and 'licensed victuallers' versus ardent teetotallers. The latter group comprised people 'who do not think a reform is worth having while they can dream of abolition' (Wilson 1894: 14). As it turned out, the Gothenburg system never became a national policy in Sweden. However, in 1917, the country endorsed an alcohol policy featuring two measures, the first of which carried through the idea that the profit motive should be eliminated in the alcohol trade. The second measure aimed to control an individual's purchases of alcohol through a system of ration books. Temperance boards with local knowledge made decisions based on social and moral behavioural standards about whether individuals could obtain ration books that gave them access to alcohol (Blocker et al. 2003: 605, Room 2012). Similar controls have operated in some Aboriginal communities in Australia: in the Northern Territory, for example, permit committees made up of local people (the equivalent of the 'temperance boards') made decisions about whether individuals were fit to hold permits to obtain alcohol.

'Gothenburg' in Britain

Like the United States, Britain was intrigued by the Swedish system because it offered a middle way through the policy deadlock between two warring factions: the reforming restrictionists and the teetotal prohibitionists (Greenaway 2003: 71, 1998). The Swedish system represented a form of liquor control that was grounded in acceptance of the use of alcohol; however, by controlling where and how alcohol was sold, 'sought to structure and influence the use so as to limit the social and health harm from drinking' (Room 2004: 330). Britain had debated

---

3   Several American states implemented versions of the Gothenburg system in the 1890s as a better alternative to prohibition, but the movement ultimately succumbed to the activities of the Anti-Saloon League and the advent of National Prohibition in 1920. Following the repeal of prohibition in 1933 (and concerned to avoid old evils), American investigators recommended regulation policies for the states, proposing a state monopoly for distribution and retail package sales or, alternatively, the development of state-based licensing systems. Most states adopted licensing systems, but 17 instituted some form of monopoly. These have lasted remarkably well; only two American states have since ended their retail distribution monopolies (Room 1993, Cook 2007: 2).

the system since the 1870s, and politicians, temperance advocates and interested citizens had visited Scandinavia to see it for themselves; these individuals helped to disseminate knowledge about the 'Scandinavian plan'.[4] Politicians who travelled to Gothenburg for a firsthand assessment included Liberal member Joseph Chamberlain.[5] Once a supporter of prohibition, Chamberlain had come to believe that access to alcohol was both 'socially necessary and morally correct, while abstinence was counter to all facts' (Brown 1972: 34).[6]

Permutations of the Gothenburg system thrived in Britain some years later when philanthropist, temperance advocate and Quaker capitalist Joseph Rowntree[7] took up, and later refined, some of its underlying principles. Rowntree and his associate, Arthur Sherwell, linked the need for licensing reform with solutions to the poverty associated with urban industrial expansion. They attributed excessive drinking to two factors: first, the monotonous lives of working people and lack of 'rational recreation' that might offer them an alternative to drink; and second, the push for profits by the liquor trade. Rowntree and Sherwell saw money raised from the trade in liquor as compensation money. They believed that liquor should be sold by publicans who were 'disinterested' in profits, and that social reform should include the provision of civic amenities that acted as counterattractions to the pub (Gutzke 1989, Greenaway 1998, 2003: 70). The idea of disinterested management represented an early example of what we now call corporate social responsibility (Talbot 2015). Across Britain, semi-philanthropic public house trusts were

---

4   For example, enlightened theologian James Wilson preached a sermon in the north of England on 'Temperance Sunday', 18 November 1894, in which he extolled the virtues of the Scandinavian plan (Wilson 1894).
5   Chamberlain (1836–1914) was a Unitarian—a social reformer but not a socialist. He was the father of future British Prime Minister Neville Chamberlain.
6   In the 1870s, Britain's Liberal party had a strong prohibitionist bloc and was closely linked with the United Kingdom Alliance, a teetotalism society. Conversely, the Tories were supported by the publicans (Brown 1972: 31). The liquor industry comprised powerful and unscrupulous businessmen who intimidated cabinet ministers and other members of parliament, magistrates and town councils, and were seen as being politically corrupting (Gutzke 1989: 52).
7   Joseph Rowntree (1836–1925) was a Quaker, businessman and philanthropist. There are many charitable trusts in the United Kingdom that bear his name, such as the Joseph Rowntree Foundation, which supports innovative and policy-oriented research, including research into temperance issues (cf. Berridge 2005, Cadbury 2010).

formed to acquire, and then improve, licensed pubs by implementing disinterested management practices: there were 60 in Scotland, usually in mining communities.[8]

The People's Refreshment Houses Association (PRHA), founded in 1896, was the most successful of these schemes. Shares were offered to the public who were eligible for a dividend of not more than 5 per cent. Surplus profit went to public utilities and officers of the PRHA were elected. Member-run public houses provided temperance drinks and food as well as beer (Rowntree & Sherwell 1903, Greenaway 1998, Burnett 1999: 132). Public houses belonging to the PRHA were mostly small village inns, some of which were described in Rowntree and Sherwell's 1903 publication on British Gothenburg experiments. A typical inn in Somerset had a monopoly on local trade and sold the full range of liquor, but had small off-premises sales, gave no credit and had no advertising of alcoholic beverages anywhere on the premises. Instead, there were conspicuous advertisements for tea, coffee and temperance drinks and a ready supply of food. The manager was paid a fixed salary and received most of the profit made on the sale of food, mineral waters, cigarettes and tobacco, but not alcohol. If the manager thought a drinker had had enough, they pre-empted harm by putting their finger up as a warning sign that they would refuse further service (Rowntree & Sherwell 1903: 23). Another description of trust house hotels emphasised the food and counterattractions available. Instead of a large bar dominated by rows of bottles, the saloon was taken up with 'sociable tables' where people consumed pea, lentil and barley soups. In Northumberland, *The Grey Arms* reportedly also sold a new item—fried potato chips 'for which a considerable demand seems probable'. The hotel had a lawn outside, a reading room and a billiard room. Another public house was run by a village council and its profits provided for a community nurse, an ambulance wagon and entertainment hall (*West Gippsland Gazette*, 14 April 1903: 5).

---

8   In Prestonpans, East Lothian, Scotland, there is a hotel known as the Prestoungrange Gothenburg, or 'The Goth', that still runs on the Gothenburg principle. It was created in 1901 by a private trust known as the East of Scotland Public House Trust. The Trust was set up by eight investors sympathetic to temperance ideals who wanted to take the profiteering out of selling alcohol while promoting the sale of food. Its profits are gifted to the Prestoungrange Arts Festival. There is also a 'Goth' hotel in Armadale, West Lothian (Armadale Public House Society 2001, Prestoungrange 2004). There has recently been a revival of cooperative hotels in Britain, as villages 'save' their local pubs by buying them (Jones 2017: 13).

The benign imagery associated with the trust house scheme provoked some lampooning at the time, epitomised in a satirical poem 'The Bishop and the Scandinavian plan'.[9] In it, a Bishop invites a customer into the 'sweetest little parlour, on the Scandinavian plan' and explains that 'the House is carried on with most benevolent intent/And on Temperance Societies the profits are all spent':

> Yes! I cannot put it clearer, in explaining our intent,
> It is to benefit mankind—and pocket five per cent.
> So please walk into my parlour, and be drinking all you can,
> You will find it very pleasant on the Scandinavian plan ...
> The Scandinavian plan, my boys! The Scandinavian plan!
> By far the strangest thing there's been since first the world began!

Despite this mockery, there was support from the Fabian Society for community-run public houses. George Bernard Shaw, a well-known Fabian, joined one of the PRHA's and, in 1901, the 4th Earl Grey became chairman of the largest of the trust associations (Warner 2006, Room 2004). If pubs could not be abolished, then they should be improved:

> British Gothenburgers wanted to reform the pub, not destroy it; broaden its patrons, not make it synonymous with plebeian culture; introduce middle-class values in behavior and speech, not ostracize drinkers; and above all imbue it with respectability, not cast it out as reprehensible. (Gutzke 2007: 238)

Gutzke saw Gothenburgers as progressives who championed order, discipline, cultural uplift and the influence of the environment on drinking behaviour; were intent on diminishing drunkenness by improving the physical and interpersonal settings in which alcohol was consumed; and hoped for the 'civilizing influence of the upper and middle classes'. By the turn of the century, there was widespread acceptance of the trust principle in Britain. This was largely because the 'public house is recognized as a public necessity, and that therefore it is desirable to convert it from a mere drinking bar into something resembling, as much as possible, a well-conducted club' (Smyth [1904] 2013: 249). As we shall see, these ideas—that drinking could be 'civilised' both by altering the physical and social environment in which it took place and by allowing respectable citizens to contribute to the management of hotels—began to appear in Australia as well.

---

9   The Bishop referred to in this ditty was the Bishop of Chester, United Kingdom, who launched the PRHA, a trust designed to run pubs based on the Scandinavian Gothenburg system (International Order of Good Templars 1890, Rowntree & Sherwell 1903, Gutzke 1994).

Gothenburg ideas arrive in South Australia

The Gothenburg system—in the form of community ownership of hotels—was especially influential in South Australia. The principles of moderated alcohol sales, citizen participation in hotel governance and the quarantining of profits for the betterment of the community, had great appeal in South Australia because respectable immigrants, not convicts, had settled there. Many of these immigrants had favoured non-conformist Christianity. The colony of South Australia soon developed a reputation for self-help and communal agricultural settlement, especially along the Murray River (Whitelock 1985, Casson & Hirst 1988). These underlying factors combined to support community ownership of hotels in Renmark in the 1890s.

The town of Renmark was part of a pioneering irrigation colony established in 1887 on the Murray River by two Canadian irrigators, the brothers George and WB Chaffey. Both were teetotallers. The South Australian Government gave the Chaffey brothers the right to use 100,000 ha of land north of the river to establish an irrigation system with private capital, which enabled them to establish a colony of like-minded people. The Chaffey brothers and local residents wanted the Renmark area to be dry and advertised it to prospective settlers accordingly. In 1891, the South Australian Licensed Victuallers Act was amended to allow the Chaffey brothers' colony to be dry; the Victorian Government made a similar ruling for the Chaffey's nearby colony at Mildura, which was also set up as a temperance colony. Ironically, the irrigation systems initiated by the Chaffey brothers made extensive plantings of vines possible, resulting in the eventual production of wine and brandy in the region, along with dried and fresh fruits.[10] Renmark and Mildura (and many other towns, particularly in Victoria) already had unlicensed 'temperance hotels' that offered board and lodging, but no alcohol. Influenced by the temperance movement, such hotels were often coffee palaces with grandiose facades and fittings designed to compete with the taverns (Room 1988).[11] Their popularity declined over the years as residents agitated for licensed

10   In 1911, Dr WT Angove and his sons created the first winery and distillery in the upper Murray at Renmark (Jones 1994: 287). After World War I, blocks of land in the region became part of the scheme to repatriate returned servicemen; they often grew dried fruit.

11   The best known of these temperance hotels in Victoria is the Windsor Hotel, Melbourne. In 1886, it was known as the Grand Coffee Palace and sold no alcohol for 10 years until a successful application was made to remove the prohibition in 1897.

premises, which is what occurred in Renmark and Mildura.[12] After several years, Renmark's form of local prohibition was deemed a failure because it was not possible to stop sly grog from flowing into the area: paddle steamers unloaded kegs of beer that were broached where they lay, creating 'a club under every ti-tree' (Johnson 1997: 8). The road from the temperance colony of Mildura to the nearest source of alcohol at Wentworth was delineated by a trail of bottles (Lapthorne 1947).

In June 1895, with a story headlined 'A hotel wanted', the editor of the *Renmark Pioneer*, Chris Ashwell, triggered debate about the need to deal with this sly grog trade. Although temperance principles had been appropriate in the early days of the settlement, the population was larger now and Ashwell asked why residents of Renmark should 'be deprived of privileges enjoyed by other communities of similar population?' He had heard about the Gothenburg system that was already being debated in nearby Mildura:

> The sister settlement of Mildura has been at various times strongly agitated on this question, and last year an informal vote[13] was taken on the subject, resulting in a very large majority voting for the establishment of houses on somewhat the same system as that known as the Gothenburgh [sic] … [We] may advocate a like scheme for Renmark without laying ourselves open to the charge of running counter to temperance principles.[14]

Ashwell believed that Renmark would be a municipality one day, and that it could form a trust to have sole control over the sale of spirits and employ a manager who would have no interest in pushing the sale of drink, the net profit of which could be devoted to improving the settlement's roads. Over the following weeks, arguments for and against the establishment of a licensed hotel were printed in the newspaper. Many of these would be familiar to Australians today (particularly those who live in the Northern Territory). Temperance advocates objected to Ashwell's idea, describing it as a weak alternative to prohibition. The local Methodist pastor, Reverend

---

12   The Grand Hotel at Mildura (originally the coffee palace) was fully licensed in 1919 along with three clubs, which helped to 'minimize the sly grog traffic which had been rife for so many years' (Lapthorne 1947: 18–19).

13   The results of this informal vote in Mildura in 1894 were as follows: continuing the existing system, 9; an ordinary hotel system, 77; Gothenburg system, 284; total prohibition, 15 (*South Australian Register* 1 August 1894: 5).

14   Editorial, *Renmark Pioneer* 15 June 1895: 2. Despite the earlier vote in favour of a Gothenburg hotel in Mildura, it never eventuated. Dissenting voices questioned the 'extravagance' of the claims made for the Gothenburg system and argued that having such a hotel would simply introduce an extra bar into the town.

W Corly Butler, insisted that it would be foolish to reverse the existing 'dry' status of the land, but his argument was countered by another correspondent who stated that:

> It is a well-known fact that there is far less drunkenness in a township with a well conducted hotel, under the careful supervision of the police, than when it is prohibited, and instead of being done openly is carried on to a far greater extent by those who are unwilling to be coerced and will therefore keep it in their own houses. (*Renmark Pioneer* 1895: 4)

Further, it was argued that if a man could get an occasional drink at reasonable hours 'he would be much less likely to make a beast of himself'.[15]

A Renmark Local Progress Committee (RLPC) was formed to pursue the community hotel idea, and the South Australian Licensed Victuallers Act was amended to allow a publican's licence to be granted specifically for a community-run business, provided a majority of local householders signed a petition requesting it. There was a counter petition, but the vote was carried. Despite his misgivings, Butler signed the RLPC's petition, believing that anything would be better than sly grog and hoping that the system would 'prove a restraint on the drink traffic' (Butler 1899: 3). The RLPC approached Mrs Jane Meissner (who had owned the town's temperance hotel since 1892) to see if she would sell her business, which she agreed to do. A local station-owner provided the funds and, in March 1897, Mrs Meissner was appointed manager of the licensed Renmark Community Hotel, the only legitimate liquor outlet in an otherwise dry district covering several thousand square kilometres of South Australia (*The Argus* 1922, Young & Secker 1984: 574, Johnson 1997): the sly grog shops reportedly closed immediately. The nearest settlement was the communal agricultural village of Lyrup, 20 km away, where the only alcohol allowed was a supply of medicinal brandy that was kept under lock and key by the doctor (Jones 1994). The Renmark Community Hotel claimed at the time, and has claimed since, to be the first community hotel in the British Empire (Renmark Community Hotel, no date, Johnson 1997).

It was decided that the hotel licence should be held by an elected committee of five community members, all of whom had to be approved landholders resident in Renmark. No member of the committee could have an interest in any retail business associated with the sale of alcohol, other than the

---

15 *Renmark Pioneer* 29 June 1895: 2.

produce of their own vineyard. The first chairman of the committee was an Anglican clergyman. In keeping with Gothenburg principles, the hotel manager was to be paid a regular salary to eliminate any inducement to 'push' sales. After expenses had been paid, the hotel profits were to be used for the cultural and general betterment of the settlement of Renmark— that is, 'in the promotion or encouragement of literature, science, or art or for charitable or benevolent purposes or otherwise as the Committee shall decide and the Honorable the Treasurer shall approve' (Johnson 1997: 14).

Critics of the Renmark Gothenburg

Notwithstanding the positive outcomes that would soon be claimed for the Renmark Community Hotel, it, and the system it represented, were not without detractors. Although Butler had signed the petition supporting the hotel's establishment, in the months following its opening, he became a critic of the way it was operating. He believed the system 'was as baneful as the ordinary licensed house'. Although it had killed off the sly grog trade, he argued that:

> The service of drink in [the Renmark Hotel] was under no more restraint than in any respectable hotel in Perth, and that for a small and impoverished community the drink bill was very high. (Butler 1899: 3)

Butler was adamant that the community-owned hotel at Renmark did nothing more to lessen drunkenness than any ordinary hotel would have done. He may well have been right, but in view of the fact that most of the hotel's customers had been used to drinking sly grog, in the open, with no constraints other than the limits to supply, it is hardly surprising that drinking styles did not change overnight. At least 13 sly grog shops had been operating for a population of around 1000, and these drinkers—many of whom were itinerant agricultural workers—had yet to be habituated to the behaviours expected of them when drinking on legitimately licensed premises. More than 100 years later, a similar crisis of comportment occurred in the Western Australian town of Fitzroy Crossing when Aboriginal drinkers, who had been used to drinking takeaway alcohol in the open air, were suddenly forced by new regulations to change their drinking style and drink on (rather than off) premises; this episode is discussed in Chapter 7.

Another critic was an English Wesleyan, Joseph Malins (1844–1926), who visited Australia on a round-the-world mission for the Order of Good Templars, a teetotal society. Two years after the opening of the

Renmark Community Hotel, he spoke in Melbourne at the Collins Street Independent Church. By this time, Malins, like many others, had visited Norway and Sweden to see for himself their liquor-control systems at work. While he agreed that the Gothenburg *bolag* had reduced the number of public houses and the hours of sale in their premises, he pointed out that other drinking houses, not under the immediate control of the *bolag*, continued to open until late; this, of course, is always a problem when restrictions only target some outlets. Malins also questioned whether paying a manager a salary instead of a commission on sales of spirits was really enough to make them 'disinterested'. He believed that the apparent drop in drunkenness charges was due to changed policing practices rather than changed drinking practices, and claimed that the city of Gothenburg was *more* inebriated than Aberdeen in Scotland or Cardiff in Wales. His final, acerbic comment (aimed specifically at Rowntree and Sherwell's trust house scheme in Britain), was that:

> When Jews open pork shops, and vegetarians open butcher's shops then teetotallers may run public houses, or elect others to run them. All true Temperance men want power granted to the people to deal *with* the traffic, not to embark *in* it. (Malins 1899: 6, original emphasis)

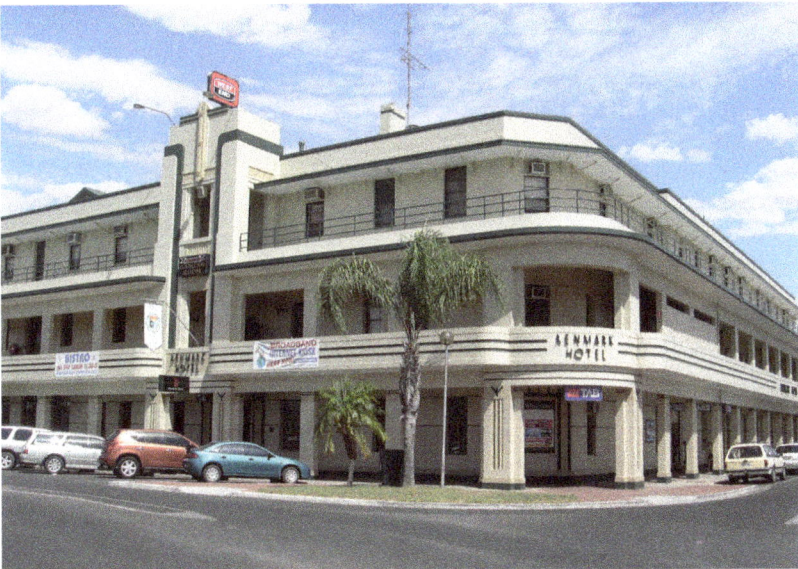

Fig. 2 Renmark Hotel, South Australia
Source: M Brady

Despite this and other criticisms, the Renmark Community Hotel continued to flourish. In 1922, it was reported that the hotel manager made every attempt to encourage sobriety; that there had been no reported breaches of licensing laws; and, on the basis of population, that the figures for drunkenness were lower in Renmark than in any other part of the state (*The Argus* 1922). The hotel announced good profits that year and £20,000 were devoted to extensions. Two years later, the hotel hoped for £10,000 a year for distribution to the township. At that time, the hotel had 70 rooms, dining for 120 people and a staff of 35; plans were in place for a new bar with marble floors, blackwood furnishings, modern pumps and ice chests. In 1936, an art deco three-storey frontage was built that can still be seen today.

Debate over community-owned hotels

As word spread among towns along the Murray River, interest in establishing community hotels moved elsewhere in South Australia and extended into Victoria and New South Wales. The story of Renmark's success was reiterated and promulgated as a model that other towns should follow. In the decades after the Renmark Community Hotel opened its doors, newspapers across Australia and New Zealand published largely positive articles about the Gothenburg system, sometimes referred to as the 'Earl Grey system'.[16] It was described as an admirable scheme:

> Every [public] house has a well-furnished tea-room, and nearly every one has a tea-garden in which customers can enjoy themselves rationally in the company of their wives and children. This is the true line of temperance reform. Offer a man something better than the privilege of getting fuddled, and nine times out of ten he will gladly take it.[17]

Inspired by Renmark, Waikerie (originally a communal village settlement on the Murray River) established its own community hotel in 1912. In the 1930s, several nearby towns followed suit, voting in favour of

---

16 'English drink question. The Earl Grey system', *West Gippsland Gazette* 14 April 1903: 5; 'Earl Grey's Trust "Pub"', *Northern Territory Times and Gazette* 2 July 1914: 8; 'Growing interest in community hotels', *Recorder* (Port Pirie) 5 January 1939: 1. *The New Zealand Herald* carried a story titled 'The Gothenburg system in Australia: Successful introduction in Renmark' on 12 May 1898: 6.
17 *Northern Territory Times and Gazette* 2 July 1914: 8. Similar optimistic visions accompanied early suggestions for licensed clubs in remote Aboriginal communities in which drinking facilities were intended to stress family gatherings, the provision of soft drinks and food and counterattractions such as pool and darts (Leary et al. 1975).

local monopolies and for the restriction of other liquor licences in their districts. Barmera opened a community hotel in 1932, and Berri opened one in 1937. The community at Loxton applied for a licence in 1934 and, in 1946, the Loxton Hotel finally became community-owned. This meant that five neighbouring towns, connected physically by the Murray River and linked philosophically through their shared history of the temperance-oriented irrigation colony, now had community-owned hotels.[18] Several small towns in South Australia opened community hotels in subsequent years: Nuriootpa in the Barossa Valley bought its hotel in 1937; in the far west, Ceduna citizens bought their hotel in 1949; Kimba residents followed suit in 1951; and the hotel at Streaky Bay became community owned in 1965. All these hotels were to be managed for the residents, with profits devoted to public purposes in the area (Young & Secker 1984).

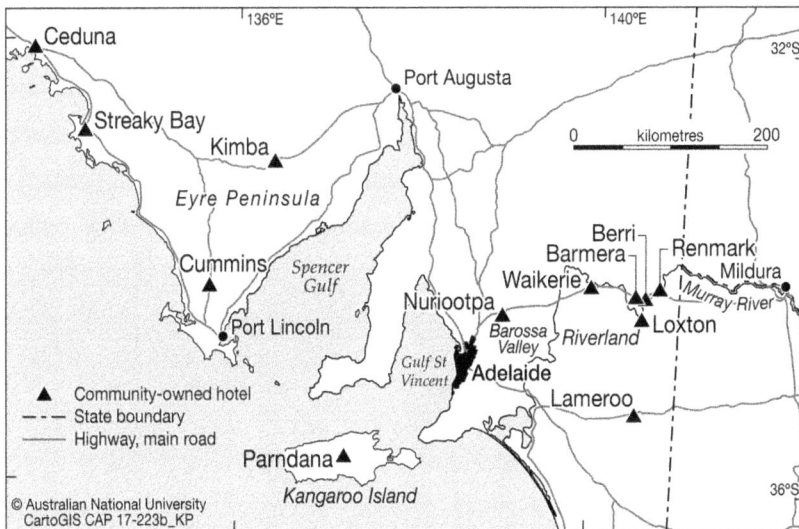

Map 1 Past and present community hotels in South Australia, 1897–2015
Source: CartoGIS, The Australian National University

In other locations, politicians, aldermen and prominent citizens advocated for community hotels in preference to privately owned establishments. Their reasons were threefold. First, there was concern about the perceived

---

18   In South Australia, the *Community Hotels (Incorporation) Act, 1938* [No. 2407] made this proliferation possible. The Act validated the incorporation of several of these hotels under an earlier one, the *Associations Incorporation Act 1929–35*, dspace.flinders.edu.au/jspui/handle/2328/24937.

growing influence of the liquor industry because of its donations to political parties: community ownership was seen as a way of countering this unwanted trend. In 1939, discussing the possibility of a community hotel in Port Pirie, local dignitaries spoke of the profitability of the liquor trade and the immense sums that were being poured into political propaganda by liquor interests:

> It should be an offence to demand from hotelkeepers a contribution to any fund or to include an amount in the wholesale price of liquor which would be contributed by the breweries to such a fund. It is said by hotelkeepers that amounts from such funds are distributed for political purposes to assist the candidature of certain persons at elections. In order that we may ultimately be freed from the thraldom of brewers I suggest that the hotels should be owned by the community and not made the vehicles of private gain.[19] (*Recorder* [Port Pirie] 1939: 1)

Second, these prominent citizens were supporters of moderation and were in favour of the harm-reduction qualities that would ideally be embedded in such hotels. Under the Gothenburg system, one alderman stated, credit was given to a hotel 'not for the quantity of liquor it sold, but for the moderation of its sales and the sobriety of its patrons'. Third, and most importantly, the local variation on the Gothenburg system appealed to politicians, local councillors and civic-minded citizens because of its revenue-raising capability. Local and state politicians were interested in community hotels because they provided a substantial stream of locally generated income that could be devoted to local needs. The community-owned Renmark establishment had become well known in South Australia, not just for the 'high standard of accommodation and service it offers', but for the '*huge sums* it has earned for expenditure on town beautification and other civil purposes' (*Recorder* [Port Pirie] 1939: 1, emphasis added).

As community groups in towns in New South Wales and Victoria began to agitate for policy changes that would make such hotels possible, their lobbying caught the attention of temperance activists and organisations such as the WCTU. Taking a hard line rather than a reformist position, these organisations were thoroughly opposed to the idea of community licences. As part of their campaign against community hotels, they argued

---

19   It is worth pointing out that liquor industry representatives still curry favour with politicians. According to the Australian Electoral Commission, in 2012–13, the Australian Hotels Association (representing hoteliers nationally) was the largest political donor in the country, with most of its donations being directed to the Liberal party (d'Abbs 2014: 21).

that good people were being led away by 'specious arguments' (Wilson 1946: 1). In 1946, remarks from the Temperance Alliance questioning the supposed successes of the Renmark Community Hotel were broadcast by a Sydney radio station. The speaker suggested that community ownership encouraged a 'mob spirit', which encouraged more drinking, and that donations to charity, which amounted to a small percentage of overall profits, allowed the hotel and the liquor trade to acquire a 'false respectability'. Temperance activists publicised details of the Renmark Community Hotel's revenue, which showed that, although a record profit of £12,000 had been made in 1944–45, of which £3,000 had been distributed to local causes, £43,752 had been spent on alcohol in the hotel's bars to secure this amount. The speaker accused the Renmark Community Hotel of donating to Christian organisations to 'buy off' the temperance cause, and claimed that donations were made in expectation of favours to come. Similarly, a WCTU pamphlet published in 1945 made use of detailed sales data from the Renmark Community Hotel to demolish its claims of generosity, observing that such gifts were merely 'a salve to the consciences of the promoters and the public, blinding them to the deterioration which takes place in the lives of their most regular customers' (McCorkindale 1945: 1).

The supposed success of 'disinterested management' was also questioned by the WCTU. It pointed out, somewhat sardonically, that there were no records of a community hotel manager being commended for reporting a *decrease* in bar trade. On the contrary, increased sales led to the manager being congratulated, commended and even paid a bonus in some instances. The author of the 1945 WCTU pamphlet, Isobel McCorkindale (1885–1971), was a Scottish-born activist who organised campaigns against liquor licences and extended opening hours. A great promoter of fruit juice, she was known for her use of scientific rather than emotive arguments against alcohol.[20] Her pamphlet warned against making community-owned hotels part of any 'community centre' set up for the benefit of a neighbourhood. She concluded, perceptively, that:

---

20 McCorkindale reported on the Carlisle scheme of state ownership in the United Kingdom, which began during World War I as a means of controlling liquor sales and thus safeguarding workers and the war effort in an industrialised area of naval bases, dockyards and munitions factories. Managers reported redesigned pubs with better facilities, sales of food and non-intoxicants and the elimination of private interests in liquor sales (Shadwell 1923). However, McCorkindale claimed that there had been no reduction in consumption as a result.

> The effect of alcohol is just the same on the individual whether it is sold over a bar owned by a private individuals [sic] or one in which the community is interested. There is something about the liquor traffic which does not fit in with an effort requiring goodwill and selflessness. (McCorkindale 1945: 4)

Many temperance activists were women. Their arguments foreshadowed a campaign by Aboriginal women who objected to the proposed establishment of a community-owned club in Alice Springs nearly 50 years later. Like their white counterparts in the WCTU, the Aboriginal women held to an abolitionist position that was intolerant of the notion of 'social' moderate drinking. While they acknowledged the good intentions of those who supported the club, they argued that even if it were owned and run by Aboriginal interests for Aboriginal customers, it would still amount to an additional liquor licence in a town already awash in alcohol. The rise and demise of the Alice Springs club is discussed in Chapter 5.

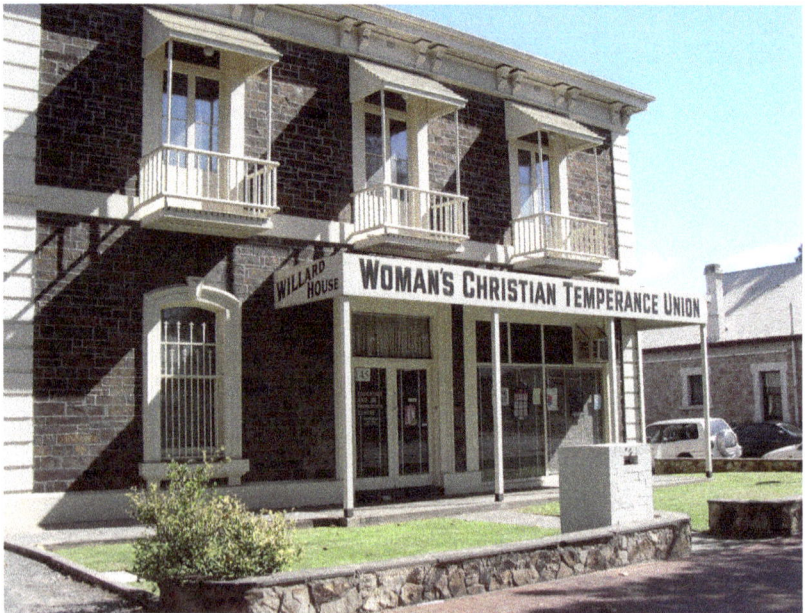

Fig. 3 WCTU Offices, Hutt Street, Adelaide
Source: M Brady

Compromising the Gothenburg vision?

The South Australian community hotels experienced their heyday in the first half of the twentieth century, after which some of their monopoly status came to an end. Increasingly subject to competition, they were placed under greater pressure to increase sales to maintain viability, as predicted by their temperance critics. Three of the original 12 community-owned premises in South Australia went broke and their leases were sold to commercial operators.[21] Community hotels became more exposed to competition after legislation was introduced in 1967 abolishing their monopoly in towns such as Renmark, Berri and Barmera. Young and Secker,[22] in their 1984 review of the South Australian Liquor Act, described Section 105, which allowed for restriction on the number of licences in Riverland communities, as 'anachronistic'. The government's decision to repeal Section 105 was the final defeat of temperance thinking in the old irrigation colony towns. Subsequently, townspeople who wanted to limit the number of hotels in their district would have to convince a central licensing authority of the merits of their position (Young & Secker 1984: 575).[23] Although monopolies still exist today, they are somewhat tenuous. As one hotel manager interviewed for this study (in 2015) explained: 'If our hotel was not a monopoly, we would have no choice but to sell aggressively, spend more on marketing [and] happy hours, as the hotel must survive. This would be contradictory to the community'.

Depending on their location, most community-owned hotels in South Australia must now compete with other alcohol outlets to varying degrees. The original Gothenburg-style principles that animated such hotels have been sacrificed and compromises made. Bearing out the criticisms and fears of temperance activists such as McCorkindale, commercial considerations now appear to be paramount. In Ceduna, for example, while the stated purpose of community ownership of the hotel echoes some of the original Gothenburg principles—such as no private individual receiving monetary benefit from the profits—other Gothenburg principles—

---

21   The nine remaining community-owned hotels in South Australia are in Barmera, Berri, Ceduna, Lameroo, Loxton, Nuriootpa, Parndana, Renmark and Waikerie. The three that have sold their leases are Cummins, Kimba and Streaky Bay.

22   At the time of the review, Andrew Secker was a public servant: he later became the Liquor Licensing Commissioner for South Australia.

23   In their review of South Australia's liquor licensing laws, Young and Secker (1984: 21) promoted what they believed was 'cautious liberalisation'. Contrary to considerable research evidence, they were of the view that liberalising trading hours and increasing the number of liquor outlets would neither significantly increase consumption, nor make alcohol-related diseases worse.

such as reducing harm by controlling alcohol sales—are not explicitly addressed. The hotel aims to be as profitable as possible so as to return profits to the local community and develop facilities to attract tourism and create job opportunities.[24] Improvements to the hotel itself have been made possible by the hotel's substantial income from its takeaway bottle shop and poker machines, both of which have arguably had negative effects on the community. In 1973, when the town's first drive-in bottle shop opened, the hotel's annual turnover 'rocketed' to $396,000; the drive-in facility boosted bottle sales by 75 per cent. Over the years, many Aboriginal people from Yalata (200 km west) purchased bulk supplies of alcohol, mostly fortified wine, from the bottle shop. In 1999, the hotel celebrated its 50th anniversary by replacing the existing modest drive-in with an enormous structure that dominated (and still dominates) a major intersection in the town. By purchasing liquor in larger quantities, the new facility could sell at lower prices (Trewartha 1999: 55, Brady et al. 2003). Several years earlier, in 1994, the hotel had introduced poker machines. Used enthusiastically by local Aboriginal people, these became a major source of revenue for the hotel.[25] While the revenue from poker machines contributes to the hotel's ability to make community distributions, the cost is high, particularly for Aboriginal people who comprise nearly 25 per cent of the population in Ceduna's Local Government Area. Poker machines draw resources from these extremely disadvantaged people, many of whom live in remote communities.

South Australian rural towns took on the spirit, if not the detail, of the ideas of disinterested management and municipal control that typified the Gothenburg system.[26] Although only the hotel at Renmark explicitly described itself as Gothenburg-style, it was this hotel that popularised the system and prompted the diffusion of community ownership. What caught the eye of other towns was the potential of profit distribution; as time passed, the distribution of monies became the paramount interest.

---

24   This was stated on the hotel's website, accessed 10 November 2014, cedunahotel.com.au/history.
25   In 1998, an Aboriginal community 200 km away from Ceduna successfully objected to an application for a gaming machine licence from a nearby roadhouse. The Liquor and Gaming Commissioner agreed with the community's lawyer that the people could 'ill afford' to gamble on poker machines, and that such machines had the potential to drain a substantial amount of money from already poor communities and to increase violence.
26   Despite the compromises that have modified the original idealistic goals for community hotels in South Australia, community-owned enterprises continue to engage with local residents in ways that normal commercially run premises do not. They publicly state they are community owned, display lists and photographs of board members, support local charities, provide local employment and training, engage in harm-reduction strategies and nurture their local customers and communities.

The community hotels idea was diffused among neighbouring towns: some were linked by shared identities as river towns or irrigation communities; some had shared histories of self-help and local cooperative enterprise; others had Lutheran origins and leanings towards alcohol regulation rather than outright prohibition. The notion of community ownership was also borne along on a wave of optimism about temperance and liquor reform and the potential to 'civilise' drinkers and drinking: in some cases, it was an integral part of the creation of towns or garden cities that were designed to enhance the wellbeing of citizens.

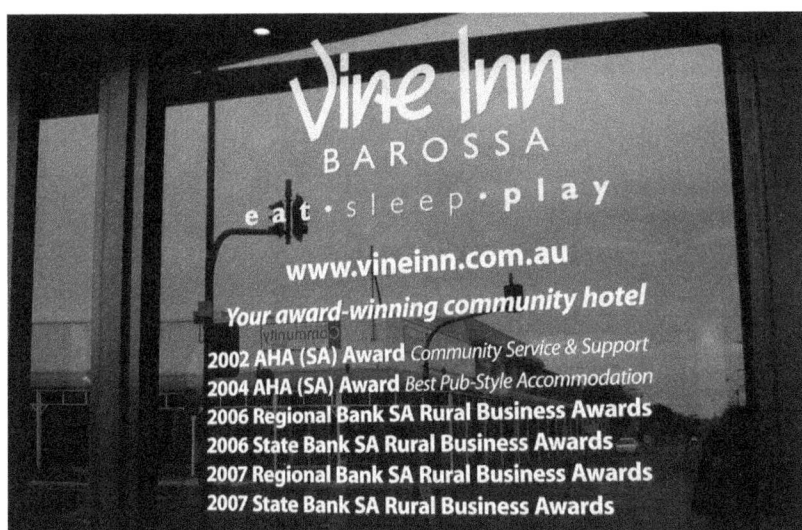

Fig. 4 Window at the Vine Inn, Nuriootpa
Source: M Brady

The community hotels of South Australia and the Gothenburg system that inspired them juggled inherently paradoxical goals and principles. The hotels and the Gothenburg system were mechanisms designed to build-up assets 'in trust', as it were, for the benefit of citizens. However, such assets and benefits were simultaneously responsible for—or at least morally implicated in—any negative effects of the socially volatile commodity involved: alcohol. This paradox was highlighted in later decades when several Aboriginal communities (and the government agencies that advised them), began to take an interest in buying licensed hotels and establishing Indigenous community boards of management.[27]

---

27   The first hotel purchased by Aboriginal interests was the Finke Hotel, Northern Territory, in 1975—a purchase made possible by the federal Minister for Aboriginal Affairs.

In the case of hotels owned by Indigenous interests, the paradoxical goals and moral dilemmas were intensified because of the unrelenting social hazards of alcohol for Aboriginal people.

Indigenous economic development agencies

Indigenous groups were interested in the idea of community ownership for a number of complex reasons. Like the politicians, aldermen and citizens who supported the Gothenburg system, Indigenous groups and several of their advisory agencies were attracted to the notion of 'keeping the money in the community'. They liked the idea of profits benefiting locals (rather than income from alcohol sales going to commercial businesses or breweries), and they used this argument to support both Indigenous hotel purchases and licensed social clubs in remote Indigenous communities. Like the Gothenburgers, they eschewed prohibition and were interested in reforming—rather than abolishing—the pub. Indigenous communities also wanted greater local control over alcohol sales, as this would enable them to bypass tortuous negotiations with reluctant publicans and licensing authorities. Finally, righteous justice motivated the purchases of hotels that had humiliated Aboriginal people by excluding them; this is discussed in Chapter 6.

In the early 1970s, self-determination policies facilitated the legal incorporation of regional Aboriginal communities, lands trusts and advisory councils. This built on earlier efforts to inspire Aboriginal 'self-help' organisations, proprietary companies and cooperatives. Public policy at this time was increasingly constituting Aboriginal leaders, elders and councillors as Indigenous 'trustees' who ostensibly took the place of the state (Smith 2002) in supervising other Aboriginal people. In 1976, a new Commonwealth Aboriginal Councils and Associations Act provided for the constitution of Aboriginal councils and for the incorporation of Aboriginal associations as vehicles of development and empowerment (Rowse 2015). This development, together with the creation of quasi-government agencies that provided structured funding programs for economic development, allowed Aboriginal associations and an emerging Aboriginal cadre of leaders[28] to obtain funds for hotel purchases and

28 Such leadership, it should be pointed out, was almost entirely male; indeed, some organisations, such as Land Councils, explicitly excluded Aboriginal women, arguing that land was 'men's business'.

other business enterprises. Unlike the non-Indigenous towns mentioned earlier, whose citizens were able to raise bank loans, mortgage businesses, or contribute private resources to buy their local hotels, impecunious Indigenous groups sought loans or grant monies from Indigenous-specific economic development agencies, such as the ADC and its successors. The Indigenous groups that received such monies were expected to abide by the policies and investment strategies of the funding bodies.

The ADC was established as a statutory corporation in 1980. Through its housing loans, business programs, small business loans and a community enterprise development scheme, it had the general aim of furthering goals for Aboriginal and Torres Strait Islander people that were broadly defined as economic and social (Commonwealth of Australia 1989a: 7, WS Arthur 1996). In a sense, the ADC operated as a means of stimulating what we would now call 'social enterprise': economic activities with social goals (Defourny & Nyssens 2006, 2010). In view of later developments, the articulation of social goals (as well as economic ones) in the ADC's founding objectives is significant. The ADC was intended to assist Aboriginal people to engage in business enterprises, including non-profit enterprises that provided facilities for social purposes. In keeping with its social and economic goals, the ADC's investment policy was broad— perhaps too broad. Its investments included housing companies, pastoral properties, a theatre company, tourist accommodation, an indoor cricket centre, cattle stations and a shopping centre in Alice Springs. It also funded the purchase of several licensed public hotels by Aboriginal community associations. Some of the ADC's investments had mixed success or were outright failures.[29] There were examples of administrative weaknesses and poor decision-making, such as the purchase of several Kimberley cattle stations that had been left in poor condition by their previous European owners.[30] As a result, in 1988, the Minister for Aboriginal Affairs, Gerry Hand, began to clamp down on the ADC and a no-confidence motion was passed against its chair, Shirley MacPherson.[31] Eight ADC commissioners were sacked (Guest 1988: 1). Tough questions were asked about the ADC at a Senate Estimates Committee, particularly about the role of Charles Perkins, and an Audit Office investigation was ordered

---

29 One notable failure was the purchase of the Oasis Hotel in Walgett (see Chapter 6).

30 This criticism was made by Fitzroy Valley Aboriginal people who believed that the ADC had been 'ripped off' when it made the cattle station purchases (Marshall 1988).

31 Shirley MacPherson was made chair of the ADC in 1986; she resigned in 1989. She was followed by Lois O'Donoghue who presided until the end of the ADC in February 1990.

into several of the ADC's investments (Australian Audit Office 1989). Despite some legitimate concerns, it is extraordinary that the Audit Office criticised what it called the ADC's 'undue emphasis' on *social* goals, such as promoting employment and creating social facilities. In May 1989, Minister Hand demanded that the ADC focus on the commercial viability of funded projects. Legislation governing the ADC was tightened with the addition of a clause preventing it from using monies from the general fund for business enterprises unless the ADC was satisfied that the enterprise would be *commercially successful* (Pratt & Bennett 2004). However, in light of subsequent developments, it is significant that the minister did not oblige the ADC to avoid commercial investment that was detrimental to the community.

Somewhat surprisingly, the ADC did not have a specific policy on alcohol. No particular safeguards were built into the loans or enterprise development grants used for the purchases of hotels—such as, for example, a proviso that an alcohol-related business should balance commercial viability with the expectation that it would cause no harm. However, the ADC did make an official comment on alcohol advertising. In July 1983, the ADC released a document entitled 'Views of the commissioners on alcohol related problems and the advertising of alcoholic beverages' that focused on concerns about the promotion of alcohol and over-glamorisation of drinking in advertising and the absence of health warnings.[32] The ADC made several perceptive recommendations, including the need for a comprehensive collation of statistical data on alcohol abuse problems in each state and territory, and an analysis of the relative costs and benefits of alcohol production, promotion, sales and the problems associated with its abuse (ADC 1983: 35). While acknowledging that the ADC was not primarily concerned with providing welfare services, the commissioners nevertheless felt that 'they would be seriously remiss if they were to ignore the problems associated with alcohol abuse'. The commissioners made it clear that they were 'well aware of and most concerned by the ravaging effects these have on Aboriginal people' (ADC 1983: 3). Yet, these concerns did not prevent the ADC from playing an integral role in the

---

32   Charles Perkins was particularly incensed about alcohol advertising. In 1985, Perkins and Bob Huddleston (an Aboriginal man who worked on alcohol issues for the Department of Aboriginal Affairs [DAA]) started a committee against alcohol advertising and placed advertisements in the press calling for restrictions on media advertising of alcohol (cf. *The Australian* 20 December 1985: 5). Their campaign, which did not specifically mention Aboriginal people, was targeted at the entire population.

purchase of three public hotels and one club with a primarily Aboriginal clientele—decisions that were enthusiastically supported by Charles Perkins (1936–2000), chair of the ADC from 1980 to 1984.[33]

The ADC and the Department of Aboriginal Affairs (DAA) were superseded and amalgamated within a new organisation, the Aboriginal and Torres Strait Islander Commission (ATSIC), in 1990. ATSIC took over the ADC's functions, such as loans for housing and commercial businesses, that had had both economic and social objectives. The ATSIC Act created the Aboriginal and Torres Strait Islander Commercial Development Corporation (CDC).[34] The CDC's primary function was 'to engage in commercial and financial activities' under strictly commercial lines; it was designed to sharpen the focus on economic self-sufficiency and economic development. Rather than facilitating social enterprises, the CDC described itself as advancing Indigenous 'economic interests'; it stressed 'sound business principles' and emphasised the importance of helping Indigenous people to 'break free from the web of dependency' (WS Arthur 1996).[35] However, from the perspective of many Aboriginal people, much of the business activity supported by the CDC was oriented towards the accumulation and distribution of *social capital*. As Martin (1995) observed (using examples from Cape York), no provision was made for targeting financial profit, nor was any provision made for monitoring the social impact of business enterprises. It appeared that the social goals and community development orientation that had been written into the ADC's original brief had, by 1990, disappeared under a renewed emphasis on accountability and profit-making.

The CDC was replaced by Indigenous Business Australia (IBA) in 2001. The IBA's investment policy continued to stress commercial and financial activities. In 2001, for example, the IBA purchased a 42.86 per cent share in the Crossing Inn at Fitzroy Crossing, Western Australia, evidently believing that it would be a solid commercial investment. As discussed in Chapter 7, it was indeed a solid commercial investment, but the hotel was also directly implicated in widespread alcohol-related harm, which caused the IBA and local Indigenous shareholders considerable public embarrassment.

---

33 ADC funds were used to purchase the Oasis Hotel, Walgett (1983); the Transcontinental Hotel, Oodnadatta (1986); the Woden Town Club, Canberra (1988); and the Crossing Inn, Fitzroy Crossing (1988). See Chapter 6.

34 The passage of the original ATSIC legislation introduced by the Hawke Labor Government was delayed because the opposition, led by John Howard, had strong objections to the notion of ATSIC, seeing it as a form of separatism (Pratt & Bennett 2004–05).

35 www.iba.gov.au/about-us/our-history/.

Kava—A short-lived monopoly

Kava is another example of a mood-altering substance whose sale was controlled by a government-sanctioned, Aboriginal-owned business. Like the Gothenburg system, a monopoly was established to regulate, rather than abolish, sales of kava, and the profits from the monopoly were used to finance projects for the benefit of the community.

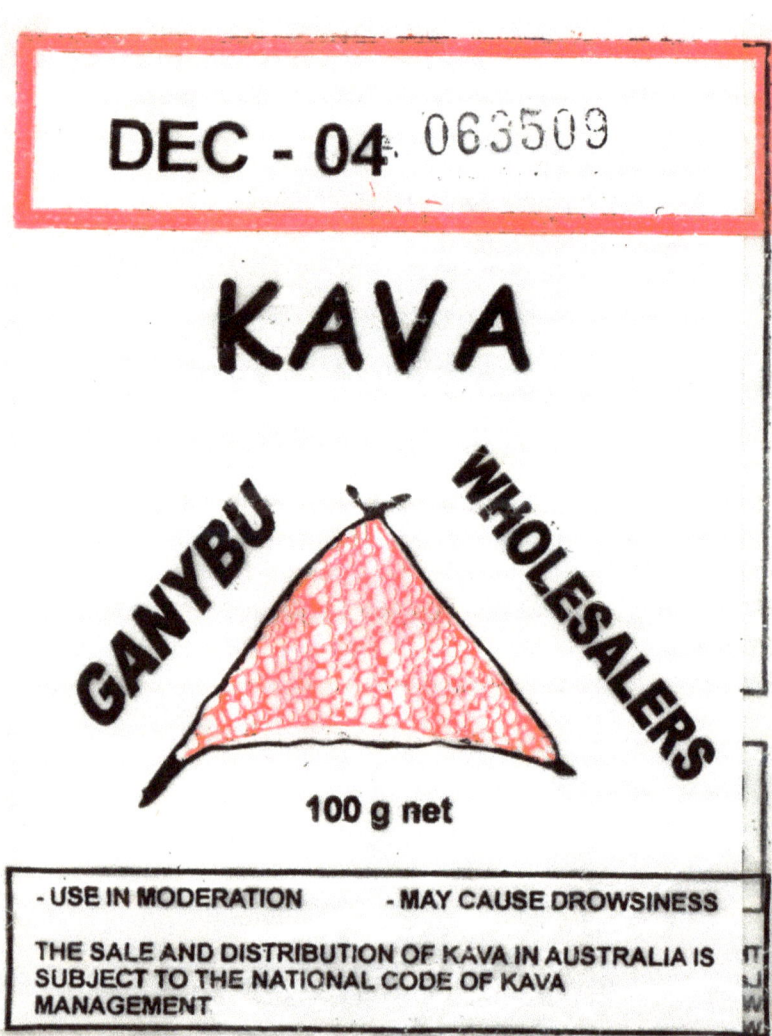

Fig. 5 Kava packet, Ganybu Wholesalers, Yirrkala, 2005
Source: M Brady

Made from the root of *Piper methysticum*, the psychoactive narcotic drug, kava, was introduced in the 1980s from the Pacific to several northern coastal Aboriginal communities. Aboriginal men visiting Fiji experienced the kava ceremony and, impressed by its tranquillising properties, saw kava as an antidote to the trouble that seemed to accompany alcohol; they asked for supplies to be made available. With the help of Uniting Church ministers, some of whom were of Pacific Islander descent and used kava themselves, the practice of drinking kava spread across east Arnhem Land communities. In Fiji, kava consumption was apparently benign and socially integrative (Lebot et al. 1992, Katz 1993). By contrast, its enthusiastic take-up by men, women and children in Arnhem Land, together with the relative absence of any drinking rules or learned self-control strategies, resulted in heavy consumption. Its popularity caused controversy about its health effects, prompting expressions of concern by Northern Territory health authorities (Alexander 1985, Cawte 1988, Gregory & Cawte 1988, Matthews et al. 1988, d'Abbs 1995, Clough et al. 2000, Clough & Jones 2004). The federal and territory governments' policy approaches to managing kava were indecisive, swinging wildly from tolerance and harm reduction to total prohibition. After originally taking a laissez-faire approach, the Northern Territory Health Department ran a health education campaign urging caution; it gave advice on hygiene, warned pregnant women not to drink kava and reminded people that kava was 'not part of Aboriginal ceremonies' (*Northern Territory Aboriginal News* 1989: 9). The trade in kava eventually prompted intense criticism of the Uniting Church, whose employees were accused of 'profiteering' from kava sales (Cawte 1988, d'Abbs 1995). In 1998, the Northern Territory parliament passed a Kava Management Act that created licensed kava areas, strictly regulated the supply and possession of kava and introduced fines for 'trafficable' quantities of the drug (Territory Health Services, no date).

An Aboriginal organisation, Laynhapuy Homelands Association Inc. (LHA), became the sole licensed wholesaler and distributor of kava for the Northern Territory. Member-owned, the LHA had a board of 12 Yolngu members and represented 16 Yolngu clans living in 19 homeland centres across northeast Arnhem Land (LHA 2008). Its kava distribution company, Ganybu Wholesalers, bought supplies from a Fijian company and sold to licensed retailers in six Aboriginal communities who were able to onsell to residents at a limit of 400 g per week per person.[36] The retailers

---

36   100 g bags of powdered kava sold for $15 (Ric Norton, pers comm, 19 August 2005).

were in communities that had, of their own volition, banned alcohol and made a conscious choice to request the sale of licensed kava instead. Profits raised by individual communities' kava sales were intended to be used for community development as well as for the mitigation of any negative health effects stemming from heavy kava use. One community used kava funds to help rehabilitate a cattle station and abattoir to create employment. Kava sales also provided the homelands resource agency, based at Yirrkala, with a valuable stream of rare discretionary income that was independent of government and could be used to support decentralised homeland communities. The LHA used the income to fund a ranger program and ranger station; a boat; housing improvements; health escort travel assistance for local people who travelled to hospital in Darwin; and donations to schools, sports and the night patrol. It also planned a number of civil works, such as a cyclone shelter and women's centre, and the purchase of tractors, generators, fencing, repairs and furniture. The LHA estimated that, after costs, the kava proceeds available for use for community benefit added up to around $900,000 per annum. With its members, directors, staff and families drinking kava to varying degrees, it was in the LHA's interests to stay abreast of claims and counterclaims about kava's health effects. It commissioned independent reviews of the medical literature that found the health risks to be minor, especially when compared with those associated with alcohol.

Monopoly trading displaced the black market to a certain extent, but the Kava Management Act did not entirely prevent illegal trading (LHA 2008: 22).[37] Seizures of illegal quantities of kava, agitation by Northern Territory politicians and an interventionist federal minister for Indigenous Affairs, culminated in 2007 in the federal government cancelling the kava import licence.[38] Without warning, all commercial importation of kava for social use was prohibited, bringing a precipitous end to the monopoly on sales held by the LHA. Thereafter, kava could be imported only for the personal–cultural use of people of South Pacific Islander descent. The LHA launched a spirited defence of kava consumption and its kava wholesale business, enumerating the many projects that were dependent on it and citing the lack of evidence of any serious health effects related to kava use. At the time, the community council at Yirrkala had $600,000

---

37   For example, it was reported that police from Tennant Creek seized 500 kg of kava, with a street value of $200,000, from a motorist travelling from Queensland (*Tennant Times* 2000: 3).

38   The ban on the commercial importation and licensing of kava was implemented by the Australian Government as part of the Northern Territory Emergency Response (NTER) in 2007.

worth of community projects that were dependent for their completion on kava proceeds and the LHA had numerous projects in train that were also reliant on kava monies (LHA 2008: 23).

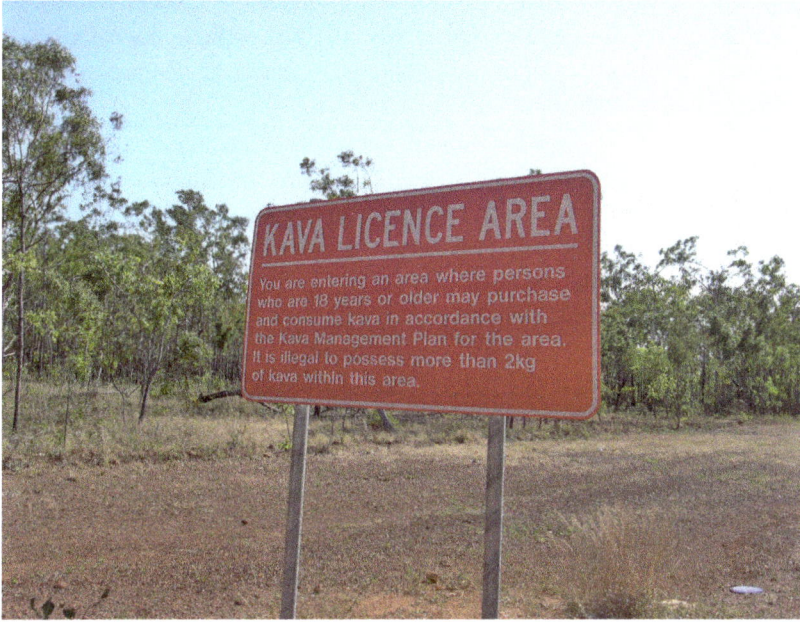

Fig. 6 Kava Licence Area sign, Yirrkala, 2005
Source: M Brady

There is no doubt that untied funds provided by the sale of kava enabled activities that benefited the community; the funds were well managed and the licensing and controlled distribution of kava through the Aboriginal-run monopoly over sales mitigated the black market in kava. Observers report that, since the ban on legal importation and distribution, millions of dollars have disappeared directly from the communities into the pockets of illegal Pacific Island traffickers. Seizures of illicit kava by the Substance Abuse Intelligence Desk doubled between 2009 and 2010 (Putt 2011). At a time when communities were also getting less financial support from government, the loss of kava income devastated their capacity to build infrastructure and provide jobs (Morphy 2008, Botsman 2015). By its own admission, the member-owned LHA was *dependent* on the kava business for a substantial part of its activities. This had been one of the criticisms voiced by temperance advocates against the fundraising capacity of community hotels: that town councils would become habituated to raising funds through sales of alcohol and morally compromised as a result. Despite being less problematic than alcohol, kava is, after all, a narcotic drug.

Unlike in parts of Sweden, there has never been a government-franchised monopoly alcohol supply system in Australia; although, as discussed here, kava was briefly a monopoly and there were (and still are) a handful of examples of municipal or community ownership of premises in both the Indigenous and non-Indigenous domains. In South Australia, where they proliferated, the interest of politicians and citizens in community-owned hotels often narrowed over time to their ability to raise revenue for local needs, rather than their supposed harm-reduction and alcohol-control functions. Indeed, with the demise of the old irrigation colonies' regional alcohol monopolies and with the rise of a competitive and less regulated liquor trade, revenue raising has become the more important goal. South Australia today has the highest per capita number of liquor licences of any Australian state or territory, and the rate of increase of licensed premises has been six times the rate of increase in population (Social Development Committee of the South Australian Parliament 2014: 44). To remain commercially viable, and to have enough profits to share with the community that supports them, the remaining community hotels have had to sacrifice some of their original ideals.

The Swedish *bolag*, and other Gothenburg-style strategies governing alcohol sales, had built-in social and public health objectives, such as making public houses eating houses, employing respectable managers who derived no profit from alcohol sales and securing strict supervision of all public houses (Pitman 1877). As mentioned, these were an early manifestation of the notion of corporate social responsibility. By contrast, the Indigenous agencies—such as the ADC and IBA—that made it possible for Indigenous communities to purchase hotels were only briefly guided by social concerns and lacked the caveats governing the Swedish *bolag*. Harm reduction was not even mentioned in their policy statements, and they ignored the glaring moral hazards associated with alcohol sales. By making economic viability such a high priority,[39] and by excluding safeguards against social or community harms deriving from alcohol sales, the Indigenous development and investment agencies failed

---

39 Arguably, these Indigenous statutory bodies—while under pressure from government audit offices to tighten their financial conduct—should have been able to create a balance between investment policies that were commercially robust *and* socially responsible.

in their duty of care to their Indigenous clients. Their policies prioritised the accumulation of Indigenous assets via business plans that were indifferent to social objectives. Particularly in the case of the Crossing Inn at Fitzroy Crossing, the commercially driven policies pursued by Indigenous economic agencies actively undermined policies that were aimed at harm reduction, sabotaging earlier ambitions for the hotel to impart moderate drinking habits. Such a trajectory runs counter to the principles that underpinned the Gothenburg system and its descendants, the community-owned hotels.

Among the remaining non-Indigenous community hotels in small rural towns, several are under financial stress with ongoing problems of staffing and management. While 'keeping the money in the community' has been a guiding principle for them, it may have had unintended consequences. In the 1930s, when towns were debating whether to create community hotels, a Methodist minister in Port Pirie presciently warned of the implicit danger of local bodies becoming dependent on the proceeds from hotel profits: he thought that community boards might not necessarily be altruistic in their distribution of revenue (*Recorder* [Port Pirie] 1939: 1). His comments touch on the dilemmas that were inherent in these enterprises from the start, and with which community hotels, whether they are owned by non-Indigenous or Indigenous entities, still grapple today.

3

The role of beer canteens and licensed clubs

The establishment of beer canteens and social clubs in remote Indigenous communities was a direct consequence of the aspiration to teach 'civilised'—or, in more modern parlance, moderate—drinking. Providing rationed amounts of alcohol was seen by many in government as a way to ease inexperienced Indigenous drinkers into familiarity with alcohol, while also helping more experienced drinkers to abandon the undesirable patterns of consumption acquired both before and after the repeal of prohibitions affecting them.[1]

Equality and the embrace of citizenship demanded that Aboriginal people should fit in and take their place in society, including at the hotel bar alongside average Australians. The leading idea was that Aboriginal people should be introduced to alcohol and *taught to drink* in a 'civilised' manner: a step along the road to integration, so that 'they' would learn to drink (and be) like 'us'. It was an idea in keeping with the thinking of civil rights activists and progressives of the time, and was also in line with the expressed desire of numerous Aboriginal leaders that their people should (somehow) learn to control wild drinking.

---

1   This chapter expands on material published by the author as a discussion paper in 2014.

Of course, some Aboriginal people already had drinking rights: these were mostly individuals of mixed descent who, by reaching certain behavioural 'standards' (such as 'adopting the habits of civilised life'[2]), had been exempted from the provisions of the various state and territory laws that prohibited alcohol possession and consumption—a status certified by an exemption certificate, otherwise known as a 'dog tag'. As Charles Rowley pointed out, such exemptions were reminiscent of French colonial practices that employed the concept of the *évolué*; in Australia, exemptions were granted to assimilated people who, although of 'native' origin, had proved themselves to be civilised and therefore eligible for full civil rights (Rowley 1970: 357).[3] Perhaps the clubs would help the previously non-exempt Aboriginal people to become *évolués* too? The idea that Aboriginal people should learn to drink like Australians who drank moderately was, arguably, an 'assimilationist' one, involving the internalisation of Western middle-class notions of individual responsibility and inner discipline. However, the idea that Aboriginal people should be able to exercise local control, shape rules and design a physical and social environment in which this moderation was likely to happen represents 'self-determination'.[4] In this respect, 'civilising' drinking was an assimilationist project that, with the advent of the idea of local control over clubs, spilled over into the era of self-determination and blurred the boundaries between the two.

Overall, it appears that broad sections of both the Indigenous and non-Indigenous polity believed that the provision of on-site alcohol facilities under the control of local people who implemented strict limits or rations was the best way to 'teach' proper drinking. Yet, the provision of canteens was by no means an Australia-wide phenomenon. Such drinking facilities only appeared in any organised way in the Northern Territory, South Australia and Queensland. Similar ideas were circulating at around the same time in Papua New Guinea, which, until 1975, was under Australian administration. Like Indigenous Australians, the people of Papua New Guinea had learned about drunkenness by observing hard-drinking colonial officers and traders, most of whom were Australian. It became legal for Papua New Guineans to purchase and consume alcohol in

---

2   This wording is from the *Natives (Citizenship Rights) Act 1944* (WA) (Chesterman 2005:125).

3   The term *évolué*, literally meaning a 'developed' or 'evolved' person, derives from the French colonial era. It was employed to describe natives who had assimilated and accepted European values and patterns of behaviour.

4   Thanks to Tim Rowse for making this point.

1962.[5] Prompted by rural men's disruptive behaviour in town hotels and a rise in motor vehicle accidents, provincial governments in the newly independent country decided to promote village clubs as an experiment in managing alcohol consumption in rural areas. It was hoped traditional social controls would swing into action and community leaders would intervene if there was violence. The clubs were envisaged as places where people could learn to drink in an environment that was comfortable for family members of both sexes, and in a manner that was based on an idealised version of the drinking habits of expatriates (Sexton 1982: 112). However, as was the case in Australian Indigenous communities in ensuing years, these hopes were found to be overly optimistic.

A sudden transition to drinking rights

Both Aboriginal people and white sympathisers campaigned for formal equal rights, including the right to drink liquor. In 1962, Joe McGinness, president of the Federal Council for Aboriginal Advancement, argued that such rights were 'important inasmuch as they at least recognise that Aborigines and Islanders are human beings' (Chesterman 2005: 25). In New South Wales, the Aboriginal-Australian Fellowship lobbied hard for prohibition to be repealed, arguing that the section of the Aborigines Protection Act (NSW) that prohibited the sale and supply of alcohol subjected Aboriginal people to 'unwarranted humiliation and segregation'. Research by prominent Melbourne barrister Elizabeth Eggleston (1976), exposed the inherently discriminatory nature of Australia's liquor laws, the enthusiasm with which police used such laws as a means of harassing Aboriginal people, and the abject failure of restrictions to prevent Aboriginal people from getting hold of alcohol. Yet, for many white sympathisers, the repeal of restrictions on Aboriginal drinking presented an ethical and moral dilemma. The people for whom this was most difficult were progressively minded Christians and temperance advocates. Such advocates supported equal rights in all areas of life for Aboriginal citizens and, aware that these would inevitably include the right to drink, feared the consequences. Dr Charles Duguid, founder of Ernabella Presbyterian mission, and his wife Phyllis Duguid, a prominent member

---

5   The Australian administration thus made the sale and consumption of alcohol legal in Papua New Guinea before the states and territories in Australia made it legal for Aboriginal and Torres Strait Islanders to drink.

of the WCTU, were conflicted about the right to drink for Aboriginal people. In 1960, Phyllis Duguid, who did not drink herself, reported to the WCTU National Convention:

> The whole question of the Aborigine and his right to consume liquor is a difficult one. In our desire to protect these people against havoc caused by alcohol, we sometimes run the risk of making them regard alcohol as a special privilege to be attained. Unhappily many do think of the right to consume alcohol as an inseparable part of citizenship. Alcohol education would make an important contribution towards the solution of the problem.[6]

Mrs Duguid's wish for 'alcohol education' was echoed by others. In 1961, a Northern Territory Missions-Administration Conference agreed that before there were any changes to the law, a public education campaign should be conducted, disseminating information on the dangers of alcohol and the advantages of temperance. The conference thought that Alcoholics Anonymous (AA) might be able to help in this endeavour (Symons et al. 1963). However, apart from sporadic efforts by charitable bodies such as the WCTU and other Christian organisations, it seems that no formal or official public education campaigns were mounted by government prior to the repeal of prohibition for Aboriginal people.[7]

When it eventually happened, state by state, the transition from prohibition to drinking rights occurred precipitously, taking many people by surprise. The repeal in South Australia in 1965, for example, was described as being total prohibition one day, complete freedom the next. The premier was accused of acting impetuously, having consulted with neither Aboriginal people nor the state Department of Aboriginal Affairs (Hansen 1972). The rapid liberalisation, it was stated, had had a 'profoundly demoralising effect' on Aboriginal people who, had they been asked, would have requested a gradual transition period 'with the *first step* being the provision of drinking facilities on the various reserves' (Hansen 1972: 6, emphasis added). On Queensland Aboriginal reserves, restrictions on supply and consumption continued until 1971 when, suddenly and disastrously, a government official was empowered to establish a beer canteen in each community (Fitzgerald 2001).

---

6   WCTU Minute Book SRG 186/1/8 1935–40, State Library of South Australia.
7   Gary Stoll (Finke River Mission, Hermannsburg) said, 'nobody knew what was going to hit them, that it would be such a big problem and that the graves would open up' (Finnane 1997: 5).

WHAT'S

IN

A

GLASS?

BEER
3 - 6% ALCOHOL

WINE
9-24% ALCOHOL

COCKTAIL
13-26% ALCOHOL

WHISKEY
50-60% ALCOHOL

THINK

and you WON'T

DRINK

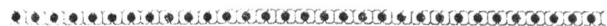

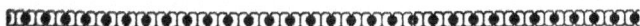

Fig. 7 'What's in a glass?' WCTU pamphlet c. 1950
Source: Woman's Christian Temperance Union

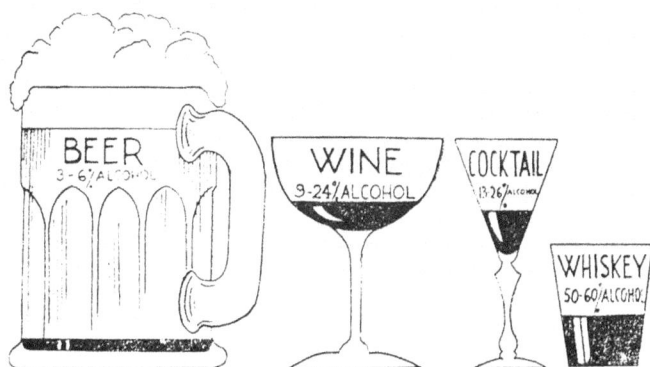

Promoting the idea of canteens and clubs

While rural and urban Aboriginal and Torres Strait Islander people could act on their newly acquired right to drink by going into hotels and drinking alongside whites, in more remote areas, access to legitimate outlets was difficult. Aboriginal residents of bush communities did not commonly frequent public hotels, and they were less familiar with alcohol than their rural and urban counterparts. Beyond the discrete and relatively protected boundaries of missions and settlements, the availability of liquor had increased with the advent of off-licence and drive-in bottle shops. These made takeaway alcohol easier to access[8] and posed a threat to inexperienced drinkers. In some regions, public opinion (in the form of non-Aboriginal townsfolk) had already broached the idea of Aboriginal people having their own beer canteens in their communities. These would not only keep Aboriginal people out of town, they would also allow for the development of 'civilised' drinking. This was suggested as early as 1954 in the Northern Territory when the citizens of Alice Springs and readers of the local newspaper were asked, in an informal opinion poll, what could be done about drunken 'natives':

> While on the one hand, we found a lot of people who believe ever increasing vigilance should be taken to see that natives do not get drink at all, we found others who favour the establishment of canteens at settlements so that aborigines can become used to civilised drinking. The exponents of the latter theory claim that a beer with a reduced alcoholic content could be sold to natives in these canteens and claim that the present troubles arise because men with no alcohol in their blood at all suddenly get hold of a bottle of wine.[9] (*Centralian Advocate* 26 March 1954: 9)

Ted Evans, head of the Native Affairs Branch (later the Welfare Branch) in Alice Springs, believed that the best way to solve the 'rotgut' wine problem in the town, was to dispense low-alcohol beer from wet canteens on all settlements, and to teach Aboriginal people how to cope with alcohol correctly. Notwithstanding the outcome of the *Centralian Advocate*'s opinion poll, he was widely criticised for this suggestion.[10] In 1961, the Missions-Administration Conference discussed the advantages and disadvantages of removing the restrictions on alcohol: with considerable foresight, a subcommittee proposed the introduction of a local option system for communities because 'well-controlled wet canteens may be needed on certain settlements' (Symons et al. 1963).[11]

---

8   The first drive-in bottle shop in Australia opened at Largs Bay, Adelaide, in 1953.
9   Twenty years later, in 1975, the anthropologist Jeff Collmann (1988: 50) reported that, following an alleged rape in Alice Springs, there had been renewed calls for wet canteens away from the town.
10   As reported by Reg Harris in *Alice Springs News* 2 July 1997: 3.
11   GJ Symonds (Uniting Church), P Albrecht (Lutheran Church) and JPM Long (Welfare Branch) were members of the subcommittee.

There was soon support for the idea at higher levels of government. Following the 1967 Referendum, the Council for Aboriginal Affairs (CAA) was established as an advisory body operating out of the newly established Office of Aboriginal Affairs located within the Prime Minister's Department. The three member body—Dr HC 'Nugget' Coombs, Professor WEH Stanner and Barrie Dexter—encouraged the government to abandon many of the programs and assumptions of assimilation and to emphasise the right of Aboriginal people to decide their own futures (Long 1992: 160). The Whitlam (1972–75) and Fraser (1975–83) governments introduced legislation that enabled Aboriginal and Torres Strait Islanders to make choices; thereafter, encouraging Indigenous Australians to take responsibility became the pre-eminent theme of government, non-government and mission authorities. The new emphasis on community decision-making extended to decisions about alcohol, and both governments and mission authorities believed that communities should discuss the 'dry' or 'wet' status of their settlements (DAA 1974, 1976: 22, Fletcher 1992).

The CAA strongly supported the idea of local wet canteens. Indeed, according to Dexter, the very idea that communities might have alcohol supplied to them in moderation at local canteens originated from the CAA.[12] The CAA was aware that bootleggers were grog running into some communities and that Aboriginal people were setting up vigilante groups to try to prevent this. It was of the view that, rather than protecting Aboriginal people, 'they had to learn to handle alcohol themselves'.[13] Although its work was undervalued (and sometimes undermined) by John Gorton, the prime minister who succeeded Harold Holt, the CAA was highly influential in Aboriginal policy until it was disbanded in 1976.[14]

---

12   The CAA believed that liquor should be available under controlled conditions on reserves and Dexter advised the minister of this in 1970. This advice was in the context of failed Aboriginal objections to the licensing of the Walkabout Hotel, which was within the reserve at Nhulunbuy and only a short distance from Yirrkala mission (Dexter 2015: 150). However, as noted, the idea of canteens had already been floated informally in Alice Springs.

13   Dexter, pers comm, 25 November 2005.

14   Gorton supported entrepreneurship for Aboriginal people, but not special rights (Dexter, pers comm, 25 November 2005).

On the ground in the Northern Territory, where the federal government had particular influence, policy was mobilised by patrol officers and officers of the Welfare Branch.[15] Many of these government representatives were critical of prohibition and supportive of the idea of wet canteens: some even 'pushed' the idea, according to church workers from several different regions.[16] John Harris (1998: 294) of the Church Missionary Society (CMS) remarked that 'under the Welfare Branch' alcohol became freely available in some communities. Reverend Bill Edwards of Ernabella Mission reported that government officers who visited the community were 'free drinkers' themselves, implying that there was a degree of self-interest in their support for wet canteens. The anticipated merits of wet canteens were certainly the subject of many discussions within government offices as settlement superintendents grappled with the problems posed by Aboriginal people from remote communities seeking opportunities to drink at rural hotels, and ending up having road accidents or facing criminal charges.

In South Australia, there was strong pressure from the state office of the DAA for one or more wet canteens to be established on what was then the dry North West Reserve, now the Anangu Pitjantjatjara Yankunytjatjara Lands. A departmental file note from 1969 explained the dilemma:

> I am certain the time is rapidly approaching when the 'liquor era' will begin in the N.W.R. [North West Reserve] area. And also I am certain the majority of the people will drink liquor. The alternative before us is to act in time by providing at least some education or to try and shut the door after the horse has bolted. For example, the West Coast area[17] ... The provision of a wet canteen is not saying that the people *shall* drink. It is providing the means by which those who desire to drink or at least experiment, may do so under reasonable circumstances.[18]

---

15   The patrol officer service ended in 1974, and the Welfare Branch became the Welfare Division of the Northern Territory Administration. Later, many former patrol officers joined the federal DAA as public servants (Long 1992).

16   Reverend Jim Downing of the Uniting Church asserted that patrol officers, members of the Welfare Branch and later DAA officers, and mission superintendents, all pushed for canteens. Father John Leary of the Missionaries of the Sacred Heart Mission (MSC) at Melville Island, Daly River Mission and Wadeye, identified specific government officers as having promoted alcohol availability in the communities (interviews with author).

17   The author was referring to the recently licensed beer canteen at Yalata community on the far west coast of South Australia.

18   D Busbridge, Assistant Director DAA, 6/1/69. GRS 6624/1/P, DAA520/68. South Australian State Records (original emphasis).

The superintendent of the North West Reserve was also in favour of the controlled availability of liquor there: he argued that a proposed recreational centre at Amata should include a bar where Aboriginal people, who he referred to, rather significantly, as *évolués,* might drink.[19]

In the context of an increase in Aboriginal drunkenness in towns such as Alice Spring, formal government inquiries (rather than simply local field officers or departmental staffers) began to recommend that alcohol should be made available in Aboriginal settlements. The Northern Territory Legislative Council conducted a Board of Inquiry into the sale and consumption of liquor in 1973. This was prompted by the Territory's weak liquor ordinance, which was allowing licensees to get away with poor-serving practices, resulting in 'scenes of drunkenness and degradation in and around the hotels, streets and creek beds … far worse than anything expected' (*Centralian Advocate* 1973: 1).[20] The inquiry, which declared that Territorians (in general) were Australia's biggest drunks and roundly condemned poor drinking facilities and the irresponsible behaviour of licensees, primarily addressed Aboriginal drinking. It recommended the establishment of social clubs for Aboriginal people, and advised that these should not be confined to settlements or missions: 'fringe dwellers' around towns such as Darwin and Alice Springs needed to be assisted to establish clubs. Summing-up contemporary explanations, the inquiry identified four underlying causes of Aboriginal drinking problems:

a. Their different stage of cultural development [and] influence of their traditional life in which alcohol played no part.

b. The lack in their culture of in-built sanctions for the control of alcohol usage [and] their being caught up in rapid social change and subsequent social disorganization.

c. Their lack of awareness of the harmful effects of drinking to excess [and] their lack of education in domestic budgeting and proper use of money.

d. Their excessive expenditure of [sic] intoxicating liquor and the poor conditions under which they consume intoxicating liquor. (*Centralian Advocate* 16 August 1973: 2)

---

19 The superintendent of the North West Reserve, David Hope, used the term *évolué* (Hope to director DAA 25/10/68. GRS 6624/1/P, DAA520/68. South Australian State Records). Jeremy Beckett (1958) used the same term when referring to mixed descent Aboriginal people in western New South Wales (234).
20 The inquiry was called for by Bernie Kilgariff, member for Alice Springs in the Northern Territory Legislative Council. It was chaired by PR Adams QC.

The idea of Aboriginal people's *choice* over the liquor status of communities was coming into play. This was articulated by Eggleston (1976: 261) who argued that granting licences to Aboriginal missions or institutions on reserves:

> Might be preferable to making liquor on reserves completely uncontrolled, particularly if it rests on a system of local option. A referendum should be held on each Aboriginal institution to see whether the resident Aborigines want the continuation of a 'dry' reserve, or the establishment of a 'wet canteen' or the abandonment of all controls on the entry of liquor.

Aboriginal people's choice on the issue of alcohol control was endorsed by the Commonwealth House of Representatives Standing Committee on Aboriginal Affairs (HRSCAA) inquiry into alcohol problems in 1977.[21] Many, though not all submissions, took a laissez-faire and generally 'wet' perspective on access to alcohol: one Aboriginal man from One Arm Point in Western Australia argued that every Aboriginal settlement should have a licence (Brady 2004: 59, Commonwealth of Australia 1977). The HRSCAA reiterated the idea that clubs would facilitate 'sensible' drinking:

> Should an Aboriginal community decide to allow alcohol to be brought into the community the Committee believes that a licensed club or beer canteen should hold the only liquor licence within that community ... A properly established and supervised club or beer canteen complying with the law relating to drinking and drunkenness and concerned with the well-being of its members presents the most practical method of encouraging sensible drinking patterns. (Commonwealth of Australia 1977: 48–9)

There would, of course, have to be guidelines, arrangements for legal responsibility and supervision, limited opening hours, rigid enforcement, the sale of nutritious food, sales of beer only and penalties for breaches. It was not clear who would 'properly establish' and supervise the clubs, what entity would hold the licence nor how best to ensure that the clubs would be 'concerned' about the wellbeing of members. While the HRSCAA believed that there was no reason why the clubs or beer canteens should not be run as commercial ventures, it had no advice about who should benefit from any profits so derived or who should decide on their distribution. It was assumed that if Aboriginal community organisations were allowed to control the outlets themselves, people would (somehow) come to terms with alcohol and moderate drinking would develop more or less automatically.

---

21   For more detail about this inquiry, see Brady (2004: 58–67).

A few years after the HRSCAA reported on alcohol problems, the Northern Territory initiated a new *Liquor Act 1981* that established a Liquor Commission as a statutory body that had flexible powers to hear public objections to the granting of licences, and that could involve local governments, including Aboriginal community councils, in liquor decisions. Since their formation, Aboriginal reserves in the Northern Territory had all been 'dry', but the Liquor Act made dry areas an option for Aboriginal communities: they now had to make a deliberate choice in the matter. The Liquor Commission toured the communities to hear their views. Communities that so desired could legitimately open community-controlled clubs with liquor served for consumption on the premises. The Northern Territory's Drug and Alcohol Bureau noted that:

> The Aboriginal councils concerned hope [in this way] to be able to avoid the potentially damaging effects of liquor in their areas while at the same time providing an opportunity for those people who wish to drink to do so in more-or-less convivial, well controlled circumstances. (Larkins & McDonald 1984: 61)

The influence of the missions

Across the world, Protestant and Catholic churches have long taken different approaches to alcohol consumption; these different approaches were reflected in Aboriginal and Torres Strait Islander communities that began as missions. The temperance movement developed from Protestantism, but there were wide variations in thinking between denominations. English Protestants were initially not as strict as Dutch ones, and Anglican ecclesiastical vineyards were once widespread. In America, it was Methodists and Quakers who spearheaded the Anti-Saloon Leagues, while in Sweden, Magnus Huss, the son of a Lutheran pastor, coined the expression *alcoholism* (Sournia 1990). By contrast, the Catholic Church tended to be more tolerant about alcohol. At the end of the nineteenth century, for example, Catholics believed drunkenness merely 'offended' the Creator, while priests celebrated communion by drinking wine. Indeed, Rome's insistence on the use of wine explains one of the major differences between Protestant and Catholic approaches to alcohol (Sournia 1990: 136, cf. Raftery 1987). These differing historical and doctrinal positions undoubtedly influenced how mission organisations operating in Aboriginal reserves reacted to the dilemma of alcohol availability in the self-determination period. The introduction of self-determination policies from 1973 onwards marked the beginning of the end of the era of Christian missions in Australia; however, missions were still influential contributors to the debate over wet canteens. Their guiding doctrinal principles and underlying philosophies were important in determining whether a community resisted or acceded to the pressure to instigate clubs. Pressure was exerted, both overtly and covertly, by members of the Welfare Branch and other government staff; the number of official inquiries, consultations and questioning of communities also served to exert pressure by drawing attention to the issue.

In the Northern Territory, the Aboriginal population had, in effect, been portioned out between the Catholic, Methodist (Methodist Overseas Mission), Congregational, Anglican, CMS and Lutheran mission societies. There were also Presbyterians, Baptists and non-denominational missionary societies, such as the United Aborigines Mission (UAM) and the Australian Inland Mission, which were strongly influenced by nineteenth-century American revivalism. As their respective missions developed, they each took different approaches to alcohol (see Table 1). Most mission organisations began to question and debate their protective role in the Indigenous arena during the 1960s, in the process, re-positioning themselves on matters of Aboriginal self-determination, land rights and the liquor question (Downing 1988, Harris 1998, Albrecht 2002). The CMS had been discussing a phased withdrawal from the training and social welfare aspects of its role in the Northern Territory since 1964. When the federal government's policy of self-determination was announced in 1973, the CMS was 'well on the way to divesting itself from positions of authority and control' (Harris 1998: 94). In 1974, the United Church in North Australia (UCNA)[22] held an inquiry into its own operations and future entitled *Free to Decide*, by which the UCNA meant that Aboriginal people were 'free to decide' their own futures. It saw itself as a 'liberating mission' facilitating the Aboriginal decision-making process (UCNA 1974). Consequently, the UCNA took an equivocal and non-aligned position on alcohol availability, believing that it had the right to oppose alcohol consumption only among its own church members.[23] In a submission to the Northern Territory Board of Inquiry into liquor laws, Reverend Jim Downing[24] wrote:

22 The UCNA was a cooperative venture between the Presbyterian, Methodist and Congregational churches. The Methodist Overseas Mission joined the UCNA in 1972. The Uniting Church in Australia was formed in 1977.
23 See the UCNA's submission to the House of Representatives inquiry into the present conditions of the Yirrkala People (1974).
24 Downing (1926–2009) was a Uniting Church minister, social worker and moderator of the Northern Synod of the Uniting Church.

Several statements have been made to the effect that wet canteens are a good thing and should be provided for all settlements. In some situations and under some circumstances they may be a good thing, but the statements still indicate that we Europeans know what is best for all Aboriginal communities. We continue to ignore the people's plea for help to control the effects of alcohol on their communities.[25]

In fact, the UCNA was opposed to the introduction of intoxicating liquors to Aboriginal communities unless the communities themselves desired a canteen or beer ration (Symons 1974).[26] It allowed the principle of supporting community decision-making to override its deeply held fears about proposals to make alcohol available in communities.

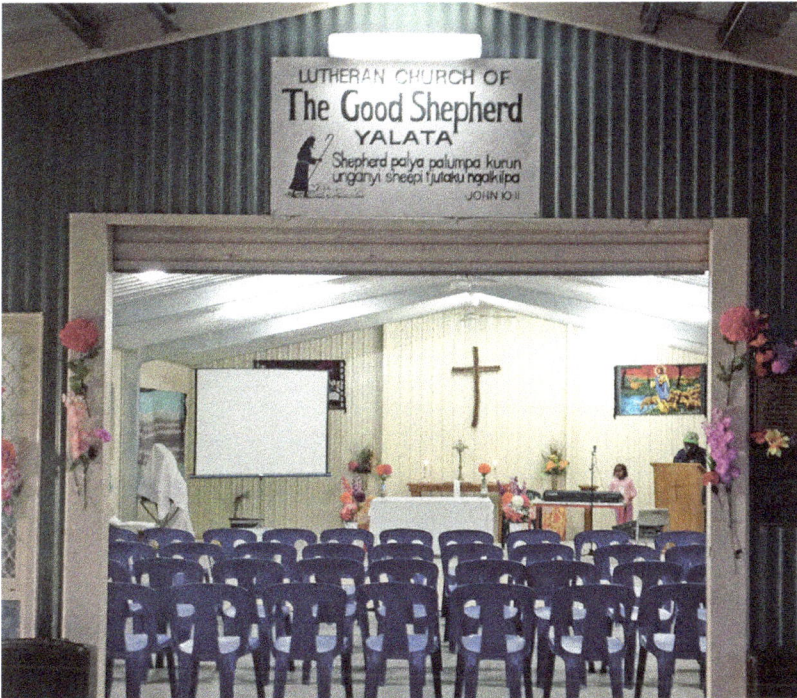

Fig. 8 Lutheran Church of the Good Shepherd, Yalata, 2015
Source: M Brady

---

25   Submission to the Northern Territory Committee of Inquiry on the Sale and Consumption of Intoxicating Liquor March 1973.
26   Jim Downing, interview, 16 August 2004.

The Lutherans generally took a tolerant approach towards alcohol and rejected prohibition (as had the Anglican synod in the 1920s). The Lutheran doctrine of the 'two kingdoms' distinguished between religious and political questions 'and, although they recognised the gravity of alcohol abuse, Lutherans declined to take a religious stance on it (Raftery 1987). The first mission organisation to obtain a licence to sell alcohol on an Aboriginal reserve was a Lutheran one—at Yalata, South Australia, in 1968.[27] Subsequently, a church member explained that the Lutheran Church was:

> Not against drinking rights for Aborigines … the sensible and correct approach ought to have been provision of drinking facilities on the reserves and missions so that Aborigines could enjoy the same conveniences as those enjoyed by citizens in our cities and country towns—drinking facilities right in their own communities. (Hansen 1969: 52)

The church should provide such facilities, 'and through precept and example demonstrate that rational drinking is compatible with responsible living, and within the demands of God and State' (Hansen 1972: 7). Concerned about models of deviant behaviour, Hansen warned that mission staff with drinking problems would not be tolerated. At the Finke River Mission, also known as Hermannsburg, the Lutheran Reverend Paul Albrecht used wine in communion because grape juice did not fit with the church's understanding of the practice of communion.[28] The mission, which took a positive approach to alcohol, instigated a short-lived experimental wet canteen for Aboriginal residents in 1972: it was not successful and was later regretted (Albrecht 2002: 45).[29]

By contrast, the Methodist and Presbyterian missions were opposed to the idea of providing even rationed amounts of alcohol and most of these communities have remained officially dry to this day.[30] At Oenpelli Mission, now Gunbalanya, the Anglican CMS was opposed to alcohol (it had also been opposed to the distribution of tobacco rations in the 1940s) (Harris 1998: 272–83). Alcohol was not ever permitted at

---

27 This was possible once a section of the *Licensing Act 1967–73* (SA) authorised 'wet canteens' on Reserves (Eggleston 1976: 219).

28 Paul Albrecht, interview, 20 April 2005.

29 This was noted in correspondence to me from Bill Edwards (10 August 2004).

30 There were exceptions to this overall tendency, such as at Mornington Island, where the Presbyterian mission instigated a beer ration in 1973 and opened a canteen in 1976. The community had a growing problem with alcohol and the minister, Reverend Doug Belcher, personally favoured the idea of a canteen (Bill Edwards, pers comm, 10 August 2004, McKnight 2002).

the Presbyterian mission at Ernabella, now Pukatja, and mission staff and Aboriginal residents all took the position that the mission should remain dry. Mission superintendent, Reverend Bill Edwards, thought that most of the staff at Ernabella came from abstinence or temperance backgrounds, which probably influenced this policy. He recalled that, in 1971–72, the idea of wet canteens was floated by government departments as a way of teaching Aboriginal people 'to drink socially'.

The debate over licensed clubs took a decisive turn in 1975 when a fact-finding committee was commissioned by the Australian Government to examine the causes and effects of alcoholism among Aboriginal people. As it happened, the team members were all associated with the Catholic Church through the Missionaries of the Sacred Heart Mission (MSC) at Port Keats, now Wadeye (Leary et al. 1975). The Leary report, which strongly endorsed the idea that providing beer to Aboriginal people in community-based clubs would encourage both good behaviour and moderation in consumption, led to the establishment of the Murrinh Patha Social Club.[31] The club's rise and demise is described in Chapter 4. Two more clubs associated with the MSC opened in Tiwi Island communities. Clubs were also established at the Catholic communities of Daly River (Nauiyu), Pirlingimpi (Melville Island), Wurakuwu (Bathurst Island) and Santa Teresa in central Australia. It is notable that five of the eight licensed clubs that still exist today in Northern Territory Aboriginal communities were previously Catholic missions. In two of these, the same Catholic brother was responsible for obtaining their liquor licences; somewhat ironically, he also set up the local AA groups.[32] Father John Leary, who ministered at several of these missions, later recalled: 'In the beginning I had the idea you could teach ... civilised drinking, two or three cans, enough ... My bishop thought *assimilation was the way that people had to learn*'.[33]

---

31 There were many other recommendations in the Leary report, and much of it was progressive. For example, the authors demonstrated an awareness of the influence of the contextual and contingent nature of much Aboriginal drinking, and the social and economic 'setting' within which Aboriginal people drank. They proposed that Aboriginal people suffered from a kind of 'environmental alcoholism'.

32 Brother Andy Howley instigated beer rations at Nguiu on Bathurst Island as well as at the Sacred Heart mission at Port Keats (Walsh 2005, Brady fieldnotes). He also travelled to the United States to investigate culturally relevant alcohol treatment approaches and instigated dry-out programs and AA-style support groups in some communities.

33 Father John Leary, interview, 16 August 2004 (emphasis added).

Table 1 Liquor status and mission associations of major Aboriginal communities, NT, 1987

Community	Liquor status Open	Liquor status Semi-restricted	Liquor status Restricted	Licensed Club	Association with mission*
Northern communities					
Angurugu		X			Anglican CMS
Bamyili (Barunga)		X		Club	–
Beswick		X		Club	–
Daguragu/Kalkarinji		X			Baptist
Daly River		X		Club	Catholic
Gapuwiyak			X		UCNA
Galiwin'ku			X		Methodist UCNA
Goulburn Is			X		Methodist UCNA
Garden Point (Pirlingimpi) (Tiwi)		X		Club	Catholic
Maningrida		X			Methodist UCNA
Milingimbi			X		Methodist UCNA
Minjilang			X		Methodist UCNA
Ngukurr		X			Anglican CMS
Nguiu (Tiwi)		X		Club	Catholic
Numbulwar			X		Anglican CMS
Oenpelli Gunbalanya		X		Club	Anglican CMS
Peppimenarti	X				Catholic
Port Keats		X		Club	Catholic
Ramingining			X		Methodist UCNA
Snake Bay Milikapiti (Tiwi)		X		Club	Catholic
Umbakumba		X		Club	Anglican CMS
Yirrkala		X			Methodist
Centre communities					
Areyonga		X			Lutheran
Docker River			X		Lutheran

Community	Liquor status Open	Liquor status Semi-restricted	Liquor status Restricted	Licensed Club	Association with mission*
Haasts Bluff	X				Lutheran
Hermannsburg			X		Lutheran
Kintore			X		Lutheran
Lake Nash	X				–
Lajamanu			X		Baptist
Papunya			X		Lutheran
Sta Teresa			X		Catholic
Warrabri (Ali Curung)			X		–
Willowra			X		Lutheran
Utopia			X		–
Yuendumu		X			Baptist

*Not necessarily an actual mission establishment

Source: Author's data

Over the years, there were further experiments with beer rations and rudimentary canteens in many communities in the Northern Territory. By 1988, there were six on-premises licensed clubs in Aboriginal communities.[34] In mid-2007, there were eight clubs licensed for on-premises consumption and two licensed for off-premises sales only.[35] By 2013, there were still eight on-premises licensed facilities in discrete Aboriginal communities in the Northern Territory.[36] In South Australia, the only licensed canteen in an Aboriginal community was at Yalata Lutheran Mission; it opened in 1969 and closed in 1981. Significantly, the closure of disastrous clubs, such as those at Santa Teresa and Yalata, did not prevent people, usually outsiders, from suggesting that they be reinstated.

In Queensland, it was government rather than mission action that prompted the establishment of 'canteens', as they were referred to in that state. Following the establishment of Aboriginal councils on settlements

---

34 These were at Daly River, Port Keats, Pularumpi, Bathurst Island, Milikapiti (Melville Island) and Gunbalanya (Oenpelli).

35 These were at Daly River, Nguiu and Wurankuwu (Bathurst Island), Milikapiti, Pirlangimpi (Melville Island), Gunbalanya, Kalkaringi and Peppimenarti. Beswick and Barunga had off-licences.

36 These were at Beswick, Gunbalanya, Kalkaringi, Milikapiti, Nguiu, Peppimenarti, Pirlangimpi and Wurankuwu.

and missions in 1971, beer could be sold in communities under restrictive licensing conditions. Subsequently, canteens were opened at Aurukun, Bamaga, Injinoo, Kowanyama, Lockhart River, Napranum, Pormpuraaw, Mornington Island, Palm Island, Woorabinda, Cherbourg and Yarrabah. Most of the mainland canteens and taverns were closed down as a result of Justice Tony Fitzgerald's report in 2001 and later decisions made by the Queensland Government aimed at reducing extraordinary levels of alcohol consumption and alcohol-related harm.[37] Only three canteens still exist (*Koori Mail* 2013: 12). In the Torres Strait, Saibai, Erub and Mer have licensed community clubs.[38]

Mixed motivations for clubs

Public opinion and official statements reveal an uneasy and contradictory mix of underlying motivations for these licensed facilities, especially in the early years of their development. In some cases, whether a community applied for a liquor licence depended on the religious denomination of the relevant mission settlement, or the attitude of a particularly influential missionary or superintendent. In other cases, there were contributing local circumstances prompting the decision, such as the desire to circumvent a worrisome takeaway liquor outlet nearby. Rudimentary voting occurred in some instances; community meetings were held that often resulted in sizeable pockets of disgruntled residents, usually women, feeling that their views had not been heard. While there were always residents, sometimes even a majority, in favour of having a club, substantial numbers were also always opposed—and women made up the bulk of non-drinkers. However, until the mid-1980s, Aboriginal women were not represented on councils and were usually left out of discussions about alcohol availability, both in the communities and in consultations with the Liquor Commission (East Arnhem Health Workers 1978).

---

37   See volume 2 of the Cape York Justice Study (Fitzgerald 2001: 50–1) where Fitzgerald notes the conflict of interest borne by community councils' profiteering from sales of alcohol at canteens for which the council is the licensee. Legislation passed by the Queensland Labor Government in 2008 prohibited any local community council from operating and profiting from canteens; this resulted in the closure of most canteens, as they were unable to find alternative suitable private licensees. The legislation banned all councils from owning a licence, not just those in Indigenous communities.
38   As at October 2017.

Stimulating sociable drinking

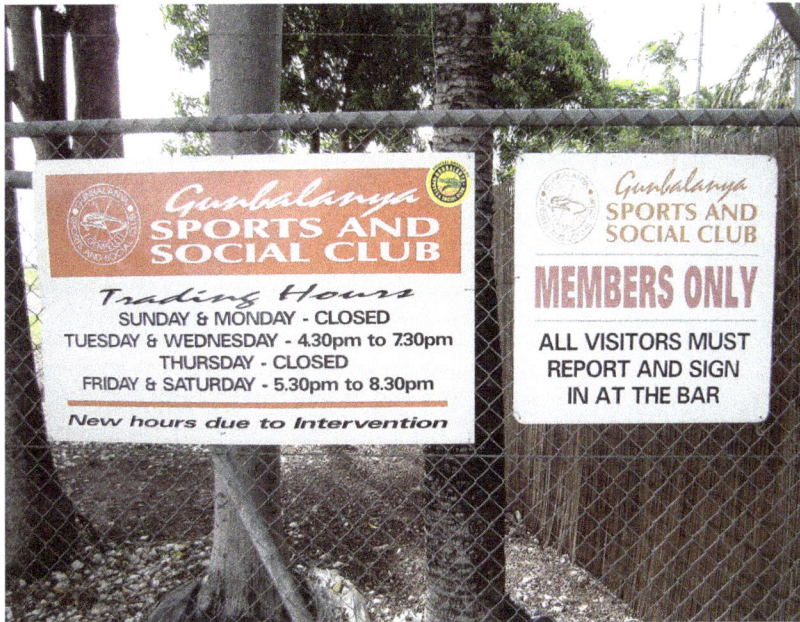

Fig. 9 Membership signs at Gunbalanya Club, 2013
Source: M Brady

The 1975 Leary report encapsulated the aspiration—the hope—for the adoption of more moderate, sociable drinking styles in Aboriginal communities. In some quarters, there were hopes that the clubs might form part of larger community centres that would counsel problem drinkers; in this way, 'the Aborigines themselves [would] have a responsibility as regards the education and rehabilitation of the problem members of their community'.[39] Clubs were espoused as the antidote to a variety of evils—uncontrolled access to takeaway liquor, drink driving and drunken misbehaviour on the streets of rural towns—and as agents in the process of learning better drinking habits. It was not only Aboriginal people who were thought to benefit from the controlled drinking environment provided by clubs: investigating the effect of increased mining activity

---

39   Powell, Police Commissioner to Symons DAA, Adelaide, 19/3/1979 [GRS 6624/1/P, DAA 520/68].

and influx of European mineworkers in Arnhem Land, the Fox Report[40] recommended that clubs rather than hotels be established.[41] As recently as 2008, prominent Territorian Ted Egan, previously of the Welfare Branch and later the Administrator of the Northern Territory, proposed that off-premises drinking should be banned throughout the Northern Territory, and that licensed premises such as bars and hotels should all be (re)licensed as clubs, where people signed in as members—'punched the bundy'—and were subject to the clubs' rules, regulations and conventions.

Control over Aboriginal movement

Early arguments put forward by outsiders in favour of clubs reveal an underlying desire to control Aboriginal people, not just their alcohol consumption. In colonial times, the practice of rationing food and tobacco replaced violence as a mode of government, largely because it was found to be more successful at rendering intercultural relationships peaceful and predictable. As a result, rationing carries with it a history of control over Aboriginal lives, as Tim Rowse documented in *White Flour, White Power* (1998). During the assimilation era, Aboriginal people began to orient their lives, at least in part, around the receipt of European goods such as flour, tea, sugar and tobacco; beer rations in missions and settlements functioned in much the same way, encouraging people to remain 'tethered' to the mission and dissuading them from ranging further afield.

Older Aboriginal people, particularly women, were positive about the fact that clubs would control the mobility of their husbands and sons: they often supported proposals for clubs in the hope that they would keep the men and boys at home, divert drinkers from nearby or distant outlets and lessen the risk of car accidents. It was also hoped that clubs would put an end to dangerous drinking camps and groups of people drinking in the scrub or the 'long grass' in towns.

---

40   Also known as the Ranger Inquiry, the Fox Report (1977) led by Justice Fox, influenced the subsequent development of uranium mining at Nabarlek and Ranger in the Northern Territory and Olympic Dam in South Australia.
41   This was a plan for the regional population as a whole, not just the Indigenous population. A licensed club was established in the mining town of Jabiru as a result of these recommendations; however, its history has been marked by repeated attempts to sell takeaway liquor and become, in effect, a hotel (d'Abbs & Jones 1996).

However, it is noteworthy that the most vociferous supporters of licensed clubs in bush communities were often the white citizens and mayors of towns such as Ceduna, Alice Springs and Katherine that have large Aboriginal populations in their hinterland. Non-Aboriginal town-based residents and politicians have been keen to dissuade Aboriginal people from visiting towns (because of their capacity to drink and make trouble), preferring instead that they be 'out of sight, out of mind' (d'Abbs 1998). In 1997, there were a rash of calls for wet canteens covering a wide geographical area. In April that year, the Northern Territory Liquor Commissioner, Peter Allen, announced that 'drunks wandering the streets with takeaway liquor could no longer be tolerated'. Wet canteens and clubs, he claimed, were an 'option that cannot be ignored'.[42] The Territory's Chief Minister stated publicly that he wanted an end to 'dry' communities. The pressure for clubs spread across the region, with communities pointedly being asked, yet again, to vote on whether they wanted to have licensed outlets. Two Territorians with long-term mission and community experience, were outraged. They argued that, by failing to appreciate and understand past failures, those who were pushing for wet canteens, including the politicians, were 'not doing their homework'.[43] Nevertheless, in 2011, the Alice Springs deputy mayor again called for wet canteens in bush communities, places where 'the family can sit down and have a meal together, and have a beer together'.[44] In May that year, numerous Territory politicians called on the federal minister for Indigenous Affairs to allow for wet canteens to be established, specifically to stop problem drinkers from 'drifting' into Alice Springs (Murdoch & Skelton 2011).

Over the years, town-based Aboriginal organisations have also joined the debate over clubs. In the early 1980s, the Central Australian Aboriginal Legal Aid Service, based at Alice Springs, called for wet canteens to be established out bush (Collmann 1988: 50). In 1982, the Alice Springs town camper's representative body, known as Tangentyere Council, wrote to communities in the catchment area asking them to consider having canteens to reduce the drinking problem in town (O'Connor 1983). In doing so, Tangentyere was trying to protect the interests of its constituents in town camps who were dealing with drunken visitors from the bush.

---

42   *Centralian Advocate* 18 April 1997: 1.
43   These were Pastor Paul Albrecht and Gary Stoll. *Alice Springs News* 4(42) 1997: 3.
44   *ABC News* 14 January 2011.

In South Australia, one Lutheran commentator took the control idea even further, advocating drinking facilities in Aboriginal settlements as the means by which church authorities could retain 'absolute control' (Hansen 1972: 7, cf. Brady & Palmer 1984).[45] In the context of statements such as these, it is salutary, and not entirely irrelevant, to remember that during the apartheid era in South Africa, the native affairs bureaucracy provided segregated beer halls for black mine labourers. The authorities saw beer halls as a means of bringing the leisure activities of the black population under state scrutiny and control. By providing beer-halls, South African authorities hoped 'to remove African alcohol consumption from white view, and thus create at least the illusion of order' (Ambler & Crush 1992: 19, La Housse 1992).

To raise revenue

One widespread motivation for the establishment of clubs in Aboriginal communities in the Northern Territory was to keep cash circulating in the communities, rather than losing it to publicans in town; the linked option of devoting profits to local causes was also attractive. This reasoning continues to be heard in arguments in favour of establishing clubs, and retaining them once established, today.

In Queensland, in the 1970s, the rationale for clubs was clear. There were no aspirations for the clubs to teach civilised drinking; instead, the clubs—appropriately referred to as 'canteens'—were instigated as a means of raising revenue. The Bjelke-Petersen Government actively and overtly promoted beer canteens as a way of generating revenue for community councils and shires to pay for local services (Martin 1993, McKnight 2002, Moran 2013). The sudden availability of alcohol in previously dry communities caused turmoil. In the beginning, the income spent on alcohol consumption was lost to communities because the profits from liquor sales 'streamed into departmental coffers through the Welfare Fund' (Kidd 1997: 302). Later, club takings became a source of substantial and highly valued 'untied' monies that local community–government councils could use at their discretion. The desire for profitability acted as a natural brake on any moves to curb sales as a harm-reduction measure. The commercial imperative for local (Aboriginal) government councils

---

45   This thinking was revisited in 2008 in light of government plans for large Aboriginal communities to become 'growth towns' with provision for 'normal' commercial enterprises such as licensed restaurants and clubs (Northern Territory Licensing Commission 2009: 8).

to maximise sales was so strong in Queensland, and the conflict of interest so great, that the Fitzgerald Inquiry recommended—and the state government agreed—that their right to sell alcohol and profit from the sales should be removed. Fitzgerald (2001) recommended that clubs be run by completely separate, private interests[46] and that local government councils be provided with compensation (cf. Martin 1998).[47]

Enacting rights to drink

While there were some less benevolent motivations on the part of interest groups, there were also mixed motivations for the establishment of clubs within Aboriginal communities themselves. Some Northern Territory communities with existing clubs demonstrated complex reasons for wanting not only to maintain their clubs, but to make them more appealing. Clubs were seen as recognising the 'rights' of drinkers; conversely, they were viewed as bargaining tools that placated the drinking members of a community by 'giving them something'. For example, in a discussion in 2005 over the potential loosening of conditions of an existing community licence, one community member stated:

> Grog is a big problem here. We are slaves to all you drunken mob … There's a lot of domestic violence and underage drinking. But we can't deny the drinkers' rights too. We gotta give them something too. Otherwise we should tell them to go to [nearest town]. We gotta balance their rights. Give them their rights too, all you sober people. So the community's got to support the drinking men … I'm starting to live with this grog problem. Balance it out, sober and drunken man. All these grog men say they agree as long as we give them something here so they stay and work. We can't frighten them by making them go to [the nearest town].[48]

---

46 Naturally enough, Fitzgerald's recommendations were immediately disputed by local councils. For example, at Bamaga, the council said that their community should not be included in the plans as 'it is a peaceful community with a well controlled canteen' (*Torres News* 3–9 May 2002: 1).

47 Following Fitzgerald, the Queensland Government insisted on transferring liquor licences away from community councils and shires to community-based boards, with canteen profits to be audited separately under strict new licensing conditions (Queensland Government 2002, Dalley 2012, Moran 2013). In 2008, the government went further, in effect closing down most canteens and clubs in Aboriginal communities. McKnight (2002: 211) pointed out that regional bodies or local boards would still see people struggling for political clout and the accoutrements of political power.

48 Excerpt from a Northern Territory Licensing Commission hearing regarding an application for a restricted area in the Maranboy district (5 May 2005: 17).

Similar comments were made elsewhere:

> We have this problem. How can we manage it in some way? Got to be realistic. They love their alcohol. If you cut off their alcohol it will drive it underground. They're not going to say 'oh, I'll just stop drinking', they'll just live like a homeless person to get a charge. I never drank. I see the impact it has.[49]

The social, cultural and political outcomes

Despite aspirational rhetoric about the ability of clubs to teach 'civilised' drinking, no one had any idea how to put this into practice. There was no systematic policy process guiding the rollout or management of clubs in Aboriginal communities; no in-house policy advice or training. Nor were there networks to link club managers, licensing agencies and health departments with health professionals and clinical psychologists. In Chapter 1, I mentioned that, during the 1960s and 1970s, researchers in Australia and overseas were examining behavioural psychology and social-learning models of drinking, training alcoholics to sip slowly and self-monitor, helping drinkers to monitor their levels of intoxication and providing lessons in alcohol and its effects. However, there is no evidence that any targeted program such as this found its way to the clubs in Aboriginal communities. The most that was offered was general information about alcohol and its effects.[50]

Misconstruing the learning model

When the clubs were first established, and for most of the years to follow, Aboriginal people were (somehow) expected to adopt moderate drinking habits simply by being provided with a limited number of cans of beer. This narrow interpretation of the proper 'setting' for alcohol consumption was not enough to inculcate a habitually moderated intake. In the 'drug, set and setting' formula designed by Norman Zinberg (1984) as a way of understanding drug-related behaviours, setting refers to more than

---

49   Brady fieldnotes, March 2013.
50   In the 1990s, the Northern Territory Living with Alcohol (LWA) program staff who visited communities to discuss safer drinking options would visit the community club if there was one, but there were no structured educational interventions in the clubs. Twenty years after the first clubs were opened, LWA published a useful guide to 'creating safer drinking environments' (Hunter & Clarence 1996).

environmental or physical settings. It also refers to the social context, or social setting, in which information is transmitted in numerous formal and informal ways. Setting is not static. Crucially, Zinberg's notion of setting *interacts* with the nature of the drug and the 'set' of the individual—their socialisation, personality and attitudes. In the case of Aboriginal drinkers, these elements often combined to value inebriation over moderation. The clubs provided a physical setting within which regulated sales would naturally limit the amount people could drink. However, they could not (at least in their early versions) influence an individual's 'set'—their pre-existing positive values associated with drinking to excess. There is no evidence that Aboriginal people who drank in clubs learned and *internalised* a restrained pattern of consumption that they practised when drinking elsewhere. Indeed, the evidence is quite to the contrary (Brady & Palmer 1984, d'Abbs 1987).

In a sense, the level of naivety on the part of mission and government authorities is surprising. By the time of the first clubs, anthropologists in Australia were publishing detailed ethnographies that described how, for many Aboriginal people, the goal of drinking was about achieving a particular kind of sociality around inebriation, rather than moderation. In the 1950s and 1960s, Jeremy Beckett (1965) demonstrated that vigorous drinking was highly valued among Aboriginal men in outback New South Wales towns. He observed that there were numerous social disadvantages in not drinking heavily, as men who failed to drink in the expected manner led 'a more restricted social life' (43). Later, Basil Sansom (1977, 1980) characterised the Darwin fringe camps as 'free grogging communities' (51) in which people unapologetically lived 'longa grog' (44) and aimed to become roaringly and helplessly drunk. Rory O'Connor (1984: 175) observed in the early 1980s that people in Alice Springs were 'clinging tenaciously' to heavy-drinking patterns that led to disease, injury, loss and family breakdown.

The notion that providing rations of alcohol alone would 'teach' moderate drinking also failed to take account of the *interpersonal* social setting— that is, the powerful influence of social modelling and the associated idea that people conform generally to what their fellows are doing. O'Connor (1984) referred to the 'contingent' drunkenness of Aboriginal people living in Alice Springs town camps; he argued that any loss of control over the amount of alcohol consumed *resided in the group*, not the individual. Dismissing accepted individualised notions of alcoholism, O'Connor (1984) represented problem drinking as group dependence or contingent drunkenness—a style of drinking that depended for its existence upon the correct physical and social environment. The Alice Springs town camps provided the ideal physical and social environment for heavy drinking. O'Connor argued that even if problem drinkers attended treatment programs or group therapy, they would inevitably conform to the influence of the group and re-adopt its behaviour on their return. His position was borne out by d'Abbs (1987), who found that the communities whose residents had the highest rate of protective custodies for intoxication in Darwin were the communities with licensed clubs at home. In other words, people who may have drunk moderately at clubs in their own communities were not doing so in Darwin: whatever they may have 'learned' was not being carried forward into another environment.

The clubs were trying to mould socially embedded behaviours, values and relationships into something else; instead, they created a self-selected group of consociates and peers who shared largely similar desires for the drinking experience and who were now consuming alcohol together, within settings that were atypical and, in effect, racially segregated. Rather than clubs moulding drinkers, drinkers were moulding the clubs to suit their own purposes. In a club environment, most drinkers share the same goal: namely, how to accomplish the desired heightened mood with a limited amount of alcohol and within a limited time frame. This has, in effect, created a remote Aboriginal community version of the Australian six o'clock swill. As one club manager put it, they are 'on a mission' to get drunk. Everyone knows when closing time is (in some clubs it is announced by an industrial-style siren). Achieving the desired heightened mood is managed in several ways: by drinking 'quick way'—that is, drinking the last beer really quickly to get a charge before leaving; saving up drinks until just before closing time; or waiting until the last minute to buy drinks (Dalley 2012). In some locations, drinkers invent subterfuges or gamble with drinks or drink tokens to accumulate more than their allowance of beer cans.

For around two decades or more, most of the clubs bore no resemblance to the places imagined by Leary and many government officials: they had no 'proper facilities for drinking' or 'family atmosphere'. At Yalata, for example, although the canteen had been intended to interrupt grog running from the nearest town and to 'help people to drink beer in a controlled and sensible way',[51] the facility comprised a large hall with a concrete floor and iron roof, a counter across one end, a concrete apron at the front and outside toilets. A team of psychologists from Adelaide University who studied the canteen observed, drily, that it could in no way be considered *comparable to the pub on the corner* (Penny 1979: 4, original emphasis). Ten years after the canteen was licensed, a DAA report stated categorically:

> There is no evidence of developing 'civilised' drinking habits. The customers drain their cans rapidly and then give the appearance of being left lost and wondering about what to do next … A shallow survey of the scene would indicate that the beer rationing scheme has little to commend it and in fact could be harmful. (Cooke 1978: 12)

There was no evidence that providing beer at the Yalata canteen had decreased the consumption of port, which was purchased from a roadhouse 60 km away, and the DAA noted that non-drinkers had no difficulty in obtaining a ration of beer, which they promptly gave to others. The beer ration was further sabotaged by drinking men who convened games of two-up outside the canteen using their beer cans as betting chips, a regular event witnessed by myself and a colleague in 1981 (Brady & Palmer 1984). As we wrote then, the beer ration merely whetted the appetites of those who wanted stronger drinks. Yalata canteen drinkers then proceeded to commission local drivers of private cars (known colloquially as 'taxis') to make trips to other sources of alcohol in town.

Learning 'civilised' drinking was not possible in Queensland either, because, like Yalata, for many years, the canteens in Aboriginal communities simply sold open cans of beer in sheds without seats, food or social amenities. At Kowanyama, in 1973, the canteen was a window through which DAA officers handed out the daily ration of cans: two, then four and later six (Moran 2013).

There are many examples of the abject failure of clubs in Aboriginal communities to inculcate moderation, especially in their early years. At Aurukun, in far north Queensland, the ration at the club in the 1980s was two jugs of beer per drinker, three nights a week. Since each jug contained 1.14 L of beer, this rationing practice effectively normalised and institutionalised the consumption of large amounts of alcohol. Under

---

51 This was stated by Don Dunstan, Minister for Aboriginal Affairs in South Australia (SRG 186, Series 174–82, SLSA).

pressure from their male kin, members of the community council were persuaded to increase these amounts (Martin 1993). Some Queensland clubs had no limits at all, and figures from one community collected in 1982 showed that each drinker consumed an average of seven jugs per night (Commonwealth of Australia 1977, Fua & Lumsden 1984). At Oenpelli, now Gunbalanya, the council objected to uncontrolled alcohol sales from a nearby store and successfully took over the licence, opening its own Sports and Social Club.[52] In 1984, Sue Kesteven, one of a team of researchers engaged in a study of the impact of uranium mining in the region, reported that sales of beer were not being rationed at the Gunbalanya Sports and Social Club, and that there was open flouting of the dry area legislation. By 1996, the club was reported to be well managed, with better security, a pleasant beer garden, entertainment and a system of banning those who misbehaved. However, alcohol-related violence was not uncommon (d'Abbs & Jones 1996: 46).

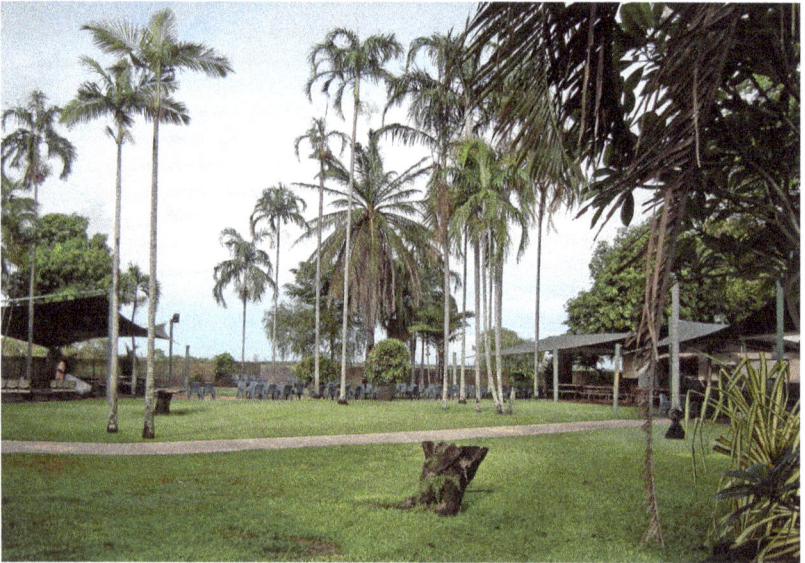

Fig. 10 Beer garden at Gunbalanya Club, 2013
Source: M Brady

---

52   After failing to have the Border Store's licence cancelled, the Gunbalanya Council bought the lease and allowed the store's licence to lapse (Kesteven 1984: 193).

In recent years, the rules have been tightened at all community-based clubs in the Northern Territory, primarily as a result of the intervention undertaken by the Australian Government in 2007 (Shaw et al. 2015).[53] Under new regulations, community clubs can only sell mid-strength or low-alcohol beer (3 per cent or less) in cans (not kegs); they can only open for four days a week and cannot make takeaway sales; and they must make hot food available. These regulations were targeted at curbing what had been, in some instances, lax serving practices and increasingly laissez-faire attitudes. For the most part, the eight existing Northern Territory clubs have made genuine efforts (often under duress) to implement safer service and to try to inculcate moderation and sociable drinking practices.

For a particular type of drinker in remote communities, twenty-first-century clubs provide a sociable venue where Aboriginal men and women, as well as non-Aboriginal staff and visitors, can relax with a few mid-strength beers and have something to eat before going home at around 7 or 8 pm. Troublemakers are banned for varying periods of time, plentiful signage lists the rules of behaviour, food (of varying quality) is available, there is music, television and pool tables, and some clubs provide free bottled water as people leave. Children are not allowed to enter; instead, they peer through the wire netting surrounding open-air beer gardens, observing everything and waiting for their parents to emerge. For determined drinkers, the club is never enough. Recent regulatory changes away from 'heavy' drinks (i.e. those with high alcohol content) to lower alcohol content beers, have inevitably prompted these drinkers to go elsewhere. This is the price of implementing strict limits on sales and trying to provide a moderation-inducing environment; all clubs have lost some customers and income from sales since the 2007 restrictions were imposed.

The vulnerable nature of Aboriginal authority

It is not difficult to suggest reasons why clubs in Aboriginal communities largely failed to achieve ascribed goals. One reason was an overly optimistic expectation that local people would be able to manage the

---

53 In October 2007, as part of the NTER, the Australian Government implemented restrictions that applied to all social clubs in remote Aboriginal communities in the Northern Territory. In Queensland, governance arrangements for the clubs and 'taverns' of Cape York were dramatically altered following the *Cape York Justice Study* that documented widespread binge drinking, poor management of community licences and rampant alcohol-related violence (Fitzgerald 2001).

clubs and enforce the rules, and that they would do so in a disinterested manner with the welfare of the community at heart. As with the village clubs in Papua New Guinea, it was assumed that if clubs were located in Aboriginal communities, Aboriginal traditional social controls, enforced by elders, would reinforce rules of behaviour and help to uphold the agreed in-house policies, thus contributing to the overall project of socialising drinkers into moderate consumption. However, by the time the first clubs were opened, anthropologists, as well as documenting the values attached to heavy drinking and intoxication, had noted the absence of individuals with clearly defined legislative functions in Aboriginal communities, and had commented on the widespread belief that ordinary men had neither the right nor the authority to make rules that others must follow (Meggitt 1975, Myers 1979). There was also the matter of whose land a club stood on and, as a corollary, who had authority over misbehaviour on that land (Downing 1988). Experienced missionaries expressed doubt about the extent of Aboriginal authority over interpersonal disputes and social disorder; church workers, such as Paul Albrecht (2002: 39), wrote of the 'authority vacuum' that lay between Indigenous cultural authority figures and the civic roles of councils or local governments. Perhaps the most thoughtful consideration of this matter was provided by Charles Rowley (1970) who questioned the common assumption that Aboriginal people had a physiological inability to resist alcohol. Challenging the often-repeated view that Aboriginal society did not develop its own controls to deal with alcohol because there was no 'law' about alcohol in 'traditional' Aboriginal culture, he argued that:

> Aborigines suffered the worst effects of alcohol, not only because it offered to individuals temporary escape from what seemed a pointless existence but also because of the vulnerability and nature of authority in Aboriginal society. That there was no 'law' about alcohol was an initial cause of vulnerability, no doubt, but the fact does not in itself explain why Aboriginal society did not develop controls to deal with it … There were, of course, as the anthropologists have shown, social controls in each group and … leadership … exerted by the men of high training and status. But social controls of a traditional nature are especially vulnerable when the whole basis of the tradition is in question; even more so when, as in this case, it has been wrecked by rapid depopulation, loss of control of the land, and the obvious disregard of indigenous religious assumptions by the newcomers … and probably the first use of alcohol had the effect it has continued to have of reducing the great man to an object of ridicule; and of giving to the doubting and tentatively dissident youth courage to defy him. (30–1)

3. THE ROLE OF BEER CANTEENS AND LICENSED CLUBS

There appeared to be a degree of ignorance among policymakers about the limited range of Aboriginal authority, and little acknowledgment or understanding of the entirely socially normative ethic of non-interference that exists within Aboriginal society, resulting in a high tolerance of the (mis)behaviour of others (Brady 2004: 60). As well as misconstruing the nature of authority, government, welfare and some mission authorities assumed, incorrectly, that even small communities would be cohesive enough to manage the clubs, determine what constituted alcohol-related harm and create strategies for reducing it (Gray 1996: 409). In reality, there was little frank debate at community meetings and people generally offered poor solutions to problems.[54]

Clubs that initially seemed to operate in the intended manner soon increased the allowable ration, causing the system to deteriorate rapidly: several clubs were halted abruptly. Rudimentary clubs and beer rations came and went in several locations. At Hermannsburg, for example, in the 1970s, a newly inaugurated Aboriginal council issued two cans of beer on three or four occasions per week, which worked well. However, Aboriginal elders were unable to enforce the rules. Bowing to pressure from kin, more and more cans were distributed and, within a year, the missionaries—having reached the conclusion that the idea of moderation made little sense to Aboriginal people—called a halt to proceedings.[55] Sue Kesteven (1984: 201–2) wrote perceptively about the difficulties of community control over alcohol sales and demands for special favours:

> This constant pressure from Aboriginal people for waiving of rules in each particular case is one of the main drawbacks to finding a congenial, enforceable set of rules which suits the entire population. Those in favour of drink seem to thwart the intentions of rules that they themselves may set up when sober or when not in need of alcohol. Until they come to terms with their contradictions, and the implications of continued heavy drinking, this problem will not be solved except by the imposition of strictly applied rules, policed by non-Aborigines.

Even when the rules for 'civilised' drinking are made by the community itself, the group pressure to waive such rules is strong. As Kesteven's research demonstrated, such problems are associated with social expectations and norms embedded within Aboriginal sociality and, as

---

54 Council members at Yalata, for example, railed at drinkers while being grog-runners themselves; drinking camps (often without water, shade or access to help) were frequently suggested as solutions to noisy drinking in the community.

55 Paul Albrecht, interview, 20 April 2005.

such, are not necessarily solvable through regulatory mechanisms. Senior men and women in a community are often unwilling to intervene and, if they do, their attempts to deal with ration-rorting or drunken behaviour often have little effect. Indeed, as illustrated in the case of Wadeye and its drinking club in the late 1980s, discussed in the next chapter, it would take a serious alcohol-related crisis or tragedy to trigger decisive leadership, and group acquiescence in that leadership.[56]

Power, money, largesse

As beer rationing systems became institutionalised into canteens, and the canteens were transformed into clubs (some of which became extremely lucrative), it became apparent that there had been a failure to consider the corrupting implications of the potentially large income that would be generated by sales of beer. The Aboriginal associations, non-Aboriginal managers or local community councils running clubs soon found that they could make significant profits from the sale of alcohol. Local discord over the proper distribution of funds notwithstanding, the money-making capacity of the clubs transformed them into powerful (some would say *the* most powerful) economic and political institutions within Aboriginal communities (Martin 1993, d'Abbs 1998, McKnight 2002). In some cases, this power came to be concentrated in the hands of one individual— the club manager—or else a very small group of Aboriginal people, who could both receive and confer favours. In 1998, d'Abbs observed that the high income generated by some clubs created a concentration of power and problems of governance; that there was little scrutiny by community members; and that numerous social and political difficulties were caused by one person (or a small group) having a virtual monopoly of control over a highly valued resource (682). Echoing the historical arguments between temperance advocates and community-owned licensed premises, d'Abbs noted that a community's economy could become alcohol-driven, with club profits representing 'untied' grants, and that clubs could create a symbiotic relationship in which drinkers became dependent on the club (for their social life and entertainment) and the club became dependent on high levels of consumption (for its continued economic prosperity).

---

56 Yalata Community Council only took decisive action against alcohol after the death of five community members in 1991 (Brady et al. 2003).

Temperance advocates in previous decades had voiced warnings about how alcohol profits could be used by community-owned hotels to 'buy off' critics and earn themselves a false respectability. By donating to community causes (such as charter aircraft, swimming pools, playground equipment, sports jerseys and facilities, and covering the cost of funerals) community leaders, the governing committees of clubs and the (non-Aboriginal) managers who run them, have done just that, thereby making themselves (somewhat) immune to criticism. Insofar as the 'business' of the clubs allowed for the emergence of a stratum of community leaders with access to a stream of money that they could dispose of without being accountable to any outsiders, these developments were arguably aligned with self-determination.[57] At Kowanyama in Queensland, for example, the council directed most of its $1 million canteen profit to a mothers and babies centre, women's shelter, school bus, after-hours security for nurses, and ranger and outstation program (Moran 2013): who could complain about that? However, these same councils in Queensland communities are also responsible for the peace, order and welfare of their populations, thus creating clear and irresolvable conflicts of interest and principle (Martin 1998: 4, Fitzgerald 2001: 42).[58] David McKnight (2002: 115) observed that whether or not the canteen on Mornington Island used its profits for 'good works', they were obtained at a horrendous social cost, and that the canteen itself often threatened community wellbeing.[59]

A convenient tool for politicians

An analysis of the history of the policies that underpinned the establishment of licensed clubs shows that there has been a major shift away from the original ideas about their role in habituating people to moderate drinking. During recent elections in the Northern Territory and Queensland, some politicians promised to re-examine and to liberalise alcohol availability through clubs.[60] Such proposals are invariably fed by

---

57 Thanks to Tim Rowse for making this point.
58 At Yarrabah, in 2002, the council chairman said that the pub (the club) was the only enterprise they had; it made $200,000 a year, all of which was channelled into housing maintenance and employment opportunities (Hodge & Emerson 2002: 3).
59 Mac Marshall and colleagues (1982: 456) suggested that similar problems in Papua New Guinea could be avoided by making provincial liquor licences government owned and removing the profit motive.
60 This happened during the election in 2012. (See *Courier Mail* 2013.)

'moral panic'.[61] An outbreak of (white) citizen outrage over a particular incident, or surge of Aboriginal visitors to a regional town, prompts the suggestion that Aboriginal people from communities would be less likely to come to town if they could drink in their home communities. Mayors of regional towns, town councillors, politicians or the police (often a newly arrived officer), propose wet canteens or clubs for those communities as the 'perfect' solution to public drinking and drunkenness among Aboriginal people. A spike of policy interest leads to a surge of public commentary and media interest and renewed political pressure for clubs to be established in communities. Coroners investigating alcohol-related deaths in remote areas become involved, receiving submissions from local interest groups that include recommendations for clubs. Free to make wide-ranging policy recommendations and politically loaded observations in their reports, some coroners conclude that wet canteens might solve the problem,[62] others warn against them as disastrous.[63]

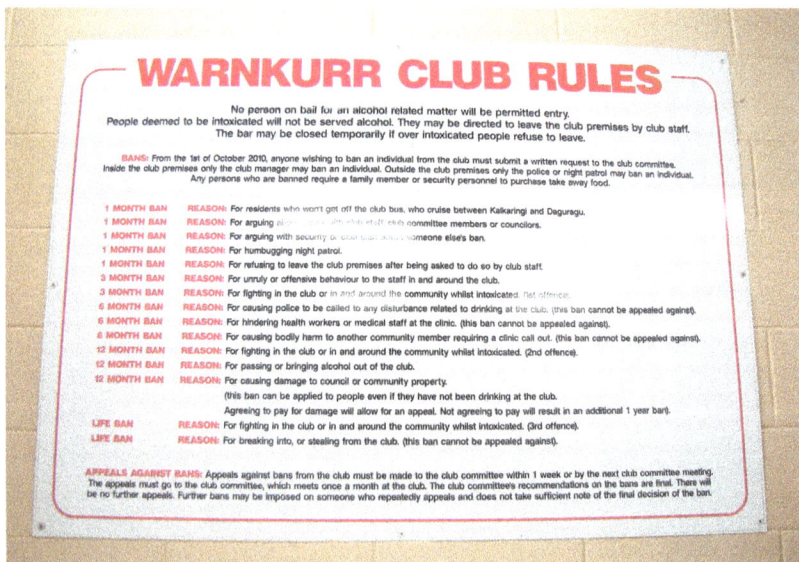

Fig. 11 Warnkurr Club Rules, 2013
Source: M Brady

---

61   The phrase 'moral panic' was coined by deviance sociologist Stanley Cohen (1972, cf. Goode & Ben-Yehuda 1994).
62   This was the case when W Donald, Northern Territory Coroner, investigated five separate Aboriginal deaths near an outback takeaway liquor outlet in 1997.
63   See Coroner's Court of South Australia (2011).

Local political struggles

Early in their history, the clubs provided the opportunity for a different kind of localised political struggle. Depriving individuals of access to a community's club has proved to be a powerful means of social control, and this power can be wielded by various groups, including local community councils, club committees and individual managers, the police, and other bodies within communities. The ability to ban individuals for poor behaviour can be a useful tool with which to attempt to condition better drinking practices; clubs can 'bar off' people for spitting, abuse, failing to leave the premises and for drunkenness. As long ago as 1980, drunkenness at the Leichhardt River canteen was punished under such rules put in place by the police.

Clubs often display long lists of names of people who have been banned and the length of the ban: some people are banned for life. Clubs also display lists of the behaviours that will result in banning (e.g. abusing staff or fighting). This enables drinkers to object if they feel they have been banned for no good reason: 'banned for cold blood'.[64] In most cases, the lists of proscribed behaviours are compiled by community members who sit on club committees and the manager. Some bans, or threats of bans, are beyond what might be considered reasonable in any other licensed premises: to some they seem overly authoritarian. Some clubs have become a de facto community policeman, pressuring community members to fulfil civic responsibilities. For example, a plumber in one community who was tired of children tampering with his building site, displayed a sign that read: 'Keep Out! Children found on this site parent's will be banned from the Club' (Shaw et al. 2015: 121).

Exasperated by parental neglect, community members often suggest that *other* community members be 'barred off' the club for neglecting their children, or not sending them to school. In other cases, family members may approach a club manager and ask for a miscreant to be banned until he or she has made the necessary reparations for an offence. A club manager may approach the community's health staff and ask for the names of perpetrators of an assault, or the names of pregnant women, to ban them from the club. Needless to say, such requests are usually politely refused.

---

64 'Banned for cold blood' = banned for no good reason.

In the absence of an existing 'traditional' authority that might extend to personal misbehaviour, the display of lists of 'banned behaviours', the fact that they frequently extend into the realm of personal conduct, and the alacrity with which Aboriginal people themselves propose deprivation of access to the club as a form of social control, represent a new form of Indigenous authority that has evolved under 'self-determination'. Beyond reasonable behaviour at the club itself, the lists reveal a desire on the part of community members and club committees for there to be some degree of order and civic responsibility in the community more broadly. The existence of the lists also suggests the degree of impotence felt by the civic-minded majority when trying to persuade their fellows to behave better, to send their children to school and to feed and provide for them (Myers 1979, Brady 1992, Purtill 2017).

The unresolved challenges of clubs

The debate about licensed social clubs in remote communities is unlikely to be resolved, as arguments for and against them appeal to politically significant constituencies. National inquiries have documented the concerns and controversies surrounding clubs, and researchers, including myself, have analysed comparative data on the injuries sustained in communities with and without clubs; the effect of clubs on health and wellbeing in general; and their effect on people's cash expenditure, especially the diversion of funds away from food and other necessities (Brady & Palmer 1984, Langton et al. 1991, Martin 1993, d'Abbs et al. 1994, d'Abbs & Jones 1996, Gladman et al. 1997, Hoy et al. 1997, d'Abbs 1998, Shaw et al. 2015). Before concluding this discussion about efforts to 'teach' moderate drinking by means of rationing, canteens and clubs, it is important to mention some of the less obvious—more ontological— implications of this somewhat compromised project.

Tethering

Irrespective of how many regulations and harm-reduction measures are in place, or how 'good' a club might be, one psychosocial outcome of clubs is that Aboriginal people living in communities with licensed clubs become 'tethered' to them. The concept of tethering derives from archaeology, where it is used to describe how the movements of ancient megafauna were tied to and bounded by the resource-rich riparian corridors, or circuits, that provided their food and water (Smith 2013: 66). By putting a brake on the movements and interests of people, and confining them to the area that provides the desired resource, social clubs act as metaphorical tethering mechanisms.[65] In the past, the provision of food rations and water supplies by government to dispossessed Aboriginal groups performed this role (Rowse 1998, Brady 1999). Now, beer clubs fulfil one of their intended goals—keeping people at home and protecting them from the dangers of drunk driving and uncontrolled takeaway alcohol—through tethering. However, this creates another, somewhat less desirable, outcome.

Clubs bring about a narrowing of focus and contribute a sense of *confinement* to life in communities (cf. Purtill 2017: 230). Clubs (and drinking itself) become the centre of people's lives—the focus of attention to the exclusion of other activities and social and cultural engagements, so that people's thoughts seem to revolve exclusively around beer. Observing the relationship between the people of Mornington Island and their canteen, David McKnight (2002: 109) commented that in their 'continuous hunt for beer almost everything else becomes secondary'. Ten years later, anthropologist Cameo Dalley (2012: 151) wrote about the same community and how people structured their lives around the licensed outlet there:

> The limited opening hours constrained the amount of time available to consume alcohol, which in turn contributed to the formation of a daily routine for some Aboriginal people structured around its operating times. During 2007, this routine began before the 4 pm opening time with those working for the local Mornington Shire Council.

To be ready by 4 pm, shire workers made sure their tasks were completed well before 'knock-off' at 3 pm. Finishing at 3 pm enabled drinkers to go home to prepare for their visit to the club, have a shower and get changed. Most customers made an effort to look clean and neat, sometimes borrowing clothes from kin (Dalley 2012: 151). This kind of planning ahead, taking into account of club opening times, affects people's contact with the land. People will abandon trips into the bush, fishing and hunting expeditions—even overnight stays to map sites on the land—to hurry back and be at the club when it opens. If the club, for whatever reason, is closed, this alters daily life dramatically. When, following the federal

---

65   I am grateful to Dr Peter Murray for making this analogy and drawing it to my attention.

government's intervention in 2007, the Northern Territory clubs were instructed to close for two days each week, community members reported that they had a 'holiday from grog' on those days: some went fishing; others 'rested their brains' (as one person put it); and some men went shopping and prepared food for their wives—all apparently remarkable activities.[66] Such comments from community members imply that they experienced a kind of relief from the usual obsessive focus on the club with its mixture of pleasures and pains.

Separatism

Most of the effects of tethering—curtailing and inhibiting people's interests and providing an obsessive preoccupation—are largely subliminal. Alongside these, the clubs are also effectively racially segregated, becoming Aboriginal domains. In achieving their goals of providing safer, controlled and sociable drinking environments, clubs are atypical in their social composition. No white Australian community workers drank at the 'canteens' when they were first introduced.[67] Despite becoming slightly more salubrious and less segregated in some places over time, Aboriginal clubs continue to be qualitatively different environments from other clubs or public hotels. In a public hotel or a town-based sport's club, an Aboriginal drinker might mingle with a range of other people and experience different drinking behaviours and settings for drinking and eating (and, perhaps, be subject to more stringent regulation).[68] This point was made in the 1960s by an objector to the licensing of a beer canteen at Yalata, who predicted that the canteen would have the effect of forcing Aboriginal people away from the hotels 'where they are equal with the white man and where they are learning to drink sensibly'.[69]

---

66   Brady fieldnotes, February 2013.

67   This has changed in recent years; non-Indigenous staff members and visitors now frequently patronise the clubs. In an intuitive acknowledgement of the notion of modelling 'good' drinking behaviour, some of these non-Indigenous patrons consciously 'set an example' by drinking moderately and not becoming intoxicated (Dalley 2012: 164, Brady fieldnotes, 2013).

68   This is not to deny that some hotel bars—such as 'animal bars'—frequented by Aboriginal people in rural Australia are nasty, dark, unsafe and subject to sometimes brutal security. Sansom (1980) refers to the 'thong bars' of Darwin: hotel bars where improper feet were those in thong sandals rather than shoes. As Sansom pointed out, Aboriginal 'fringe' dwellers drank thong-side, not shoe-side (180).

69   The objection came from a Methodist minister, Reverend Oates. State Library of South Australia, SRG 186 Series 174–82.

Papua New Guinea faced similar dilemmas in the 1980s when there was government pressure to expand the number of drinking clubs in the (often remote) villages. Well-informed policy researchers and alcohol policy experts cautioned against such a proliferation and recommended that:

> It is far better to maintain a limited number of readily accessible public houses that can be inspected at least once a month, easily policed when problems occur, and kept physically separate from village areas where drinking may have a bad effect on women and children and disrupt other aspects of village life. (Marshall 1982: 456)

In Australia, the clubs in communities have always been atypical venues; they are neither proper 'membership' clubs like those of the towns (servicemen's clubs, RSL clubs, bowls clubs and sport's clubs—which often have extensive dining rooms), nor are they pubs. Unlike rural towns with clubs and pubs, for decades, the missions and communities had minimal or no policing, no safe place for the intoxicated and no hospitals (only primary care clinics) to deal with alcohol-related injuries. Aboriginal clubs are remotely located, in communities that are isolated from normal monitoring and checks and balances; in the early years, they were run by inexperienced staff. For all these reasons, they were cut off from changes taking place elsewhere: they were left behind. When the liquor laws in Australia were liberalised and deregulated in the 1960s, people believed that the drinking environment—the physical setting—was important. With the extension of licensed service hours, hotels began to change their layout and facilities; the long bars that had been built to accommodate the pressure of six o'clock swill drinkers gave way to smaller bars with adequate seating. 'Vertical' drinking[70] was known to produce excessive consumption, as was crowding: were these basic principles ever applied to the canteens and clubs in Aboriginal communities? The answer is no—or, more correctly, not until recently. Yet, even if clubs in Aboriginal communities now have good policies in place—even if they manage the drinking environment well—they remain strangely anomalous venues, more akin to the drinking facilities provided for remote mining camps, with their tethered and skewed clientele, than anything else.

Australia has only recently begun to implement 'civilising' and harm-reducing strategies in Indigenous community clubs. The process remains ad hoc and has met with strenuous resistance at times. It is regrettable that

---

70   Vertical drinking (standing up) arose from a lack of seating; it encouraged greater amounts of alcohol to be consumed and thus was targeted by pub reformers (Talbot 2015: 29).

clubs were allowed to operate for so many years without these strategies in place. Arguably, this strategic and policy error has set back progress on the daunting task of encouraging change in the culture of drinking. As the Northern Territory Licensing Commission (2009: 7) chair thoughtfully observed:

> In the longer term there will need to be a focus on developing more cogent and appropriate policies in relation to safer, more orderly and supervised alcohol consumption for many of the [town] residents and visitors … Greater efforts therefore need to be made to improve drinking practices of those whose consumption and exposure to the use of alcohol is 'at the margin' … Better drinking habits will occur with regulation combined with harm minimisation education, with the key aim of reducing binge drinking and fostering socialised and more temperate consumption.

4

The wrecking of the Murrinh Patha Social Club: A case study

During the 1950s and 1960s, many of the mature-aged Aboriginal men from Port Keats, or Wadeye as it is now known, worked on cattle stations between Timber Creek and Kununurra. When they were away from home, Aboriginal people drank freely in towns; however, such drinking was not permitted in their home communities. Aboriginal reserves had remained 'dry' since their formation, even though in 1964, the right to drink had been granted to individuals off reserves in the Northern Territory. By the late 1970s, it was clear that men from missions and other communities were travelling elsewhere to buy alcohol; this prompted some women from Wadeye to support the idea of local availability to 'keep the men at home' (HRSCAA 1976: 669). Wadeye, the site of the Catholic Mission of Our Lady of the Sacred Heart, became one of the first Aboriginal communities in the Northern Territory to experiment with a licensed 'social club'.

The development of the club

The decision to apply for a licence to establish a club at the mission was based on the idea that Aboriginal people would learn to drink 'properly' if the amount of alcohol was controlled and the physical environment was appropriate. It was not a contradictory notion that a Catholic mission in charge of an Aboriginal settlement should allow drinking; the Catholic

Church and its missions were largely liberal-minded in their approach to the use of alcohol (Sournia 1990). The Catholic priests and brothers at Wadeye drank alcohol themselves in the Presbytery.

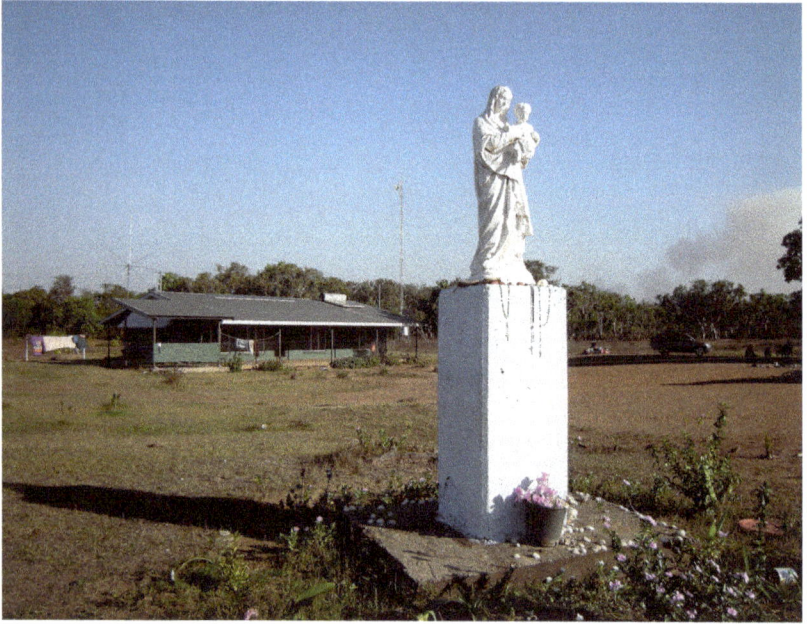

Fig. 12 Statue of Virgin Mary at the old Mission site, Wadeye
Source: M Brady

Apart from the desire of some community members to have a club, the decision was influenced by a report, published in 1975, that was written by a team of researchers who were all Catholic. Three of the authors, Father John Leary, Father Patrick Dodson and Luke Bunduk, were intimately associated with the Sacred Heart mission at Wadeye: Leary was the mission superintendent over two periods; Dodson, recently ordained, was posted to Wadeye to become Leary's curate (Keeffe 2003); and Bunduk[1] was an Aboriginal man of the landowning Kardu Diminin clan at Wadeye who later became president of the Kardu Numida Council.[2] Another team member, Bernie Tipiloura, a Tiwi Islander, was also a Catholic.

---

1   Bunduk took the place of an earlier team member, Bernie Tipiloura.
2   The Kardu Numida (meaning 'one people' in Murrinh Patha) Council was incorporated in 1978 to be the administrative body for the community once the Catholic mission ceased to perform this role. Between 1992 and 2000, the Kardu Numida Council entered a phase of administrative and financial restructuring to resolve the mixture of inappropriate governance arrangements and inadequate financial support that had developed in the context of a rapidly growing population (Desmarchelier 2001: 41).

The research was commissioned by an intergovernmental committee and the research team was tasked with investigating the causes, effects and amelioration of alcohol problems among Aboriginal Australians. The first inquiry of its kind in Australia, the team toured the country in a kombivan, visiting rehabilitation centres and interviewing people in parks and bars. Their report was decisively anti-prohibitionist:

> History has shown that prohibition does not work. Isolation does not safeguard prohibition, it simply puts off the day. We must face reality and human nature and the fact that sooner or later alcohol will come into the lives of these people. Aborigines (and everyone else) if they want to drink and retain their dignity and identity must acquire the ability of being able to control their drinking, otherwise it will be their destruction. To help gain this control there must be:
>
> a. a realistic educational programme on alcohol.
>
> b. provision of proper facilities that help towards the formation of good drinking habits. (Leary et al. 1975: 5)

The authors proposed that in tribal areas and 'self-contained' communities, licensed clubs would suit residents, and they made suggestions for the type of licensed premises they had in mind: it should have pleasant surroundings, music and entertainment, good food, soft drinks, provision for families, and rules and encouragements for good behaviour on open display—all designed to 'create pride in something good'. The authors envisaged that such a club might also be a place where people with drinking problems could be detected and helped: an optimistic suggestion that reflects something of the idealism of the era. The emphasis given to the idea of *learning moderation* suggests that some members of the team were aware of the thinking of the time about social-learning models:

> Much attention must be given to the formation of proper facilities for drinking. The learning process for drinking among Aborigines has been a sad one. Prohibition taught them to drink as much as possible, in the shortest possible time, in the worst possible surroundings. Lack of funds got them on to cheap fortified wines, the quickest way to achieve results. They so frequently continued [sic] their education in drinking with destitute alcoholic Europeans, or being encouraged to drink to excess by Europeans with ulterior motives. Drinking, we have been told, is a learnt process. Let us change the teachers. (Leary et al. 1975: 27)

The Leary report provided momentum for the mission at Wadeye to make a successful application for a liquor licence. In the late 1970s, what became known as the Murrinh Patha Social Club was inaugurated.

It aimed to provide a safe drinking environment where people could learn to drink responsibly, and to ensure that they spent their money within the community. Building on the Leary report's recommendations, three members of the Catholic clergy at Wadeye were instrumental in getting the club started: Father John Shallvey, Brother Andy Howley and Brother Kinnane.[3] Leary, interviewed many years later, explained the decision:

> In their society they never had alcohol and because of this they never developed ways and means of handling it. So when we had Port Keats we started the first club there. In the beginning I had the idea you could teach them civilised drinking, two or three cans—enough. But mostly if you had a big supply, the whole lot went.[4]

At the time, alcohol was available elsewhere in the region. At the Peppimenarti store,[5] 91 km away, Aboriginal people could buy a case of beer at any time, provided it was not consumed near the town during working hours (Stanley 1985: 80). Wadeye people could also obtain alcohol at the Fairweather Hotel on the northern side of the Daly River crossing, 189 km north of Wadeye; in the wet season, they often swam across the crocodile-infested waters to reach the pub.

The drinkers

Once the mission gained a liquor licence, the initial arrangement was simply to enable people to buy two cans of takeaway beer from a store: several outstations were also permitted to sell alcohol to residents.[6] Subsequently, the club was established in a recreation hall at Wadeye. In the early years, the club seems to have worked well; there was music and entertainment, and grassy shaded areas and outside tables, as envisaged. Behaviour at the club was governed by a complex series of rules set by the (Aboriginal) management committee, and misbehaviour was promptly dealt with according to the committee's cultural guidelines. There was

---

3   Xavier Desmarchelier, pers comm, 11 January 2013. In the early 1980s, Brother Howley also applied for a liquor licence for Nguiu on Bathurst Island, which was also a Catholic mission (Walsh 2005: 68).
4   John Leary, pers comm, 16 August 2004.
5   Peppimenarti, a cattle station of about 200 Aboriginal people associated with Daly River mission, was run by Harry Wilson. Daly River Mission also had its own Nauiyu Nambiyu Beer Club, which had two drinking sessions a day, rationed at three cans for men and two for women. Profits were directed to a social development fund (Stanley 1985: 68).
6   Bill Ivory (pers comm, 6 May 2015) recalls drinking with John Chula and family at Yeddairt in 1978 at a bush bar they had constructed on the outstation. The beer was supplied by the Catholic mission and was consumed in a 'convivial and friendly' environment.

a four- or six-can limit on full-strength beers, and drinkers bought the requisite number of tokens to exchange for beer.[7] Women sat on the grass and quietly played cards for beer tokens. The club was a social hub: it was open six days a week, Monday to Friday between 5 and 7 pm, and on Saturdays between 4.30 and 7 pm. Takeaways were available to permit holders from 3–4 pm. It was said to be 'a good place, the whole community, black and white went there. [The first manager] was good, no humbugging'.[8] Another Aboriginal patron commented:

> Phil S was the first manager, a good one. It was well run with snacks and music in the early 80s. At first it was all cash, then Phil S had the idea of tokens [four tokens each person] … They tried light beer … no-one liked it.[9]

There were many responsible drinkers at Wadeye; older people arrived dressed in their best and people enjoyed being able to have a few beers without having to leave the community.

The club was financially viable and contributed socially and financially to the community. As was the case in other communities, the revenue from the club was the only untied income available in Wadeye; it provided funds that could be spent on local needs free from government control. To utilise the club's 'facilities' (a euphemism for purchasing beer, as there were no other facilities, such as food, water or security, until later), a person had to become a 'member' (at no cost). Young people turning 18 were often coerced by family members to sign up for membership (even though most 18 year olds did not drink), as a way of providing more beer to family members, usually their fathers. The club became 'the epicentre of everyone's lives', as one observer put it. However, it soon varied between being a great asset and being a great problem. The drinking adversely affected the singing and performance of ceremony, which was of great concern to many senior men.[10] Over time, there were changes in management and management policies, resulting in a decline in the

---

7   The limits changed from time to time. By 1987, the limit was six cans per person. One informant remembered one resourceful young man who made counterfeit tokens by punching holes in a saucepan: 'We had to have a meeting about that', commented Anthony Dooling.
8   Mark Crocombe, pers comm, 14 July 2009.
9   Bill Ivory, pers comm, 14 July 2009.
10   Kim Barber, pers comm, 5 March 2014. Thanks to Kim Barber and Xavier Desmarchelier for these descriptions of the club and its patrons.

scrutiny of alcohol distribution and undermining of the various rationing systems; drinkers started swapping cans and some non-drinking women gave their allowance to their husbands, leading to violence.

The club was controlled by a management committee or board (all men, all drinkers, some of them dependent drinkers), who instructed the manager in the rules of engaging with local people. The manager and management committee were thus enmeshed in a close reciprocal alliance, aspects of which probably did not always comply with the Liquor Act. One Aboriginal community member recalled later that:

> The board of six or seven drinking people and the club manager—they were confused, 'brainwashed' people. They were supposed to have a four-can limit but used to bring wives, grandmothers [to use their allowance]. Aboriginal people worked there.[11]

The committee was responsible for selecting six local men (not women) to fill the highly desirable jobs at the club; selection was based on family and cultural preferences. Once everyone had gone home after the club closed at 7 pm, these men could stay on and consume their six cans of beer without being importuned by family members. Other perks for employees included cash advances, charter flights to Darwin and attendance (all expenses paid) at the annual Northern Territory Football League grand finals.

Meanwhile, the customers played cards and gambled with beer tokens.[12] As anthropologists have observed in relation to other settings, alcohol at Wadeye became a form of legal tender, and the club was the place where business was conducted (cf. Sansom 1980, Brady & Palmer 1984, Collmann 1988).[13] Groups of men reached agreements about who would accumulate more beers through what were known as 'sixpack clubs'; members took turns to drink three cans only, giving the rest to another person to enable that person to get 'full drunk'.[14] These arrangements became part of a 'hidden world' in which social, cultural and financial debts were accrued and repaid. If nothing else, these strategies demonstrate how determined many individuals were to drink to inebriation. At the

11   WP, interview, 14 July 2009.
12   Carol Watson, pers comm, 16 August 2009. Watson was in Wadeye conducting interviews for a major Northern Territory drug and alcohol use survey (Watson et al. 1988).
13   Xavier Desmarchelier, pers comm, 11 January 2013.
14   This was documented in a letter from Kardu Numida Council to the Liquor Commission written in September 1995.

time, apart from drinking on premises at the club, hundreds of people at Wadeye also held liquor permits that allowed them to drink alcohol at home (Australian Institute of Aboriginal Studies 1984: 214).[15]

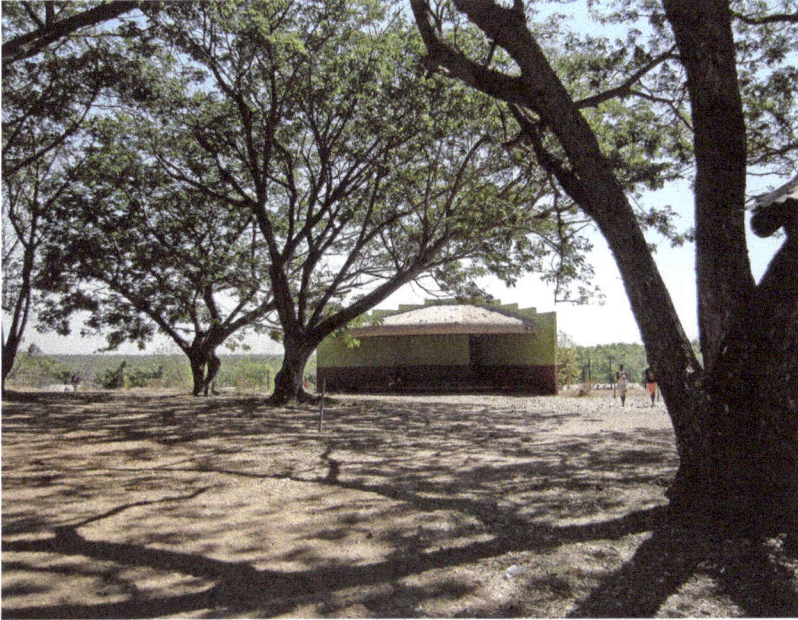

Fig. 13 Sound shell at Murrinh Patha Social Club, Wadeye, 2009
Source: M Brady

The non-drinkers

While the club was always well attended, Wadeye also had a significant non-drinking population, which included individuals who had given up alcohol after having been heavy drinkers. These people were encouraged and supported by an active AA-style group that had been set up by one of the mission brothers, Andrew Howley (who had also applied for the liquor licence). Howley had received a travelling scholarship to the United States to investigate sobriety groups and American Indian approaches to alcohol abuse. On his return, he visited the Holyoake Institute in Perth and was impressed by its approach to counselling and training using

---

15   In 1984, the number was 374 permits at Wadeye: some of these permits were held by white staff.

a 'family disease' treatment model for addiction.[16] He subsequently initiated Alcohol Awareness and Family Recovery (AAFR) programs in Darwin and Wadeye, the principles of which were based on the Holyoake model. This model promoted the idea that the families of alcoholics were 'co-dependents' whose actions inadvertently enabled drinkers to keep drinking: for example, by sending money to support drinkers, taking over essential roles neglected by drinkers and by making excuses for them.[17] According to the Holyoake model, welfare and other agencies were 'enablers'; they provided money that enabled families to survive while breadwinners drank away the primary income. Aboriginal legal services were implicated too, for by providing legal advice in alcohol-related cases, they protected drinkers from experiencing the full consequences of their actions (d'Abbs 1990: 21). The Holyoake model advised that, to counter what amounted to tacit support for drinkers, families needed to show 'tough love' to dependent drinkers, and not 'cover up' for them by lying on their behalf, paying their bills or providing for them, since all of these things allowed alcoholics to deny and escape from their problems.

Apart from the AAFR group at Wadeye, the Catholic brothers and nuns and committed local Aboriginal men, George Cumaiyi and Cyril Ninnal, also ran a residential rehabilitation program near Daly River at Five Mile.[18] This supported families dealing with alcohol abuse and provided a referral service and a focus for local self-help groups using the AA and Al-Anon Family Group models. An evaluation of the program at Five Mile found that attendance had a modest but real effect on drinking behaviour (d'Abbs 1990: 5). Between 1987 and 1989, more than 100 Wadeye family members attended the alcohol awareness courses at Five Mile or Darwin (d'Abbs 1990: 40). In fact, more than half of all admissions to the Five Mile AAFR program were drawn from either Wadeye or Nguiu on Bathurst Island. Notably, both communities had licensed clubs. The AAFR program at Wadeye was incorporated later as Makura

---

16 Holyoake, in turn, was influenced by the United States Minnesota-based Hazelden Institute's philosophy and methods, using the idea of addiction as a chemical dependency. Howley took Wadeye men Cyril Ninnal and William Parmbuk to the United States to attend the 55th AA–Al Anon International Convention (Williams 1990). See Chenhall (2007) for a detailed ethnography of the operation of an AA-based Aboriginal residential treatment program.

17 The term 'co-dependency' has been contested, with one professor of psychology stating that it had been expanded way beyond its useful role to encompass virtually the entire population (Lisansky-Gomberg 1989: 120).

18 Five Mile ran from the late 1980s to early 2000s. Its program was based on the family disease concept linked to the 12-step model that is used by many Canadian First Nations treatment programs, as well as Holyoake in Perth.

Wunthay,[19] a support and alcohol-education group that drew together a strong core of non-drinkers, women and other community members concerned about alcohol. It was this group at Wadeye, combined with ideas about 'tough love', that triggered the action that was taken against the club.

The group met at the Presbytery; a key figure was Freddie Cumaiyi, a senior man who had lived through his own personal struggles with alcohol as well as those of his family. William Parmbuk, a key player in the demise of the club, was also in the group. He spoke of his perceptions of drinking:[20]

> I never drank. My mum was an influence: she told me, 'it will kill you'. I grew up where I saw different areas like Darwin, Katherine, Kununurra, where I saw my people affected by grog, in the long grass. I never tasted it. Straight from school I was a health worker. A teacher and her partner worked in the health clinic and I learned from there how alcohol affect your life—I see people with domestic violence, family being sad. The club was operating while I grew up. In the 80s men would go up to the club and there was some violence, family around, break-in, smashing church window because of the last night [the night before]. Next morning a fight would be on. I saw that for 12 months or more and I felt sad and I joined AA, I wanted to learn from other men how it affected. I listened to them all. There were six or seven men in the group started by Brother Andy Howley and Freddie … I was only teenager. It started with two men sitting under a tree, talking about their life as a sober person.[21]

Membership of Makura Wunthay was made up of people drawn from across the many different clans at Wadeye. As was (and is) the case in many Aboriginal communities, there was a major split between the drinkers and the non-drinkers: Wadeye was polarised. As it grew, Makura Wunthay came to represent the only alternative (and wholly Indigenous) perspective on alcohol that could pose any kind of challenge to the dominance of the club committee, which was composed entirely of drinkers. Non-drinkers did not consider it appropriate to sit on the committee; for example, when

---

19   Makura Wunthay (Murrinh Patha language): *makura* = 'no water (beer)'; *wunthay* = 'restriction' ('don't drink' or 'good water').
20   The non-standard, vernacular style of Aboriginal English has not been edited or corrected throughout the book.
21   William Parmbuk, interview, 14 July 2009.

two committee members decided to stop drinking, they resigned from their positions. As a result, there were no non-drinking representatives on the committee.[22]

Social unrest and the club

Notwithstanding the efforts of the non-drinkers, the late 1980s saw increased alcohol consumption associated with the club and a build-up of social unrest. The club's licence was suspended on 26 occasions over a nine-year period—signalling what turned out to be a tumultuous history.[23]

Misbehaviour *at* the club was dealt with swiftly and according to the cultural guidelines established by the management committee; however, once the club closed at 7 pm, the committee's authority ended and its members had no desire to take responsibility for antisocial behaviour enacted beyond the club's boundary. This job fell to the two police officers stationed at Wadeye. The high incidence of crime at Wadeye was almost exclusively related to the consumption of alcohol at the club (Tangentyere Council 1991: 91, note 2). In July 1988, five months before the wrecking of the club, there was a fatal stabbing (both the perpetrator and victim had been drinking at the club and the victim was unarmed). The Supreme Court judge who presided over this manslaughter case characterised the community as being in a state of domestic conflict; he referred to clan conflict, general social upheaval, widespread aimlessness, drunkenness, unemployment and a lack of effective leadership and governance.[24] Hostilities were so strong after the stabbing that the perpetrator had to be flown out of Wadeye for his own safety.

There was increasingly vocal opposition to grog in the wake of this incident: Aboriginal residents recalled, 'we felt like its killing our people. A lot of medical evacuations then'; and, '[it's] killing our culture'. Several community members reported that, late in 1988, the community was 'on a knife edge'; 'things got worse and worse'. When the council tried to ban a number of young troublemakers from the club, their family

---

22 Xavier Desmarchelier, pers comm, 11 January 2013.
23 Colin McDonald, interview, ABC Radio 6 December 1989.
24 Angel J, Supreme Court of the Northern Territory, *The Queen v Phillip Daniel Berida*, 5 April 1990; see also Madigan 1988: 1.

members, instead of supporting such a ban in the interests of the community, confronted the council and demanded to know why their sons had been banned. In October, the *Northern Territory News* (1988) reported rioting at Wadeye: gunshots were fired in the main street and brawls took place involving 200 people. Police reinforcements were sent in and 12 men were arrested. The club was closed for a week. In the six months between July and December, monthly police returns showed that there were 56 arrests or summonses for offences at Wadeye (Legislative Assembly of the Northern Territory 1991: 167). People were afraid to venture out at night, as many youths were armed with knives; health workers were frightened to go to the clinic without an escort. At times, up to 30 women and children sought overnight refuge at the Presbytery and convent.[25] School attendance was low, and there were numerous break-ins and property damage to the school, clinic, store, private houses and vehicles. The unrest culminated in an act of unprecedented civil disobedience:

a group of young men broke the windows of the church.[26] This act served as the trigger, finally, for decisive community action.

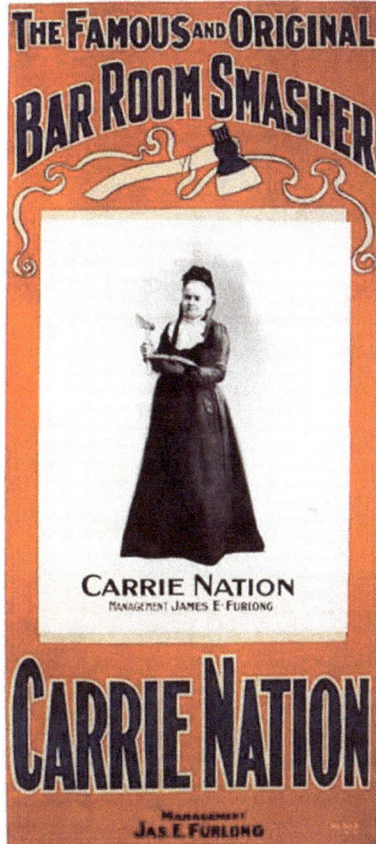

Fig. 14 Carrie Nation Lecture Poster, c. 1901
Source: Kansas State Historical Society

25 Xavier Desmarchelier, pers comm.
26 Several interviewees stated: 'There was trouble with drink! They knocked all the louvres out of the church!'; 'Young fellas smashed and stole cars, breaking windows in church'.

Smashing the club

On the afternoon of Saturday 3 December 1988—in a scene that rivalled the activities of the saloon-smashing activist, Carrie Nation, whose Anti-Saloon League campaigners 'hatcheted' bars and liquor stores in the United States[27]—a group of Aboriginal non-drinkers assembled outside the club, wielding axes and star pickets. They stormed onto the club premises and proceeded to demolish its interior. The Wadeye club smashers were led by Freddie Cumaiyi of the Rak Kubiyirr clan,[28] who wore a ceremonial red *naga*[29] and carried a shovel-nosed spear and a woomera. The group was soon joined by a large number of other participants who smashed the fittings and equipment inside the club, while 200 people reportedly stood outside cheering. The club's attackers asked the attending police to keep away while the destruction took place, and they agreed; no one was injured. It was an unprecedented, dramatic and well-orchestrated intervention.

In 2009, I collected accounts of the incident from many participants or observers who, while they agreed on the overall sequence of events, varied on some of the detail. William Parmbuk, aged 22 at the time of the attack, was one of the protagonists. He gave the following account:[30]

> In 1988 we destroyed the club. We had a meeting; at the meeting [were] seven men and some women. Old Freddie Cumaiyi—an ex-drinker and part of the AA group [said]: 'This thing's killing us, separating families, everyone sad'. We decided on Saturday afternoon, when the club open. We stopped in front of the club. I had a fighting stick. Club manager came to open the gate. I stopped him and said 'We're gonna bash your club'. He didn't believe! Inside my body was boiling anger, outside I was happy. Old Freddie [was] painted up, with a spear, wearing a red naga. He said, 'smash it!' I fired a 303 into the lock of the steel door and then we started to destroy whatever the club owned. We used axes. I had an axe as

---

27   In the early twentieth century, Carrie Nation famously carried a small axe (a hatchet) with which she and her followers smashed up liquor supplies and saloons in actions she called 'hatchetations'; they often stormed into bars singing hymns (Cook 2007). Nation was particularly outraged by the effect of drunkenness on women and children.

28   Freddie Cumaiyi (1926–89). The Rak Kubiyirr clan owns land adjoining the area of Wadeye.

29   *Naga* = loin cloth or waist cloth usually of red cotton. In the early twentieth century, a fabric known as 'turkey-red' was often distributed to Aboriginal people in payment for work (cf. Searcy [1909] 1984: 81).

30   Like Freddie Cumaiyi, William Parmbuk was not a member of the landowning clan. I interviewed Parmbuk and others at Wadeye in July 2009. He was then 43 years old and a member of NORFORCE (an Australian Army Reserve regiment engaged in surveillance and reconnaissance). He ran the army cadet unit.

well. I was saying 'I'm going to smash you'. I made a hundred holes in the club-owned boat! The police came and I stopped them. I said, 'We want to destroy this club—come back and arrest me later'. We destroyed everything: TV, boat, big TV screen, smashed VB cans with star picket. I drove a tractor! Big crowd came around. Word went round quick, then whole community got involved, helped to smash it. All the women and kids, young men.

The following accounts come from various Aboriginal community members:

Young fellas smashed and stole cars, breaking windows in church. They [other, non-drinkers] thought the problem might be coming from the club. So G with a 6.5 rifle shot the lock [of the club], smashed the fence with Hilux [Toyota]. Some women were involved. When they entered the club everyone stood back and the AA people came rushing in. Freddie had an axe and a shovel nose spear and a naga. The old man had got wild with drinkers who belt their wives and kids.[31]

I was there when Freddie smashed the club. I was still at home, but people were lining up for ticket [beer token]. That old man, Freddie, was in a red naga and a shovel spear. People had been drinking and getting violent. Men with tickets were already inside the club, they pulled back against the fence and everyone, kids and women too, everybody was there [attacking the club]. Freddie said [he was] feeling sorry for women and children, kids were hungry, women get family payment for food and husbands take that money for themselves, kids went to school hungry. Freddie spoke in language.[32]

There was trouble with drink, they knocked all the louvres out of the church. Old Freddie got wild. He got all the non-drinkers. I was still drinking [in 1988], I gave up early June 1989, but I was in there. I didn't see what was happening. In the afternoon we were waiting for 5 pm to open, soon as we got back we see big mob all round club. We thought it was fighting going on, but it was all getting beers. They knocked all the fence out. Nobody got angry; they helped themselves to beer. Opened the door where the beer locked in, got fence out, threw beer out.[33]

They had a meeting before all this [the wrecking of the club] to discuss it, because women wanted the non-drinkers to be safe. The club wasn't quite open; people were waiting to go in. Freddie [was] worried that women

31 RC, son of Freddie Cumaiyi.
32 SB, previously a Makura Wunthay worker.
33 AD, of Wentek Nganayi outstation.

were frightened of their husbands. Every night women get frightened of their husband. When we saw Freddie painted up, he was very angry, 'mad'. With rocks and axes they all smashed the cans. 'Come and get your last drink!' they called out. They drove a Hilux into the fence, and pulled the beer down.[34]

Non-Aboriginal residents also witnessed the event. One recalled:

I heard two shots of a rifle and blokes racing past. People flashing past! Straight to the club! The manager turned up and the non-drinkers said 'no, mate. We won't hurt you' ... George Cumaiyi fired the shots. They damaged the office, broke into the walls; there was a grader running around. It was a *community* statement.[35]

Leary's associate, Xavier Desmarchelier,[36] was also there that day. He remembered how:

After months of increasing violence, at about 4.30 pm on December 3 there was a shotgun blast that came from the club area. At that time such blasts were not unusual within the community however they normally occurred after club hours. I went down to the club. There were about 20 people outside the club fence. On the inside of the fence facing the club doors stood Freddie Cumaiyi in ceremonial attire—nagga, body paint and wommerra [sic]. Freddie was directing the group of people outside the fence who proceeded to break down the fence with chains, ropes and vehicles. Once inside the fence these people went to the main door of the club and smashed it open with crow bars and axes. Meanwhile a crowd outside the club was growing. I spoke with Freddie indicating that perhaps there was another way. He said: 'This is our way, this is the only way left to us' ... [T]he main door to the club had been smashed open and access to the coolrooms had been obtained. Cartons of beer were being brought outside where non-drinkers (men, women and children) broke open the cartons and begun smashing cans of beer on the concrete and against the brick wall. There was cheering from people outside the fence as cans were smashed ... However not only cartons of beer were targeted. Those inside the club began smashing the interior—pool tables, fans, chairs, counters etc. Nothing was left standing. Meanwhile outside the club members were focused on the cartons of beer that were being piled on the concrete. They

---

34 Group discussion with ND, GJ and JJ.
35 Mark Crocombe, historian at the Wadeye Knowledge Centre, 14 July 2009.
36 Xavier Desmarchelier, 11 January 2013. In 1988, Desmarchelier was helping Leary to establish an Indigenous leadership centre at Daly River; he now works with Jesuit Social Services.

entered the club and began breaking them open to drink. This was the beginning of the free for all and then the behaviour that has been referred to often as 'the riot'.

According to a Catholic Sister who was also there that day:

> They were sick and tired of trouble from grog, bringing in non-drinkers to the club who got grog. Once it closed, there was chaos and noise until midnight. The community was in a big split between drinkers and non-drinkers. The lead-up to the 1988 smashing was the clinic … and the church was perpetually getting smashed. The club had been badly managed. [On the day], the drinkers were at the club at 5 pm. The non-drinkers were having their AA group. 'We will smash everything' Freddie said, 'We won't hurt anyone'. They told the police they were going to do it.[37]

Dr Elizabeth Moore, District Medical Officer, recalled that: 'Freddie had said at a council meeting that "any more trouble at the club, we'll smash it down". And they did! Pushed fences, knocked out walls, poured out grog. They did $300,000 worth of damage'.[38]

Press reports were accompanied by sensational headlines: 'Aftermath of a rampage. Families flee riot' (Jackson 1988: 1); 'Port Keats in alcoholic turmoil'; 'Beer at centre of NT riot' (Cooke 1988: 1). However, all eyewitness accounts concur that it was a well-planned, premeditated action that involved no violence against people, only property; that the police were informed; and that key people peacefully gave themselves up to police afterwards. Desmarchelier stated that:

> As an eyewitness to the actual event the one word I would *not* use to describe [it] would be a riot. Freddie provided directions to his people as to what actions to do; they looked to Freddie for direction; at all times Freddie was in control of what was happening. No person was hurt. The target was the club premises and the beer.

Another commentator described the atmosphere as being like a midnight feast at boarding school, with people helping themselves to the cartons of beer liberated from the club. The 'free grog' was taken by drinkers to the community living areas and there was heavy drinking over the next few days; however, according to witnesses, there were no inter-group fights or injuries.

37   Catholic sister, Yvonne, 14 July 2009.
38   Dr Elizabeth Moore, District Medical Officer, 12 October 2009.

NORTHERN TERRITORY News

Phone 62 8200 DARWIN: Monday, December 5, 1988 40c*

Aftermath of a rampage

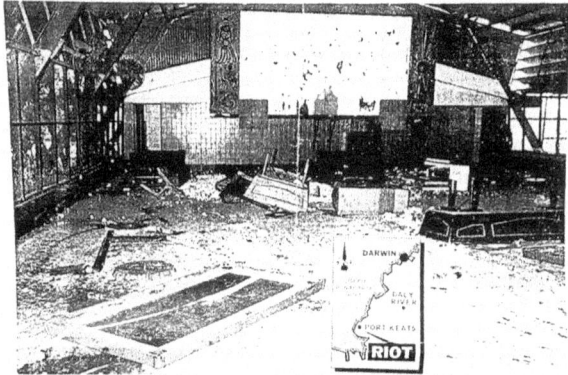

Overturned pool tables and other debris is strewn around the floor inside the Port Keats Club after the weekend riots.

FAMILIES FLEE RIOT

By PAUL JACKSON, GENNY O'LOUGHLIN and DEBBIE GRIMWADE

Police with batons are patrolling the remote settlement of Port Keats today after a weekend of rioting.

Five white women and 11 children were evacuated to Darwin yesterday.

Nearly 300 people were involved in the riots which began on Friday night after a man rampaged through the settlement smashing the church, hospital, police station and vehicles with rocks.

A woman at the township today said people had feared for their lives as the club was ransacked and people's homes were raided.

Damage to the club was said to total more than $100,000.

Police said the rioting had been quelled and the situation was quiet. ● Continued Page 3

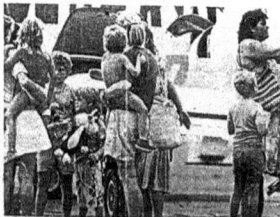

Women and children arrive at Darwin Airport after fleeing Port Keats. Picture: CHERYLYN CAINES

Fig. 15 'Aftermath of a rampage'

Source: *Northern Territory News* Monday 5 December 1988

The aftermath

A few days later, a group of 10 Aboriginal health workers at the local health centre clarified their position in relation to the wrecking of the club in two letters to the Liquor Commission. In the first letter, they explained why they supported the actions of the protestors:

To the NT Liquor Commissioner, 6/12/88

Dear Sir

Our reasons are

People causing trouble at our Health Centre

Always damaging our Hospital vehicles and windows

Childrens get sick from hunger because of the father and some mother's are spending money on grog. The childs 'Road to Health' chart always on the red line. Because there's not enough food.

When someone is hurt and taken down to the Health Centre, people come around here and starting getting mad at the Clinic and at the health workers, and swearing and all that. Every night they come around here for medicine when its not the right time.

Some mothers don't bring their babies at the right time, [but] wait for their husbands to come out of the club, and bring the sick baby to the clinic. And husband starts to get mad at us and cause of troubles. When they enter the clinic door husband starts to talk rough talk. So we the health workers [get frightened], shaking and droping everything. Sometimes we in a hurry we might give them wrong medicine and we might kill someone and get into big trouble. Drunk people write dirty words on our health centre and vehicles.

If the club reopens again we'll do the same thing again smash up everything, and that's our promise. Because of the grog lots of our people are getting sicker and sicker, high blood pressure, diabetes and liver damage.

Signed: Aboriginal health workers

Phillipine Parmbuk, Stephanie Berida, Annunciata Dartinga, Lillian Tcherna, Ethelreda Dartinga, Sabina Parmbuk, Philomena Crocombe, Therese Nemarluk, Agnes Tchemjairi, Lucia Ngarri.[39]

---

39 I have photocopies of these letters in my possession.

The health workers who signed the letter were all Aboriginal women with close connections to the Catholic nuns; they had been brought up in the dormitory system at the mission and had worked for many years in the old mission hospital. All became senior spokespersons in their groups as they grew older.[40] Disturbed by talk of reopening the club, the women wrote a further letter on 20 December. The second letter stated that, following the club's closure, illegal grog had been flown into one of the outstations and, as a result, a Wadeye truck had rolled, injuring eight people, two of whom had had to go to hospital. The women wrote:

> Some people say they want the club open at Port Keats because they don't want the men to go away to Darwin or Kununurra drinking because they might get killed. Well there has been more men killed at Port Keats from the grog than away from Port Keats … We think grog should be stopped forever. From the health workers at Port Keats.

Two of the club's attackers, William Parmbuk (aged 23) and Maurice Mullumbuk (aged 25), were charged with illegal entry and criminal damage. The case was heard in Darwin by Senior Magistrate Alistair McGregor in October 1989. Parmbuk and Mullumbuk were defended by solicitor Colin McDonald.[41] By then, Freddie Cumaiyi, the senior man who had led the action against the club had died. Freddie's son, George Cumaiyi, told the court that his father had warned the community: 'If the church, school and hospital keep getting damaged, then we will damage your place [the club]. That was the warning the old man made'.[42] The District Medical Officer gave evidence that health conditions, including alcohol-related injuries and child malnutrition, had improved significantly in the months since the club had closed. The magistrate drily observed that the social club at Wadeye could more accurately be described as the 'antisocial club', as it had contributed to a drastic deterioration in the quality of life at Wadeye, which now endured alcohol-related trauma and chronic bad health due to considerable and sustained high alcohol intake. McGregor heard evidence that the club took around $72,000 a month: money, he observed, that was probably derived from social security payments.

---

40   Three of the signatories were of the same clan (Rak Kubiyirr) as Freddie Cumaiyi (Bill Ivory, pers comm).
41   McDonald is now a QC.
42   The following quotations are drawn from transcripts of ABC radio broadcasts at the time (tape supplied by Colin McDonald and Jonathan Hunyor, 8 September 2010).

The magistrate dismissed the charges against Parmbuk and Mullumbuk. He dealt with the element of riot by stating that the men had right of entry to the premises, and found only the damages charge to be proved. McGregor had no doubt that both men were guilty of this offence, but he accepted that their motives were honourable. Rather than a case of violence, it was a case of restoring peace. Despite acknowledging the risk of precedent that might extend to other communities, McGregor ordered that no convictions be recorded and the men were released. This unprecedented decision provoked a welter of media coverage.[43] McDonald, Parmbuk and Mullumbuk's lawyer, told ABC radio that:

> It was a social revolution in the true sense of the word, however it was a disciplined revolution where the ground rules were no-one was to get hurt and in fact no-one was hurt. And it's interesting in this case that the two charges dealing with the element of riot were withdrawn because the Crown could not find, amongst 500 persons present, one person who was afraid. The evidence was that people were cheering and celebrating the destruction of this source of evil in their midst.[44]

Twenty years later, Parmbuk described the court hearing and the dismissal of the charges:

> I had a good lawyer, Colin McDonald. We had back-up from doctor, visiting doctor. In the magistrate [court] Alistair McGregor—I was a bit nervous—he said, 'Stand up William! William! You are like Rajiv Gandhi! I will accept what you have done for the sake of the community. I now drop this charge. You may go'. Before that he asked me: 'If the Club reopen again, would you do it again?' and I said 'Yes. It's not for me it's for the sake of the community'.

Perhaps inevitably, the closure of the club meant that those who wanted to drink alcohol, including some senior men, left Wadeye, sometimes for extended periods. One consequence of this was that council meetings no longer had the ratification of several key people. Another consequence was an increase in the number of intoxicated people on the road, which resulted in several deaths.[45] Unfortunately and coincidentally, the road from Wadeye to Daly River had been upgraded that year, meaning that

---

43   'Club wreckers who "saved people from alcohol" freed', *The Australian* 7 December 1989: 4; 'Port Keats: charges proved, no conviction', *Northern Territory News* 24 October 1989: 5; ABC Darwin radio news broadcasts December 1989.
44   ABC News Radio Darwin 6 December 1989.
45   However, as the second letter from the health workers stated, there had been deaths at Wadeye itself because of alcohol-related violence.

vehicles could travel faster than previously. Sly grogging increased as men grouped together to charter planes from Kununurra to fly alcohol into some of the outstations. 'Family money' was also depleted. These side effects of the club's closure naturally led to grumblings, with some in the community questioning Freddie Cumaiyi's 'right' to have brought about the club's demise.

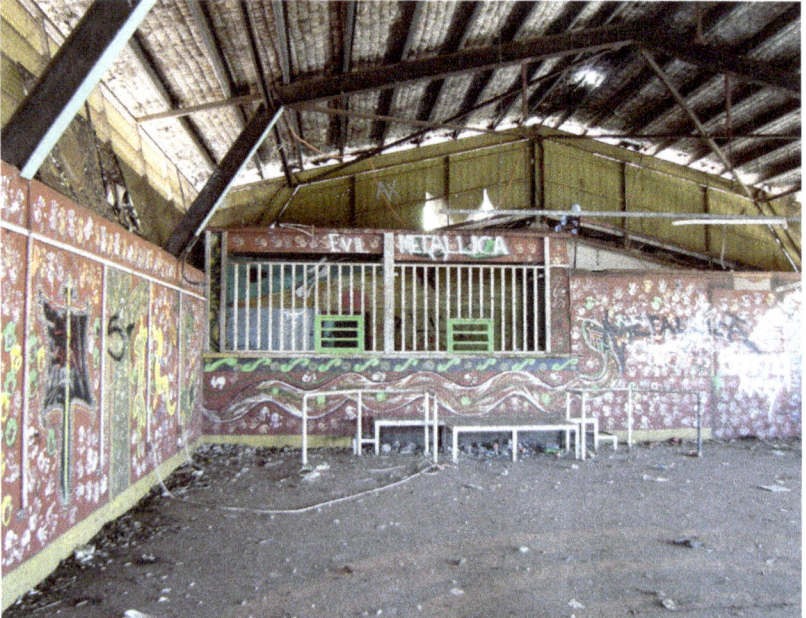

Fig. 16 Remains of the Murrinh Patha Social Club, 2009
Source: M Brady

Reopening the club

Only three days after the wrecking of the club, Liquor Commission representatives from Darwin visited Wadeye and held meetings with the community about whether the club should be reopened. Clearly, there was pressure to do so (as evidenced by the follow-up letter from the health workers): in fact, there was so much pressure that the secretary of the Northern Territory Department of Health and Community Services wrote to the Commission advising it to take a 'hands-off' approach—rather than continually asking the community when it wanted the licence to be recommenced (Tangentyere Council 1991: 93, note 5).

In the early 1990s, the club reopened and closed on several occasions. In March 1995, the reopened club was attacked, culminating in a large brawl; the Licensing Commission became involved and the club was closed and the manager sacked. In September 1995, Kardu Numida Council at Wadeye made a determined effort to reform the way the club operated. They approached the Liquor Commission to reopen it, this time under a new name: the Kardu Numida Social Club. Changing the name of the club was significant. Its former name, Murrinh Patha, represented only one of the many different language groups living at Wadeye and in the surrounding area, and other groups felt disenfranchised—'living in their shadow'. Renaming the club Kardu Numida, meaning 'one people', appealed those who sought unity in the community. A letter to the Liquor Commission, signed by the council's president and executive officer, laid out a new policy that contained a number of changes and a more formal code of discipline than previously.[46] The club committee was to be composed of members of the Kardu Numida Council, and the manager or licensee was to be employed by the council (rather than the club being a separate entity, as previously).

The council's plan for the 'new' club made no allusion to the notion of learning to drink in moderation, as had been the case in the 1970s. However, it did suggest that light beer should cost less at the club, to make it more attractive to drinkers, and that a proper cafe be opened, rather than a 'greasy spoon'. The council and elders stressed their intention to eradicate the 'sixpack clubs' that allowed chosen individuals to drink large numbers of cans. In terms of policing the club, the plan stated that council members and elders would take an active role, and that a group of respected persons from different tribal groups wearing armbands would police the discipline of members during trading hours. The proposal also explicitly addressed the issue of revenue from the sale of alcohol. Whereas in previous years, club profits had been ploughed back into the club itself, ignoring the interests of the 'large number of teetotal members of the community' and providing benefit only to its patrons (the drinking population), the council stated that under its new plan, the club would be valuable as a means of directing thousands of dollars into the local economy. Specifically, under the new policy, the council planned: 'to use

---

46   Letter to the Liquor Commission signed by the Kardu Numida Council executive officer (Boniface Perdjert, a senior member of the landowning Diminin clan) and president (Leon Melpi) reporting on a council meeting at Wadeye on 8 September 1995.

the earning power of all commercial ventures at Wadeye to construct an Olympic size swimming pool, upgrade housing and allocate funds to government initiated work training schemes'.

In September 1995, the Liquor Commission agreed that the club could reopen. It gave Aboriginal women at Wadeye 10 days to look at the new rules and make changes, if desired. Presumably they did not object, because a licence was issued to the newly incorporated Kardu Numida Social Club Ltd. that allowed for opening hours from 5 to 7 pm Monday to Friday, and from 4 to 7 pm on Saturday (or 8 pm, depending on the football season).[47] The licence specified that four 375 mL cans could be sold per person, and that any proposal to change the limit would require a full report on social behaviour. Purchasing on behalf of another person was prohibited. The licence listed the rules of behaviour that had been drawn up by the council, including that anyone apprehended for an alcohol-related offence in Wadeye would be automatically suspended from the club for six months; women were not allowed to buy beer during pregnancy and for three months after giving birth; and there was to be a women-only area, designed to prevent men from taking beer from their wives or girlfriends.

These strategies constituted a determined attempt by all involved to make the club into the sort of drinking environment originally envisaged by Leary and his co-authors in 1975. The proposal coincided with the Northern Territory's Living with Alcohol (LWA) program, an ambitious prevention and education scheme funded by a small levy on alcoholic beverages that (as its title suggests) stressed the need for Territorians to accept and manage alcohol with moderation. The LWA program offered to help at Wadeye by training club staff and by giving the council ideas on safe management of clubs, drawn from a handbook then in preparation (Hunter & Clarence 1996). The Northern Territory's Chief Minister, who took a personal interest in the program, and the program's director were both supportive of sensible drinking policies for Aboriginal social clubs.[48]

The optimism accompanying these planned safeguards to governance and social control was short-lived. As it turned out, the Kardu Numida Council collapsed around this time—a result of its inability to respond to

---

47   Licence Number 80801358, Kardu Numida Social Club Ltd., 21 September 1995, Nominee Stanley Robert Gibson.
48   Dr Shirley Hendy, pers comm , 13 August 2009.

the needs of the rapidly growing town (Desmarchelier 2001)—ushering in a long search for a more appropriate community governing structure. Soon after its rebranding and reopening in September 1995, the club closed again due to drunken brawls; customers had been receiving more than their four-can limit. In December, only three weeks after yet another reopening, young men broke into the club in the early hours of the morning and stole between 800 and 1,200 cartons of beer. A violent brawl erupted involving spears, boomerangs and firearms (Alcorn 1995): health clinic staff were evacuated and other community service providers were nervous. The chair of the Liquor Commission, John Maley, suspended the social club licence indefinitely and, despite sporadic calls for it to be reopened, the club remained closed.[49] Following this final closure, police reported a surge of public drunkenness in Darwin, which they attributed to Wadeye drinkers away from home.[50] In an extraordinary reaction to this development, the Assistant Commissioner of Police suggested that an Aboriginal licensed club should be developed in Darwin (Bane 1996).

Analysing the events

Numerous historical, social and cultural factors contributed to the difficulties faced by the people of Wadeye as they tried to inaugurate and sustain a social club that was based, ostensibly, on the idea of 'learning to drink' in a manageable way. 'Learning to drink' might have been the goal articulated by the Leary team, and by the Catholic brothers who applied for the licence, but it was not (necessarily) the goal of the bulk of Wadeye drinkers. Learning new ways to drink was always going to be challenging at Wadeye.

Social and demographic factors

The Port Keats–Wadeye region was known to be socially volatile. Although the Indigenous inhabitants had had friendly encounters with Macassan trepang fishermen in the eighteenth century (Hercus & Sutton 1986: 47), early European commentators, such as Alfred Searcy and WEH Stanner,

---

49   In April 1998, Wadeye council proposed yet another new liquor licence of some kind, a plan supported by the Liquor Commission registrar, David Rice. However, this never eventuated (*Northern Territory News* 1998).

50   It is difficult to establish the reliability of the claim that the 'surge' of public drunkenness in Darwin was caused by Wadeye people rather than drinkers from anywhere else.

described them as fearless, 'ferocious' and hostile to interlopers.[51] With six Indigenous language groups and 20 different clan estates in a region rich in natural food resources, battles and raids between the various language groups were not uncommon (Taylor 2004). The original Port Keats mission was founded in 1935. In 1939, it moved to Wadeye, a few kilometres away on the land of a Murrinh Patha-speaking people, the Yek Diminin. As happened elsewhere, the mission attracted Aboriginal people from a wide region, concentrating them, over a relatively short-time span (around 70 years), into one densely settled area. Although ceremonially allied, these groups had always been spatially dispersed.[52] Hence, relations between the different groups were often fraught. To lessen conflict and keep the peace, the first missionary introduced a rotation system in which only half the 'outside' groups could be in the community at any one time (Falkenberg 1962: 18). This demonstrates the extent to which Wadeye was, and still is, a complex community. Composed of a mixture of large and small clan groups, all of whom have affiliations requiring them to make compromises and to negotiate social arrangement and interactions with each other (Ivory 2009: 79), there were fractious social relationships to be managed at Wadeye long before the arrival of alcohol.

A dramatic expansion in the population complicated matters. There was a steady rise in population in the post-mission, self-management era. During the 1980s, there were an average of 50 births per annum. In 1985, when the community made its rather sudden transition from governance by the Catholic mission to self-management under the Kardu Numida Council, the population was estimated to be 1,156. By the mid-1990s, when the council collapsed, the population was estimated to be nearly 2,000 people (Taylor 2004). Not only had the population grown, but the ratio of young to old people had increased dramatically.[53] Stanner had warned of the implications of the growth of a youthful population for social disadvantage at Wadeye back in the 1960s; however, as John Taylor (2008: 217) observed, his prescient advice about increasing disadvantage went unheeded by government.

---

51 The coastal area is dotted with tamarind trees planted by these visitors from Sulawesi.
52 In 2010, Wadeye had an estimated population of up to 2,500 people (Taylor 2010: 3).
53 This shift to a youthful population has continued due to improvements in child survival, a high fertility rate and high adult mortality: around half the population is now aged less than 18 (Taylor 2010: 10).

This meant that, at the time of the last concerted effort to open a viable social club in 1995, the older generation in the community were confronted by a crisis of authority and leadership. As Taylor's (2004, 2010) work on the demography of the region has shown, the considerable population momentum and rise in the number of youths and young adults overwhelmed community institutions such as the Kardu Numida Council. The weakening of customary means of community control, usually enacted by senior men and women, further complicating the situation (Desmarchelier 2001). From around 1987 onwards, youth gangs, or 'mobs', who named themselves after heavy metal bands and adopted their iconography, proliferated at Wadeye (cf. Brady 1992, Mansfield 2013: 154).[54] These pressures, and the demographic imbalance between young and old, created two colliding forces: a burgeoning youth sub-culture that included young men whose behaviour was antisocial (e.g. smashing the church windows), and who frequented the club and were unresponsive to adult remonstrations; and older people, such as Freddie Cumaiyi, who were able to invoke the necessary authority to recruit and direct participants in the risky plan to wreck the club.

Legitimising intervention

It is neither common nor culturally acceptable for Aboriginal people (even senior people) to intervene as directly in the affairs of others as did Freddie Cumaiyi and his companions on the occasion of the club-wrecking. Numerous social scientists working in Aboriginal communities, including myself, have documented a distinct reluctance to interfere in other people's business, criticise their behaviour or attempt to persuade them to do something they do not wish to do—such as stop drinking or sniffing petrol (Myers 1979, Sansom 1980, Brady 1992, 2004). People resist being bossed around and have a strong sense of personal autonomy. The prevailing feeling, as David McKnight (2002: 206) observed, is that if someone wants to get drunk, they have the right to do so, and no one can stop them. This makes the action taken by Freddie Cumaiyi and the 'AA people' even more extraordinary.

---

54   At Wadeye, the upsurge in metal 'mobs' coincided with the arrival of television and broadcasts of the music video program *Rage* (Mansfield 2013).

Although he was a senior man, Cumaiyi was not a member of the Kardu Diminin clan that owned the land on which the community, and the club, was located.[55] Arguably, in orchestrating the wrecking of the club, he was acting beyond the limits of his authority. Therefore, he had to strategically demonstrate that his actions had legitimacy. There were several events that provided him with sufficient justification for his action, but these still had to be socially and culturally sanctioned and legitimised. Cumaiyi had repeatedly and publicly expressed anxiety about the safety of women and children in the community: these were incontestable concerns that provided him with a socially acceptable justification for the action that he and others took. Expressing concern about the health and safety of children, especially, was unchallengeable, even by the drinkers or those in opposition to Cumaiyi's position. It is significant that the health workers' letters to the Liquor Commission also focused primarily on the effect of drinking on children.

As mentioned, the breaking of the church windows by drunks seems to have been the decisive insult that provided the final trigger for action to be taken. The assault on the church building was both actual and symbolic: it constituted a physical assault on a building that had been constructed by community members and it also represented an attack on the (Catholic) spiritual practice and values that permeated the lives of the older generation. For these reasons, it was a critical incident. Coming after a downward spiral of violence, unrest and homicide, it provided Cumaiyi and the non-drinkers with a recognisable excuse for action. In attacking the club, Cumaiyi and the members of the alcohol awareness group were inspired by the 'tough love' they had learned about in meetings: they were literally performing tough love through their actions, which demonstrated that they would no longer play the role of 'enablers' or 'co-dependents' in their relationships with drinkers.

Further legitimising his right to intervene in other people's business in this way, Cumaiyi reminded onlookers that he was a ceremonial man: a senior Law man held in high regard for his ceremonial involvement. He deliberately arrayed his body with signifiers of seniority and ceremonial significance: he wore body paint and a red loincloth (the *naga*) and he carried traditional weapons. In short, he created a performance. At Wadeye, the red *naga* is worn primarily for men's ceremonies, although

---

55   However, Freddie's mother's country was located at a site called Wentek Nganayi, now an outstation, which was the location of the original Port Keats mission in 1935.

it is also worn at public dance performances.[56] Some observers recalled that Cumaiyi carried an axe and a woomera—the latter signified that he was a senior leader of a clan group. Significantly, the main weapon he carried was a shovel-nosed spear. The shovel spear, as opposed to the lighter, three-pronged 'wire' spear, is a serious weapon. Sometimes as 'much as ten feet long', it was the main hunting and fighting weapon:

> It is bamboo-shafted and has a lanceolate blade laboriously rubbed down from iron fence-droppers or heavy-gauge roofing … its efficacy is a function of the strength of the thrower's arm, aided of course by his skill. (Stanner 1979: 75)

It was the spear with which Wadeye people had settled their differences in the past, and it still carries authority today. In wielding this spear, Cumaiyi effectively communicated his intention to fight, or at least to make a very strong statement. The spear demonstrated that he meant business.

The wrecking of the club showed that the community had reached a tipping point. The behaviour of young men had pushed others in the population beyond their customary level of tolerance. Like many other Aboriginal communities with alcohol in their midst, Wadeye residents had long tolerated high levels of disruption, sleeplessness, violence and abuse, dealing with it through unconfrontational and indirect means. Thus, intra- and inter-community factors (which included the long history of disparate and fractious groups, the rapid population rise, the number of young people and their unrestrained behaviour, and the fragile local government) contributed to the decline in standards at the club and to high levels of social unrest and fearfulness in the community.

Management and regulation issues

Apart from social volatility, there were other, proximate influences on the club's fortunes and stability that led to its demise, such as the quality of various managers. In conversations about the club, Wadeye people often referred to the role of club managers; many volunteered the names of managers who they thought did a 'good job' as opposed to poor managers who put profits before people—'more grog, more profit'. The wrecking of the club in 1988 occurred during the time of a profit-oriented manager.

---

56 The red *naga*, or loincloth, is worn by Aboriginal people in many top end NT communities for ceremonial and public dance performances. The term '*naga*' was documented in 1879 as being the Woolner language term for 'clothing, covering'.

In 1995, at the time of the attempted rearrangement of the club's governance structure, several interviewees recalled a well-liked manager, referred to here as 'GD':

> [We] had pool tables when it was GD. He used to make sure boys only came once for their 4 cans. GD was best manager, he made a stage for band, had funds to go to the church and school, he helped them. When I used to work for GD, if people tried to get a second round, it wasn't fair, they would ban them and put their name on the board. There was a committee [the speaker was a member] met every fortnight to see how much money in there, how much they paid for barge [bringing supplies]. [It was] his own idea. He reckon, 'it's all your money, from the people'.

Other than undertaking the necessary checks required under the Liquor Act to ensure that a candidate was a 'fit and proper person' for the job, it seems that neither the Liquor Commission nor any other agency assisted the community to hire appropriate managers by advising them of the qualities to look for. The job of managing the club at Wadeye—indeed, managing any club in a remote Aboriginal community—arguably required much more than simply being a fit and proper person.

Clubs in Aboriginal communities are unusually demanding liquor licences to manage. They are often located in geographically isolated areas, which makes normal monitoring and inspections by authorised bodies more difficult. Wadeye is situated on the edge of coastal mangroves, 320 km southwest of Darwin, and is accessible by rough roads for only six months of the year. The club manager at Wadeye had to navigate competing pressures and interest groups within the community, and liaise with the local Aboriginal council (his employers) and the management committee of the club, while dealing firmly with a highly contentious and volatile commodity: alcohol. Making decisions about the revenue from alcohol sales, including the extent to which revenue could be sacrificed to minimise alcohol-related harms—matters that required a high degree of integrity and nerve—gave the club manager considerable power and influence. Liquor Commission policy and outreach did not extend to giving 'troubleshooting' advice on how to negotiate these local, social and cultural aspects of licensing in an Aboriginal setting. As far as the day-to-day matters of club management and operation went, the community was on its own. It did not always choose wisely.

Regulation issues were the responsibility of the Territory's Liquor Commission. The fact that a significant segment of the community had to resort to 'self-help' to deal with the club, reflected badly on the Commission.[57] Despite the accumulation of warning signs at Wadeye (i.e. violence, social unrest, homicide and the selection of inappropriate club managers), in the years and months prior to the wrecking, the only strategy brought to bear by the Liquor Commission was the relatively crude mechanism of closing the club, which it did periodically. According to Tangentyere Council (1991), the actions of the Liquor Commission revealed its 'indifference to the community's alcohol problems'. With its narrow concentration on administrative detail, the Liquor Commission represented a 'regime that was really remote from the lives of [the] people' (91, 94). Media representatives covering the Darwin court hearings in 1989 asked pointed questions about the Liquor Commission's role in the decline in standards at the Wadeye club, suggesting that the court case would bring 'new attention' to the Commission. One reporter asked McDonald whether he thought the Commission had been 'a little bit too easy going in keeping the Wadeye licence going?'[58] The solicitor replied that, while it was easy to criticise the Liquor Commission, it faced a huge problem:

> Over nine years there were 26 suspensions of the licence. And in that time a person's hoped that things would get better. The track record is that it didn't. There were homicides, there were brawls, huge ugly and violent incidents. Finally, a large group of people said we've had enough, we can't take this anymore and took it upon themselves to close the club peaceably but effectively and I think the Liquor Commission really has got to think, 'now what do we do? Is the social evil caused by this club so great that we should contemplate a different course, or simply as the people said, we want the club closed down for ever?'

Throughout much of the period in question, the relationship between the Liquor Commission and Aboriginal communities (in general) was characterised by a 'lack of effective communication and ongoing consultation' (Race Discrimination Commissioner 1995: 54). In the years between 1986 and 1989, the Commission made numerous controversial

---

57   After the trial of the club wreckers, one of the acquitted men urged other communities to follow their example and destroy their drinking clubs, implying that the situation in other communities' licensed outlets was also less than ideal (transcripts of ABC radio broadcasts 6 December 1989, Tangentyere Council 1991: 92).

58   ABC News Radio Darwin 6 December 1989. Transcribed from taped interviews provided by Colin McDonald and Jonathan Hunyor.

decisions that were perceived as unduly favourable to the liquor industry (Race Discrimination Commissioner 1995: 49).[59] Adding to its poor image, the chair of the Liquor Commission resisted suggestions that there should be greater Aboriginal representation on the Commission (Race Discrimination Commissioner 1995: 51).[60]

Apart from highlighting the inadequate responses of the Liquor Commission, the rise and fall of the Murrinh Patha Social Club provides some salutary lessons for the well-meaning Catholic fathers, brothers and nuns of the Mission of the Sacred Heart at Wadeye, as well as for the various branches of government dealing with health, alcohol management and liquor regulation. The history of the club demonstrates that good intentions and agreed upon rules of behaviour are not enough to influence what happens outside club hours and beyond club boundaries, especially in a fractious community in which interpersonal violence has become normalised, and community members have limited powers of persuasion over the behaviour of fellow residents.

Grassroots activism

Notwithstanding a culturally embedded ethic of non-interference in, and tolerance of, other people's activities and freedoms, an accumulation of traumatic incidents or 'spark factors' may serve as a catalyst, pushing people beyond their limits (May et al. 1993, Edwards et al. 2000). The orchestrated attack on the club at Wadeye is a vivid example.

The incident happened at the beginning of series of community mobilisations—mostly led by Aboriginal women—that took the form of public demonstrations outside liquor outlets, petitions and marches against grog. Beginning in the late 1980s as a truly grassroots movement, and gathering momentum in the 1990s, Aboriginal community

---

59 Controversial decisions under Liquor Commission Chair KG Rae included the granting of a bottle shop licence to the Gap Hotel in Alice Springs in 1986, despite numerous objections from the community; in 1989, the Commission renewed the Curtin Springs takeaway licence (near Uluru), in the face of a barrage of objections. The hearing was later the subject of a Northern Territory Supreme Court appeal, after which the Commission's decision was reviewed (Race Discrimination Commissioner 1995: 45, note 181). In March 1989, the Commission, under Rae, granted a takeaway licence for Erldunda roadhouse, despite evidence from numerous witnesses of the enormous alcohol-related problems faced by Aboriginal communities in that region of central Australia (*Centralian Advocate* 23 March 1989).

60 Tangentyere Council suggested that the Liquor Commission should appoint one person with Aboriginal health expertise and have some Aboriginal advisory committees (Westman 1989).

activism around alcohol abuse can be likened to an Aboriginal women's temperance movement (see Chapter 5 for a fuller discussion). Women's participation in the attack on the Murrinh Patha Club served to embolden Aboriginal women elsewhere. On Bathurst (one of the Tiwi Islands), Aboriginal women began to agitate against drunken behaviour in December 1988. At the request of the mother's club there and the Nguiu Council, the Liquor Commission cancelled all personal permits to possess alcohol on Bathurst Island, making it illegal to drink anywhere other than at the Nguiu Club (O'Loughlin 1988). When it became apparent that this strategy was not working, Aboriginal women on Bathurst Island threatened to close down the club, citing 'big trouble' there, fighting, drunkenness and the continued service of intoxicated people (Bonner 1989: 3). Bathurst Island and Wadeye shared close associations and communication networks: both were (former) Catholic missions and Aboriginal residents and Catholic brothers frequently moved between the two locations.[61] The diffusion of direct action ideas against drinkers was, therefore, not surprising.

Eighteen months after the Wadeye club attack, in July 1990, several hundred women from Pitjantjatjara communities on the South Australia – Northern Territory border, marched on a remote roadhouse at Curtin Springs, made speeches in opposition to its liquor licence and presented a letter to the Liquor Commission calling for restrictions on sales of takeaway alcohol. Their activism continued for several years until restrictions were eventually achieved. The three Aboriginal women leading the action were aware of what had happened at Wadeye, and were inspired by the active role taken by female health workers and members of the AA group there.[62] In March 1993, Aboriginal women from Hermannsburg travelled to Alice Springs to demonstrate against the granting of a liquor licence at a delicatessen. This relatively small action was followed by a highly publicised and much bigger 'march against grog' in Alice Springs, which involved hundreds of Aboriginal men, women and children from five remote communities (*Northern Territory News* 1993: 6, Brady 2004: 84). Like Freddie Cumaiyi, these women expressed fears about the future of their children and grandchildren, thereby deploying culturally acceptable reasons to justify their interventionist stance. These events are explored more fully in the next chapter.

61 Brother Howley and Father Leary spent time at both missions.
62 These leaders were Tjikalyi Colin, Nora Ward and Mantatjara Wilson (Maggie Kavanagh, pers comm, 26 September 2014).

The ruins of the Murrinh Patha Social Club still stand today, inscribed with identifying tags and graffiti of the different gangs that are prevalent in the community, primarily the Judas Priests and the Evil Warriors. Many Wadeye residents travel to the club at Peppimenarti to drink: others travel further afield to obtain grog; some drinkers have road accidents, and some die as a result. People at Wadeye continue to debate whether to have a club again. In 2009, one of Freddie Cumaiyi's descendants observed:

> Don't reckon we'll have a club again. Lot of trouble. It's better this way. Young boys—trouble. Bonnie [Boniface Perdjert] was talking about getting the club back but we said 'no club'. [We] might as well just go to Darwin.

5

The rise and fall of the Tyeweretye Club: A case study

While most of the lobbying, political and otherwise, for Aboriginal people to have their own licensed canteens or clubs envisaged facilities in remote bush communities—'out of sight, out of mind'—some people proposed town-based social clubs designed for, and owned by, Aboriginal people. One was the Woden Town Club in Canberra, which catered largely for Aboriginal public servants (see Chapter 6). Another was the Tyeweretye Club, a licensed premise south of Alice Springs that opened in 1993 and closed in 2005. '*Tyeweretye*' in Western Arrernte means 'people being together'.[1] The Tyeweretye Club polarised opinion in the town and beyond, affecting Aboriginal groups, their representative bodies, the Northern Territory Government and the Liquor Commission. Arguments for and against its explicit strategy of 'teaching' moderate drinking lasted for more than a decade.

Lobbying for a club in Alice Springs

The idea for an Aboriginal club in Alice Springs was first floated in 1975 by Aboriginal men who were interviewed as part of a study of alcohol use sponsored by the Regional Council for Social Development. The report's title, *40 gallons a head,* referred to the author, Liz Wauchope's (1975)

---

1   *Tyeweretye* = 'getting together' or 'people being together'. This information comes from Betty Pearce, then a key member of Tangentyere Council (pers comm, 8 August 2008).

estimate that the population of the southern region of the Northern Territory consumed 40.9 gal of beer, per person, every year—almost twice as much as any other heavy-drinking community for which data were available (3). Wauchope made this estimate before it became possible to calculate alcohol consumption using the percentage of pure alcohol in drinks.[2] Questionnaires were circulated to residents of Alice Springs, and 300 randomly selected households were interviewed with the help of a young Aboriginal field officer from the Aboriginal Medical Centre, Geoffrey Shaw.[3] At the time, there were approximately 20 Aboriginal 'fringe camps' on the outskirts of town, with people living in shanties, tents and humpies; 30 of these residents were also interviewed for the study—mostly young Aboriginal men, all of whom were drinkers. The young men spoke of the social pressures to drink, their personal problems, bad living conditions and the fact that they had no viable employment or entertainment as alternatives to drinking; they were especially concerned about the drinking of methylated spirits in the camps. They thought they should have better living conditions and, perhaps surprisingly, they believed that there should be fewer liquor outlets and more control over sales. Asked what would help them to stop or better control their drinking (all but one said they wished to do this), Wauchope noted that:

> Most replied that *there is a need for an Aboriginal club with pleasant facilities* where they can be among friends in a relaxed environment. Opinion was divided as to whether this should be licensed or not. Most believed that meaningful employment, particularly out bush, would lessen alcohol consumption. (14, emphasis added)

The following year, the HRSCAA was asked by the Minister for Aboriginal Affairs, Ian Viner, to examine the effect of alcohol on Aboriginal communities. Chaired by Philip Ruddock, the HRSCAA conducted hearings throughout the country in 1976 and 1977, and received submissions from interested parties. The Central Australian Aboriginal Congress (CAAC), a new community-controlled health service based in Alice Springs, sent in a lengthy and detailed submission. Written by its senior medical officer, Dr Trevor Cutter, the CAAC's (1976) submission also raised the issue of a social club:

---

2   The Regional Council for Social Development was chaired by Mr EA Robertson, Labor Senator for the Northern Territory, 1975–87. The study was prompted by community concerns over alcohol abuse and the decriminalisation of public drunkenness: as of 21 October 1975, intoxicated people could be taken into protective custody without charge.
3   Twenty years later, Geoff Shaw became the general manager of Tangentyere Council, representing Aboriginal residents of Alice Springs.

One of the most urgent needs within Alice Springs is the development of an effective and social club where Aboriginal People can meet and socialize utilizing alcohol as a social cohesive factor rather than an obstructive one. At present, Aboriginal People are forced to use one Hotel in Alice Springs (the Alice Springs Hotel); this is the only hotel which provides a service to tribal Aboriginal people. Other Hotels due to mainly dress regulations provides alcohol only to whites and urban Aboriginal People. This social club could be effectively developed linking to the Football and other sporting bodies which could provide meals and family activities. *It would develop an important educative role* and provide some cohesion to the Aboriginal communities … Whites generally are fully housed, live within urban Alice Springs and Tennant Creek, have motor vehicles and have a large number of clubs and hotels that they can drink within. Aboriginal People having only one Hotel[4] and the river bed and having to come to town to drink. (1196–97, emphasis added)

At that time in Alice Springs, there were 51 licensed outlets: 17 stores, which included supermarkets, 16 restaurants or private hotels, seven clubs, eight liquor merchants and three public hotels (Wauchope 1975: 3). Notwithstanding the number of licensed outlets, it was a time when Aboriginal people were often served from 'dog windows' at the rear of premises (Commonwealth of Australia 1977, Hansard, 4 June 1976: 1289). Aboriginal people were excluded from many on-licensed premises by dress regulations: 'the blacker your skin the tidier you have to be', one Aboriginal man explained (Harold Furber, cited in Simmons 1988: 6). This restricted access to on-licensed premises was one cause of the uncontrolled consumption of takeaway alcohol, which was increasingly accessible in hotel bottle shops and supermarkets.

Nothing came of these early suggestions for a town club until the 1980s, when another Aboriginal organisation, Tangentyere Council, began to push for the establishment of such a facility. With responsibility for, and representation from, residents of the town camps, Tangentyere took the initiative on a growing public drinking problem in Alice Springs by commissioning several research reports. By the early 1980s, Alice Springs was becoming something of a tourist town, and keeping drunks away from the public eye was an ongoing concern of the civic authorities. Despite the advent of the Northern Territory's 'Two Kilometre Law' in 1982, which

---

4   There was also the Riverside Hotel, licensed in 1959 (now known as the Todd Tavern). It had a bar, known as the 'Snake pit', which was gradually abandoned by non-Aboriginal drinkers, and became predominantly an Aboriginal bar. The licensee eventually took all the furniture away because the chairs were used in fights (Brady fieldnotes).

made public drinking illegal within 2 km of a licensed establishment, unconstrained drinking in the open, and in the town camps, was a significant problem. The law was a clever government strategy designed to covertly target Aboriginal drinking by imposing spatial, rather than racial, constraints (d'Abbs 2012). One researcher counted 17 open-air drinking spots around Alice Springs, excluding the riverbeds; in a single weekend, over 180 Aboriginal people used the dry Todd River for social drinking (Simmons 1988: 7). The Two Kilometre Law drove Aboriginal drinkers into the town camps, causing 'severe repercussions' (Buckell 1986: 9) for the residents there. The law provoked an 'unprecedented period of violence' (O'Connor 1983: 8), as non-drinkers now had to deal with increased numbers of drunks and associated problems of domestic violence. Bill Ferguson, a non-Aboriginal man who was a town camp resident and who later became the manager of the Tyeweretye Club, witnessed the poverty and drunkenness provoked by the Two Kilometre Law. He recalled that violence in the camps was 'terrible, houses would be knocked down as quick as built, women bashed. No-one was game to go to the camps'.[5]

In 1983, Tangentyere Council convened a subcommittee to oppose the Two Kilometre Law, which grew into the Tangentyere Liquor Committee, a grassroots planning hub on alcohol issues in Alice Springs and the town camps.[6] The Liquor Committee[7] concentrated its efforts on two strategies: it opposed applications for new takeaway liquor licences, especially those associated with food outlets and shops (Lyon 1990), and took up the idea of having Aboriginal-controlled venues for drinking. As Buckell (1986: 9) observed:

> Drinking was not going to disappear, and the establishment of many strong Aboriginal organisations in town during the 1970s ... had given people an opportunity to organise. These organisations also encouraged a sense too, perhaps for the first time in living memory, of something to fight for in the battle against grog abuse.

---

5   Bill Ferguson, pers comm, 6 August 2008.
6   Tangentyere Council supported grassroots initiatives such as 'Grog Forums', local alcohol workers, an alcohol planning unit and a Social Behaviour Project designed to improve rules of behaviour for visitors to town camps.
7   The Tangentyere Liquor Committee had representatives from each of the town camps and included Eli Rabuntja (Chairman of Tangentyere Council), Doug Abbott (President of Congress), Tony Booth, Doug Walker, Bill Ferguson and Sue Craig.

The Tangentyere Liquor Committee's main concern was the absence of:

> Retail bar outlets at which [Aboriginal people] can drink legally and harmoniously in Alice Springs … Aboriginal people are not accepted in hotels or the clubs in town and therefore everything possible should be done to give them facilities where they can socialise together in an environment that they can control. (Hungerfords 1986: 4)

In 1986, the Stuart Arms Hotel was demolished to make way for a shopping complex, depriving Aboriginal drinkers of a popular drinking spot; its corner bar was affectionately nicknamed the 'burri bar'[8] (Buckell 1986). Tangentyere Council used the occasion to publicise its concern that, without controlled drinking venues, there was little hope of making inroads into alcohol abuse. Aboriginal social clubs, they said, 'would be places not only for drinkers, but for all the family, with wet and dry bars, recreation facilities, health, transport and social support services' (Ferguson 1986: 9). The Liquor Committee proposed the establishment of Aboriginal-controlled social clubs 'where "safe" drinking patterns can be developed and modelled for younger people' (Simmons 1988: 18, Coughlan 1991). The proposal was designed to create 'healthier, socially acceptable drinking patterns in the Aboriginal community' (Tangentyere Council 1991: 95). Tangentyere Council became the driving force behind what was to be a long struggle to establish an urban Aboriginal club. The process coincided with widespread polarised debate in the Northern Territory about alcohol and Aboriginal people, and the emergence of a grassroots anti-grog movement.

Plans and consultations

With the help of academic researchers, Tangentyere Council used clinical research literature on 'social learning' and 'controlled drinking' to support its case, much as the research team led by John Leary had done in 1975 (Leary et al. 1975: 27) (see Chapter 4). While acknowledging that there were problems in using clubs as a means of educating people into better drinking styles, Tangentyere Council (1991: 95) cited behavioural research on changing dependent drinkers into social drinkers. One of the references they cited questioned earlier positive findings that alcoholics had learned to engage in moderate or controlled drinking (Pendery et al.

---

8   *Burri* = 'brother' or 'friend'.

1982), and while most of the studies reported on behaviour modification during treatment, none demonstrated that a licensed venue could bring about lasting change to drinking styles. However, Tangentyere Council argued a subtler point: that Aboriginal ownership and control of the outlet would, in itself, change people's drinking behaviour. They explained:

> We are expected to drink it and we are expected to die from it, but we are not expected to have agency in it. I am not advocating the wholesale selling of alcohol to Aboriginal people by Aboriginal people, but that is what is happening from the broader community and we do not have any agency whatsoever in the liquor side of things. I think what I am saying is that we need agency. Having agency, we can bring about control … Learning to associate alcohol with food is something that has never been tried. Learning to use alcohol in an environment in which you own and control it or it is owned and controlled by other Aboriginal people is something that has never been tried. (Tilmouth 2001: 436)

Geoff Shaw, general manager of Tangentyere Council for over 20 years, framed owning the club in political terms: 'The Club is about Aboriginals making their own way through life, it's for people to find comfort drinking with their own people. Self determination requires self management' (Northern Territory Liquor Commission 1997: 12).

The original (optimistic and over-complicated) plan was for four licensed clubs located in different parts of Alice Springs (north, south, east and west) that would cater to different language or social groups (i.e. Pitjantjatjara, eastern and western Arrernte and Warlpiri). Initially, two clubs were to be built (the North Club and the South Club), to be followed by two more at a later stage. With this in mind, the official name of the incorporated body was 'Tyweretye Clubs', and its constitution stated that it aimed to establish, operate and maintain 'licensed social clubs at which Aboriginal people may consume alcohol in a controlled environment'. The organisation was 'always of the opinion that there should be more than one club in and around Alice Springs' (Ferguson 2003: 88). One prominent Aboriginal woman stated:

> We decided the best thing was for four clubs, east, west, north and south. So that people would have ownership. If [it's] not ours, [there's] no respect. The east and northeast mob didn't get on with the Warlpiri mob.

An Aboriginal man reiterated this, stressing that when people drink they like to choose their drinking companions:

> North side people, you can't even come through the Gap![9] Couldn't even trust to come through the Gap! People would think '[I will] stay here, where I can look after myself'. You get the feel of the town, the feel of the grog, so you stay here, drink with mates, stay with their [own] crew, can't go somewhere else. (Tony Booth, pers comm, May 2009)

Reinforcing the desire for more than one club as a way of minimising trouble, several local people (Aboriginal and non-Aboriginal) spoke about changes to hotels in the town in the 1970s and 1980s, which they felt had exacerbated conflict within the Aboriginal community. Hotels in Alice Springs had been, in some respects, more welcoming to Aboriginal people back in the 1960s: in those days, there were lax dress requirements, larger bars, beer gardens and 'plenty room' to move around; Aboriginal people could reconnoitre, see who was there and whether there were people to avoid. Tony Booth, an Aboriginal man who worked at the Central Australian Aboriginal Alcohol Planning Unit (CAAAPU), recalled:

> When they started off in '64 [when drinking rights came in] they [Aboriginal people] had a pub, big rooms, food, plenty room. Pub had a beer garden too. Them two, Stuart and 'Underdowns' [The Hotel Alice] they had a beer garden.[10] Stuart Arms had different saloon bars. Not many people in pub then, 10 here, 10 there, different mob, moving around, changing round the pub. Now it's closed in. You might not want to meet up with someone [you could choose where you drank and who with in those early days compared with now].

While proposing four clubs 'raised the eyebrows of bureaucrats' (Buckell 1986: 9), some commentators stated, candidly, that the idea 'was to have four clubs where different language groups could go without running into each other' (Tilmouth 2001):

> The Clubs must reflect traditional Aboriginal identity, and provide suitable places for the separate language groups … They must firstly attract drinkers who are in the creek beds and on the camps, and secondly encourage them to seek alternatives to binge drinking. The Liquor Committee believes this can only happen if the structure and organisation of the Clubs reflects and supports traditional systems of authority. (Buckell 1986: 9)

---

9   Heavitree Gap is known as the entrance to Alice Springs from the south; it is named after a gap in the McDonnell Ranges. It is an Arrernte site.
10   The Hotel Alice had a big square yard at the back dubbed 'Madison Square Gardens' because of all the fights that took place there (Dick Kimber, pers comm, 1 August 2008).

The Liquor Committee consulted widely. It hired accounting firm KMG Hungerfords to prepare an operational and financial proposal for the clubs. KMG, which had its own club and hotel management services unit, advised Tangentyere Council on the staffing levels and costs involved in training Aboriginal staff in hospitality, literacy and numeracy, and provided advice on issues of alcohol abuse and rehabilitation.[11] KMG staff spent a week in Alice Springs meeting with Tangentyere Council representatives and assessing the financial viability of the clubs. Based on the population of Aboriginal people in Alice Springs and surrounds, they estimated that approximately 1650 people would use the clubs on a regular basis. The consultants estimated (over optimistically, as it turned out) that a pricing structure like that of other clubs would yield a 45 per cent gross profit.[12] They also estimated that income from poker machines could be in the vicinity of $72,000 per annum.[13] Overall, their report was positive. They concluded:

> Based on a suitable level of support from funding bodies, a continuation of the energetic support and initiatives from senior members of the Aboriginal community, and an acceptance by the general body of local Aboriginal people, the clubs: should be largely self-funding; and will provide a tangible opportunity for the community to address several social difficulties in a sensible concerned manner. (Hungerfords 1986: 18)

Tangentyere Council approached potential funding bodies, interested government agencies, the police and the Alice Springs Town Council (Buckell 1986), and received support from influential bodies including the DAA, the ADC and the Northern Territory Department of Community Development. A Northern Territory Legislative Assembly (1991) inquiry into the use and abuse of alcohol was supportive, as was the Northern Territory Government's LWA program. Initiated in 1991, LWA was a progressive and bold public health strategy directed at reducing alcohol-related harm in the Northern Territory; it was personally supported by the Northern Territory Chief Minister, and answered directly to him.[14]

---

11 This was to be provided by the Gillen House School of Tourism and Hospitality, part of the Central Australian Community College.
12 The KMG report priced drinks at other clubs in Alice Springs, such as the Verdi Club and sporting clubs, and it listed the membership fees charged by other clubs in Alice Springs at the time.
13 The inclusion of poker machines in the club appears to have been uncontested at this time.
14 LWA was originally funded through a levy on alcohol products containing more than 3 per cent alcohol, which raised millions of dollars. However, in 1997, the High Court disallowed the states and territories from raising revenue in such a manner and the LWA program had to develop alternative funding mechanisms. LWA has since lapsed (National Drug Research Institute and Lewin Fordham Group 1999).

LWA focused on changing drinking styles—reining in and transforming the big-drinking Territory culture to a less damaging drinking style: the Tyweretye Club fitted with this aim. Chief Minister Marshall Perron and Dr Shirley Hendy, Director of LWA, offered in-principle support for Aboriginal social clubs, provided their conditions benefited communities.[15] Both sides of politics supported the Tyeweretye Club.[16] The deputy commissioner of police and the Aboriginal health service in Alice Springs were also supportive, as were several prominent Aboriginal people including, Geoff Shaw, Lutheran pastor Eli Rubuntja, Pat Turner and Betty Pearce. Charles Perkins, an advocate of Aboriginal-owned licensed clubs, gave early assistance to the Tangentyere Liquor Committee in the form of a DAA grant to help with consultations.[17]

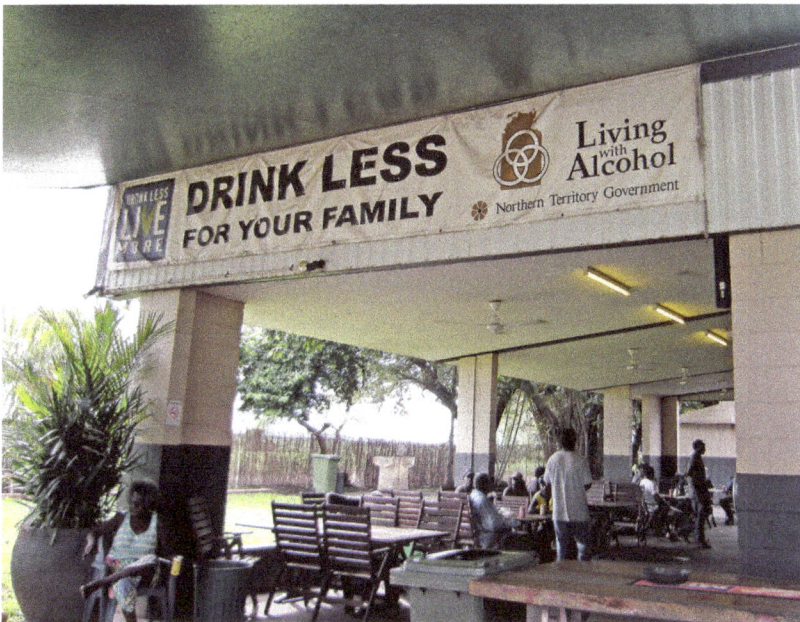

Fig. 17 'Drink Less for Your Family', Living with Alcohol banner
Source: M Brady

15   Dr Shirley Hendy, pers comm, 13 August 2009.
16   On the Labor side, local members Neil Bell, Peter Toyne and Brian Ede were supportive, as was Dr Richard Lim, the CLP member for the electorate of Greatorex, which is where the club was eventually located.
17   Brady fieldnotes, Bill Ferguson, pers comm, 6 August 2008.

However, the harm-reduction model was unpopular among advocates of abstinence, such as Aboriginal sobriety groups, supporters of AA and some Aboriginal women's groups. Believers in abstinence usually reject the notion that 'alcoholics' can ever learn to drink in moderation (cf. Brady 2004: 69–73), and some opposition to the club was ferocious. Unusually, the Liquor Commission,[18] then chaired by Kelvin Rae, was opposed to the club. Prominent Aboriginal ATSIC commissioner Alison Hunt also spoke out against the club, as did Alison Anderson, chair of Papunya Council, and Aboriginal actor and activist Rosalie Kunoth-Monks. Some Aboriginal women from town camps on the south side of town also objected. The Alice Springs Town Council was against the club.[19] By far the most organised opposition to the idea of a licensed Aboriginal club in Alice Springs came from Aboriginal women beyond Alice Springs: the Ngaanyatjarra, Pitjantjatjara, Yankunytjatjara (NPY) Women's Council, and the women of other regional communities, such as Hermannsburg. In an unlikely alliance, the NPY Women's Council and the Liquor Commission managed to prevent the Tyeweretye Club from obtaining a liquor licence for over two years.

The Northern Territory Country Liberal Party (CLP), then in government, supported the club. Hoping that it would help to minimise violence and alcohol problems in Alice Springs (Bottral 1990: 3), it granted Tangentyere Council 5 ha of relatively rural land, south of the town through Heavitree Gap and near the Little Sisters town camp. The site was Tangentyere's third choice (out of 16 potential sites); in the end, only one club was built, with a $250,000 loan from the ADC (which was later taken over by ATSIC).

The struggle to get licensed

The Tyeweretye Club submitted its first application for a licence to sell the full range of liquor in August 1990. Three months later, the Liquor Commission refused the application, citing the objections of respondents who had had negative experiences of community clubs (Tangentyere Council 1991: 95).[20] By this time, the club had been built and was open,

18   Then known as the Liquor, Racing and Gaming Commission.
19   The Alice Springs Town Council, at the time and since, has supported 'canteens' and clubs for Aboriginal people, but only if they are in bush communities, away from the town.
20   Racing, Gaming and Liquor Commission, Northern Territory, Liquor Division, Tyeweretye Club Incorporated Public Hearing, 21–23 August 1990.

but was only selling non-alcoholic drinks, prompting the headline: 'Pub with no beer offers hope'—which referred to the manager's ambitions for educating future customers towards moderate drinking (Simper 1991: 4).

In May 1991, a second application was submitted to the Liquor Commission, this time for a beer-only licence.[21] Ten months later, this application was also rejected, the Liquor Commission stating that it was concerned about the club's financial capacity. However, the decision was also influenced by opposition to the club voiced by Aboriginal women from remote communities in central Australia. These objectors thought it wrong for Aboriginal people to 'involve themselves in the sale of liquor to other Aboriginals', as they might perceive that 'it is quite in order for liquor to be consumed to varying levels of intoxication *because it is being supplied by Aboriginals*' (Northern Territory Liquor Commission 1997: 2, emphasis added). The Liquor Commission determined that, even though these objectors lived some distance from Alice Springs, they were part of the 'community' whose views needed to be considered, and it concluded that the 'needs and wishes' of the community were unfavourable to the club licence. Having previously ignored the needs and wishes—and consistent petitioning—of these traditional women over the issue of roadside takeaway licences, the Liquor Commission was perverse in taking account of their views on this occasion.

In a submission to a Race Discrimination Commission inquiry, Tangentyere Council mounted a spirited attack on the Liquor Commission's rejection of its application for an on-premises licence. Seeking to demonstrate the Liquor Commission's mishandling of Aboriginal alcohol-management issues, it cited three recent examples: indifference to the growing problems of the Murrinh Patha Social Club at Wadeye (described in Chapter 4); unresponsiveness to proposals put forward by the Imanpa – Mt Ebenezer community (to establish a community club, to upgrade policing and to resist takeaway applications from local outlets); and current rejection of the Tyeweretye Club's licence application. This rejection, Tangentyere Council claimed, exposed the Liquor Commission's preference for 'mediating judicial combat rather than contributing to a major project in alcohol rehabilitation'. Tangentyere Council asserted that, when turning down the licence application, the Liquor Commission had made no attempt to discuss the merits of the club's educational influence (i.e. in teaching

---

21 Supporters of this application included Geoffrey Shaw of Tangentyere Council, the police, a local MLA and Elliott Johnson QC, head of the Royal Commission into Aboriginal Deaths in Custody.

moderation); it had not investigated how the club dovetailed with other local programs and strategies; and had not considered the needs of fully employed Aboriginal people, some with tertiary qualifications, who had no 'congenial and non-racist' place to drink, or the needs of 'controlled' drinkers who wished to avoid the predations of their drunken relatives (Tangentyere Council 1991: 96).

Later, after thoughtfully analysing the Liquor Commission's policy, Tangentyere Council appealed the Liquor Commission's decision in the Northern Territory Supreme Court. Their appeal was successful. In March 1992, Justice Sally Thomas quashed the Commission's decision to refuse the licence, stating that the Liquor Commission had presented no evidence to back up its claim that the club lacked financial skills. She found that the views of Aboriginal women in remote communities were not shared by residents in Alice Springs,[22] and argued that the 'community' whose views mattered most was the community of people living or working within the township of Alice Springs (Northern Territory Liquor Commission 1997: 3). In a further rebuke, the Race Discrimination Commissioner commented that the Liquor Commission's earlier 'unreasonable' objection to the club was potentially discriminatory (Race Discrimination Commissioner 1995: 34). In 1993, the Chief Minister dismissed the incumbent Liquor Commissioner.[23] In March that year, the Liquor Commission—with different members, a new mission statement and policy direction, and new chairman—reconsidered the second application and granted the Tyeweretye Club a beer-only licence.

Putting in-house strategies in place

To allow time to conduct induction workshops, the Tyeweretye Club refrained from selling beer for six months after the licence was granted. The workshops sought to educate board members, most of whom were drinkers, about the rules of the Liquor Act as they applied to drinking on licensed premises. According to club manager Bill Ferguson, board members had been ignorant of the law, and of the expectations of behaviour on licensed premises. Ferguson recalled that some club members were shocked to discover that patrons who were clearly drunk

---

22 *Centralian Advocate* 30 March 1995: 3.
23 Kelvin Rae was removed; Marshall Perron appointed John Maley to the position in March 1993 (*Centralian Advocate* 1993b: 3).

could not be served more alcohol. This had not been their experience in other licensed premises, and many had only ever consumed takeaway alcohol in the scrub around Alice Springs.[24] Ferguson recalled how the rules and regulations of the club were translated into different languages and played over loudspeakers in the club 'so people could learn'. The club also advertised its rules on local television. Having had minimal formal education, and no training in responsible service or management, Ferguson learned the rules by reading the Liquor Act: 'I had to use my head', he said.

The club's constitution was unequivocal (if rather ambitious) about its aims, which were to alleviate the effects of social disadvantage, deprivation and cultural loss by:

> Establishing, operating and maintaining [licensed] Aboriginal social clubs at which Aboriginal people may consume alcohol in a controlled environment, enhanced by the provision of ancillary services … designed to promote a more enlightened attitude to the issue of alcohol and Aboriginal people and/or to mitigate the social damage occasioned by alcohol abuse in the Alice Springs community and surrounding areas of Central Australia. (Tyeweretye Constitution 1999: 3)

Club management put in place a number of policies designed to moderate people's intake and create a pleasant social environment. Food was always available, and there were self-service barbecues for people to cook meat purchased from the club. There was a mini-mart where people could exchange food vouchers,[25] and people could buy frozen kangaroo tails and pre-packed meats. Groups of women and children often came early for breakfast, and there was no pressure on people to drink alcohol. The dress rules were not too strict and bare feet were allowed; this was different from other clubs and hotels, where, as one customer explained, you had to 'dress up like white people'.[26] There was a comfortable grassed area outside the club, a bandstand and beer garden, a pool table and jukebox, and bingo games and raffles. There were six poker machines, but these were

---

24   The Tyeweretye Club continued to hold 'educational' meetings with its members; for example, in 1998, there were sessions about the operation of the Two Kilometre Law at which it was discovered that the majority of members were unaware that drinking within 2 km of a liquor outlet was unlawful: 'How far was 2 km?' The Two Kilometre Law had been in force since 1982 (Tangentyere Council 1998).

25   Tangentyere Council had its own form of voluntary income management in which people signed on through Centrelink for a food voucher system. The system was put in place over 25 years ago by senior town camp residents. www.tangentyere.org.au/services/finance/food_voucher/ [accessed 29 July 2014].

26   Jackie Okai's evidence (Northern Territory Liquor Commission 1997: 9).

rarely used and were eventually sold. Initially, the licence allowed for sales of beer only, and beers were sold in opened cans. The club encouraged people to drink light beer (which was half the price of 'heavy' beer). Club policy was to close on big entertainment days in Alice Springs, such as the Camel Cup or the Rodeo, as these events had their own special short-term licences. Friday night was band night; on these nights, the club would close at 3 pm to allow a four-hour break before the concert. Tickets cost $10 and between 250 and 300 people usually attended. The club made valiant efforts to prevent trouble among its clientele; on band nights, for example, only low-alcohol beer was sold from 9 pm until midnight. One staff member reported:

> If a donnybrooks[27] started up in the congregation in the club, they'd sort it out. We had concerts and had security at the gate with Aboriginal men and women security. We had one incident (a stabbing) outside the club in ten years.[28]

Another staff member recalled:

> There was a music stage, invited bands to come and play, not to make money but to give people what they couldn't get in town. But a rag-tag mob tried to get in and made trouble outside the gates and the media got onto it. At one time we employed three full-time properly accredited security people to take weapons off people and they removed any drunk and disorderly.[29]

Club members signed in at the front gate, and security workers would search people for alcohol and weapons. This was evidently required, as sometimes women tried to enter the club with cask bladders in their bras, and men with injuries tried to hide bottles in their plaster casts. Ferguson could remember only one incident on a Friday night when the police were called; however, the police and the night patrol were frequently called to attend to disputes among people gathered *outside* the club. Strict adherence to the liquor regulations (in the form of refusing service to and evicting intoxicated people) often created problems at the gate, partly because many drinkers had not been socialised into the behaviours expected of them, and did not understand why they were being refused service. This level of ignorance was a reflection (and indictment) of the serving practices that Aboriginal people had become accustomed to at

27 'Donnybrooks' = brawl, fracas.
28 Bill Ferguson, pers comm, 6 August 2008.
29 Gordon Fawcett, pers comm, 7 August 2008.

the few remaining Alice Springs bars frequented by Aboriginal people, particularly the (insultingly named) 'animal bar' at the Riverside Tavern, which evidently rarely enforced the law.

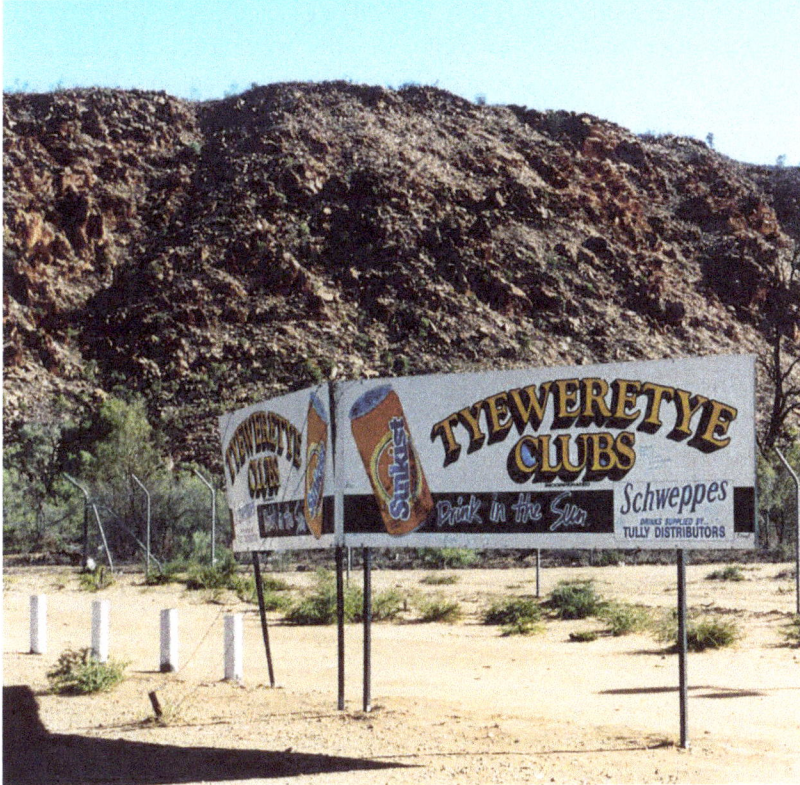

Fig. 18 Tyeweretye Clubs billboard
Source: M Brady

The challenges of running the club

The manager, a non-Aboriginal man, ran the bar with the help of a barman, a position that, for many years, was held by a Maori man. Non-Aboriginal club officials reported that it was impossible for Aboriginal men to work behind the bar; predictably, they found it difficult when their relations demanded free grog. The manager kept a close eye on supplies and the till. Nevertheless, as with all such ventures, critics suggested that the rules were occasionally bent, as the manager 'didn't know how to say "no"', and committee members were 'bought off' with alcohol.

The Tyeweretye Club had to deal with challenges and social issues that lay beyond, as well as on, its premises. An ongoing and difficult problem to manage concerned the habit many club patrons had of walking on, or across, a railway line that, unfortunately, was located near the club's front entrance. After several deaths involving freight trains, the national rail authority was forced to come up with better warning systems in consultation with Tangentyere Council. Another challenge was the press of people attracted to the general area of the club on band nights, who brought takeaway supplies, purchased elsewhere, to drink on the vacant land near the club. This allowed people to be part of the 'action' without entering the premises. Among those who entered the club were some who left their children waiting outside in parked vehicles. The club acted as a magnet to Aboriginal people who had nowhere else to go, and the manager frequently had to call the police and the Tangentyere night patrol:[30]

> [He] often rings ambulances for people outside the front of the Club, but ambulances have only very occasionally attended for persons inside the Club, for cases of medical emergencies ... people outside the Club on a Friday night organise their own liquor supplies. Each Saturday morning [the manager] cleans up rubbish from outside the Club premises ... [That Saturday] he picked up ninety empty wine casks, together with many empty bottles of spirits. (Northern Territory Liquor Commission 1997: 6)

Data from the Alice Springs sobering-up shelter showed that, while people were picked up intoxicated from the club area, the numbers were small in comparison to the number of people brought to the shelter who had been picked up from the Todd River bed (Gaff et al. 1997).

Despite all the social activities (e.g. band nights and barbeques), by 1997 (just four years after it was licensed), the club's alcohol trade was in decline, primarily because of competition presented by cheap takeaways, and the easing of restrictions on sales of 4 L wine casks. By the late 1990s, the club averaged around 30 customers a day, with trading usually confined to two hours in the morning: around lunchtime, most drinkers left for the takeaway outlets.[31]

---

30   The sources for this information include Peter Toyne (Minister for Central Australia in the 1990s); Chris McIntyre (Licensing and Regulation, Liquor Commission); Bill Ferguson (club manager); and Gordon Fawcett (club accountant).
31   The three takeaway outlets mentioned were the Heavitree Gap Hotel store, Piggly Wiggly (licensed supermarket) and BP (licensed roadhouse) (Northern Territory Liquor Commission 1997).

The Tyeweretye Club suffered the unintended effects of a series of genuine attempts to ameliorate the high levels of alcohol-related harm in the town. Trial periods of reduced trading hours and experiments in the types of alcohol sold negatively affected the club, as Bill Ferguson (2003: 87) explained:

> The Northern Territory Liquor Commission introduced restrictive trading hours for take-away outlets, Clubs and Hotels. The only alcohol sales permitted on licensed premises were light beer from 10 am and full-strength beer from 11.30 am. Our experiences have shown that this was not a real success. The patrons only waited around playing pool and watching television until 11.30 am when full beer sales were permitted. The experience of the Tyeweretye is that an organisation without take-away facilities has only a 'True Trading Time' of 11.30 am to 1.45 pm. There is a mass exodus from 1.30 pm onwards to the licensed take-away facilities.

In an attempt to stem this flow and improve the club's viability, management applied for a variation to the licence to allow sales of the full range of alcoholic drinks, not just beer, and Sunday trading. They hoped that if patrons had a choice of drinks, they would stay longer. Despite open discussion of the clubs' travails at the licence-variation hearing, the Liquor Commission accepted the 'sociological rationale' for the application. It heard evidence that the club had proved itself capable of controlling drinking; that it was a viable alternative to sitting in the riverbed with takeaway Coolibah;[32] and that Sunday trading would 'lessen … the swilling congregation' at the two takeaway outlets open in town (Northern Territory Liquor Commission 1997: 25). The club's 'only real problem' was the crowd of people who gathered outside the gates on Friday nights. In March 1997, the Liquor Commission granted the licence variation along with a trial period of extended trading hours on Sundays from 10 am to 6 pm. Customers welcomed the change, stating 'now we got a *real* pub'; a few club members switched to spirits, with young women drinking pre-mixed spirits (also known as alco-pops or UDLs).[33]

---

32   Coolibah = a popular cheap white cask wine.
33   It is worth noting that the type of liquor one drinks can be a key component of social identity and a source of prestige—or debasement (Collmann 1988, Sansom 1980).

Not only cheap takeaways threatened the club's viability: other commercial outlets also actively poached the club's customers. One hotel[34] in the vicinity of the Tyeweretye Club opened a new bar that was overtly designed to attract an Aboriginal clientele. Another hotel, which had previously been unwelcoming to Aboriginal customers, changed ownership, and the new management drew Tyeweretye's customers away by giving out stubby coolers, hats and putting on barbecues. The hotel also had a TAB, Sky and takeaways, all of which were attractive to Aboriginal customers; it even copied the Tyeweretye Club's idea of having Aboriginal bands play on premises. Local politician Peter Toyne, a supporter of the Tyeweretye Club from the beginning, described this competition as a 'grog war' (Chlanda 1998).

With the Tyeweretye Club doing no better in terms of customers and revenue, despite having a full range of alcohol on sale, in desperation, the club decided to apply for a takeaway licence in 1998; predictably, the move caused a furore. Tangentyere Council, the organisation that had sponsored the club, had objected to all new takeaway licences in Alice Springs as a matter of policy and principle over the previous 15 years. The club itself had argued that, by providing a particular social and cultural environment together with community-instigated rules of conduct for drinking on licensed premises, it was creating something special, not just another booze outlet to add to the already crowded market in Alice Springs. Club proponents had successfully used these arguments to fend off considerable opposition from women's groups and the abstinence treatment lobby. The commercial argument, that providing takeaway sales would enable the club to survive, was not enough; the club's application for a takeaway licence sparked a 'political war of words'. Prominent politicians, spokespersons and organisations, both Aboriginal and non-Aboriginal, took sides and voiced their opinions. In favour of the takeaway application were Labor politicians Maggie Hickey and Peter Toyne, who said that it would allow the club to compete with other liquor outlets for business, and that it was a necessary part of the future viability of the club (*Centralian Advocate* 1998a: 2, 1998b: 5). Toyne knew that the club owed $250,000 to ATSIC, which was not disposed to forgive the loan.

34　The Queen of the Desert Hotel.

The Alice Springs Town Council opposed the licence application. The mayor was against another takeaway licence in the town; if the club was in financial difficulties, he argued that it should approach ATSIC or LWA for help. As a health provider, the CAAC (or Congress) formally objected to the application, arguing that a takeaway licence would adversely affect women and children, cause more deaths, and contravene the club's philosophy as well as its goal of educating the Aboriginal community in responsible drinking (*Centralian Advocate* 1998c: 8). The club applied for a takeaway licence again in February 1999, but the hearing was abandoned when objectors discovered that the club's own constitution barred it from holding a licence to sell packaged alcohol (Kuilboer 1999: 13). The club suffered a loss of moral credibility in the eyes of its supporters; its repeated attempts to obtain a takeaway licence to save it financially—indeed, for the whole project to survive—was the final straw for those who had wavered in their support for the club. In April 2005, the club's licence was suspended, and in 2010, it was cancelled (Department of Justice 2010).

Analysing the demise of the club

The club's manager and key proponent, Bill Ferguson, explained the club's demise in a few simple words: 'there was too much opposition'. There is no doubt that the club was highly contentious, but it was also more than this. The club crystallised and brought to a head a long-term ideological split that had begun to form in the 1970s[35] between drinkers and non-drinkers in the Aboriginal community—the wets and the drys: between those who thought it was possible to 'live with alcohol' and those who were convinced that complete sobriety was the only route. More than individual diversity accounted for the differences of opinion among Aboriginal people; Aboriginal people's positioning on these matters determined the organisations they worked for, the strategies and policies those organisations supported, and their attitudes to the entire Northern Territory Government and its programs and initiatives, such as the LWA program.

---

35   See Aboriginal submissions to the House of Representatives inquiry into Aboriginal alcohol problems in 1976 and 1977 (Brady 2004: 59, Peele 1993).

Philosophical differences

Members of the Tangentyere Liquor Committee started to pull in different directions quite early on. The committee had originally comprised a mix of drinkers *and* non-drinkers, and these individuals became increasingly at odds with one another. In 1989, a non-drinking member of the committee, Doug Abbott, started the first Aboriginal Alcoholics Anonymous (AAA) group. This group grew into CAAAPU, an abstinence-oriented community-controlled residential treatment program (Lyon 1990: 110, Rowse 1996).[36] Conversely, the chair of the committee, Bill Ferguson, was the person who became the club's manager. Ferguson was a drinker; he was also experienced in the running of hotels, having previously managed the Finke Hotel. One non-drinking member described the committee's split:

> We started together ... Bill pulled away from us. They tried to get people teach 'em how to drink. Can't teach people to drink! Can't be both ways same time. How can we counsel anyone when you still drinking? ... I break off from there [to work at CAAAPU]. A tug of war. Trying to pull this way to keep sober and Bill pulling the other way to keep them drunk![37]

A Tangentyere Council spokesperson tried to deflate the significance of this ideological split, stating:

> Our organisation was the founding organisation for two models. The CAAAPU model is a total abstinence model. That came from the Tangentyere alcohol committee. The other option we have is to learn to live with alcohol so, out of that alcohol committee, came the formation of an Aboriginal social club called the Tyeweretye Club. (Tilmouth 2001: 17)

---

36   This informal group was renamed Aboriginal Alcohol Awareness (AAA) after the official Alcoholics Anonymous organisation objected to the original name. AAA was originally supportive of moderation messages, but later toughened its position to promote abstention. On CAAAPU see Rowse 1996.

37   Brady fieldnotes, 6 May 2009. Indeed, Tangentyere Council (1991) pushed for the club *and* it continued to support the AAA group (28). As Paul Spicer (1997) pointed out with respect to Native Americans, this epitomises the profound ambivalence within Aboriginal thinking about drinking. He wrote that Native American drinkers do not exemplify one opinion about drinking: 'Instead, their attitude is a product of the tension between two mutually incompatible positions: those that favour alcohol use and those that condemn it' (317). They recognise that alcohol can be used to demonstrate the core cultural values of sharing and relating with kin, but they also vilify it as an alien and degrading influence.

This division created defensiveness on both sides, especially between the AAA people, who eventually became counsellors at CAAAPU, and the individuals associated with the club. When CAAAPU workers visited the club to see what was going on—what sort of place it was—they encountered resistance: they felt that club staff were uninterested in providing CAAAPU contact information to customers. There is no doubt that, rightly or wrongly, the club became associated with the Northern Territory Government's sensible drinking campaign: the LWA program. In fact, proponents of the club sometimes seemed to have adopted the program's slogan. One stated:

> You can't get rid of grog. You gotta learn to live with grog. If we can learn those things, we can learn to live with alcohol, no reason why not.

Similarly, another supporter of the club remarked:

> Teaching people to *live with alcohol* was the main objective [of the club]. There was a split in views between the 'no alcohol' people and the 'Living with Alcohol' type of thinking'. (emphasis added)

The fact that the Northern Territory Government's LWA program supported the club merely reinforced the negative attitudes of those who believed that moderate consumption was neither possible, nor desirable for Aboriginal people.[38] Even the Race Discrimination Commissioner (1995: 33) cautioned that the policy of moderation espoused by the LWA program 'should not be imposed indiscriminately on all Aboriginal communities'. In truth, LWA stressed that there were drinking *choices* available to Aboriginal people other than being either a (heavy) 'drinker' or an abstinent 'non-drinker'.

In the region as a whole, the pro-abstinence, anti-moderation position was boosted between 1991 and 1993 by the arrival in Alice Springs of First Nations abstinence-oriented alcohol-treatment activists from Canada. Several of these charismatic indigenous treatment entrepreneurs spoke at conferences, networked with Aboriginal organisations and lobbied government officials, stressing the need for sobriety, supporting AA-style approaches and condemning harm-reduction policies (Brady 2004, Rowse

---

38 Such thinking is prevalent among Native Americans who often also assert that there is no way their people could drink 'like a Whiteman' in a moderate way (Spicer 1997: 307).

1996). The arrival of the Canadians reinforced the existing divergence of views about the nature of drinking problems and the best way to manage them; there is no doubt that they contributed to opposition to the club.

Gurrum'thun ŋunhi yurru ŋänitji-ŋatha manapan ļuka, manymaktja rom ŋilimurruŋgu.
These people are drinking safe amounts of grog and eating food while they drink. The kids have plenty of food.

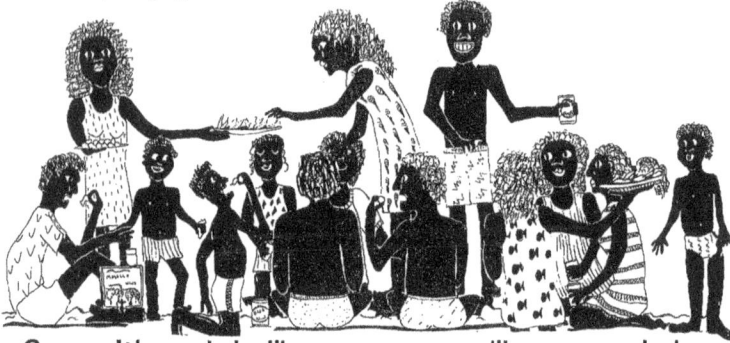

Gurrum'thunmirri ŋilimurruŋguway ŋilimurru ga bulu djamarrkuļiwu, djäka walalaŋgu ga wirrki wekama ŋathayu walalanha.
This is a careful way to drink grog.

Fig. 19 'These people are drinking safe amounts of grog'
Source: Living with Alcohol responsible drinking resource from northeast Arnhem Land

In addition to these stresses (i.e. internal fissures, growing antipathy towards the LWA program and the arrival of the Canadians), the club faced opposition from a new Aboriginal women's temperance movement in Alice Springs. Women demonstrated in public to protest the uncontrolled sales of takeaway alcohol and the devastating effects alcohol was having on their families, and they campaigned vigorously against the opening of any further outlets for liquor.[39] The movement, which had begun in bush communities, had been gathering momentum over several years. It commenced in 1988, when women of the Pitjantjatjara region southwest of Alice Springs objected to the renewal of a takeaway licence for the Curtin Springs Roadhouse, which sold alcohol to Aboriginal

---

39   The Northern Territory, at the time, had more liquor outlets per capita than any other state or territory in Australia, and Alice Springs had 37 per cent more liquor outlets per capita than the rest of the Northern Territory, 19 of which had takeaway licences (Coughlan 1991: 151).

people returning to bush communities.[40] In July 1990, with no progress on their complaints, the women marched and demonstrated outside the roadhouse. In mid-1990, there was a large, and much publicised, 'walk against grog' through the streets of Alice Springs, involving hundreds of Pitjantjatjara, Warlpiri and Arrernte people from five remote communities. Organised largely by prominent local woman Rosalie Kunoth-Monks, contingents of traditional women walked bare-breasted, 'painted up' and wearing feather and hair-string headbands (Schulz 1990: 3). Although Kunoth-Monks was reported as saying that this 'declaration of war on grog' was aimed at visitors from the bush who came to town to drink and lived in the riverbed, she was known to oppose the Tyeweretye Club; the march took place within months of the club's first licence application. In March 1993—in the same month as the Liquor Commission was reconsidering the Tyeweretye Club's licence application—30 women from Hermannsburg marched on a delicatessen in Alice Springs in opposition to its licence. When they heard that the Tyeweretye Club had been granted a licence, several Hermannsburg women[41] picketed the venue to show their displeasure:

> We are very, very sad about the grog problems. The Tyeweretye Club will mean trouble for our families. It will bring death … We want grog shops to stop selling alcohol to Aborigines but now they have opened a club especially to sell grog to Aboriginal people. It is wrong … and a waste of Government money and Aboriginal land. (Tondorf 1993a: 2)

Bill Ferguson invited the women in for a tour of the premises and answered their questions. One month later, on 23 April 1993, Aboriginal women from Hermannsburg, Papunya and Yuendumu held another big anti-grog march through the streets of Alice Springs.[42] Like members of the WCTU in the nineteenth century, the Aboriginal women placed banner-holding children ('No grog in delis' and 'Save our people. No grog') at the head of their demonstration. The anti-grog campaigners were joined

---

40   The objections to Curtin Springs were heard before Kelvin Rae (Chairman of the Liquor Commission), 22–24 November 1988 and 14–16 February 1989 in Alice Springs. Objectors were Maggie Kavanagh, the Pitjantjatjara Council Inc. and Mutitjulu Community Inc. The objections were overcharging, failure to follow an informal agreement and selling to people travelling to dry communities. They were dismissed as being 'marginal', 'hearsay' and because of uncertainty over the definition of 'the needs and wishes of the community'. It took nine years of complaints, lobbying and a coronial inquest into five deaths before an agreement was reached for trials of restrictions on takeaway sales in 1997.
41   The Hermannsburg women were led by Mavis Malbunka.
42   This march was organised by Koorine Williams from Hermannsburg.

by women from the Yuendumu night patrol (Tondorf 1993b: 3). This mobilisation against alcohol in the form of pickets and marches was, in effect, an uprising by Aboriginal women asserting their right to speak out about domestic violence, alcohol-related homicides and the welfare of their children and future generations (McGrath 1993).[43] Such a level of ferment over alcohol was unprecedented and, to some extent, incidental to plans for the Tyeweretye Club. However, some supporters of the club believed that anti-grog campaigners had been responsible for quashing the original plan for four Aboriginal clubs. Certainly, after the grog marches had taken place, several previously supportive agencies and organisations 'washed their hands' of the club. As the club's accountant explained: 'The anti-grog movement came in and they dropped us like a hot potato'.

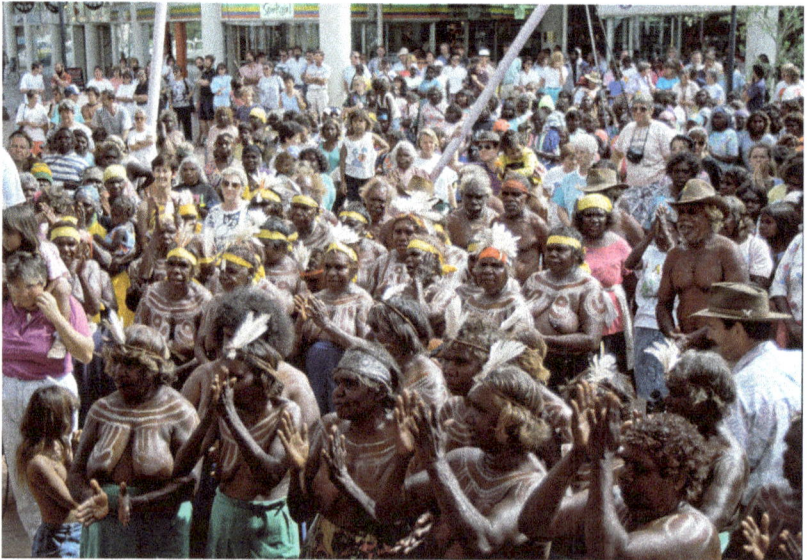

Fig. 20 Women Against Alcohol march, Alice Springs, 1990
Source: S Strike

---

43   Nineteenth-century WCTU members, members of the United States Anti-Saloon League and evangelical reformers all used the effect of drinking on women and children as ammunition in their campaigns, as did the Aboriginal women of central Australia (Grimshaw 1999).

The meaning of drinking

Another huge difficulty for the club was that it tried to tackle an inherently wicked and probably insoluble problem: changing the drinking styles of people who were thoroughly unversed in drinking on licensed premises and whose normal practice was to aim for intoxication. For some Aboriginal people, drinking to intoxication was an expression of personal power: for others, it was simply normative and had become habitual (Collmann 1979, cf. Room 1992).

A country-club style hotel–casino opened in Alice Springs in 1981. Redeveloped as Lasseter's Casino in 1986, this glitzy venue (rather than the Tyeweretye Club) attracted many middle-class Aboriginal locals. In making a case for the club's establishment, Tangentyere Council had argued that tertiary educated and employed Aboriginal residents needed a 'non-racist' setting in which to drink; however, the bulk of drinkers the club hoped to attract were people who had spent a lifetime drinking in the open, in the Todd River or the town camps. Before they switched to cask wine, many of these people were port, sweet sherry and methylated spirits drinkers. Anthropologist Jeff Collmann lived in a town camp in the 1970s; he observed that most town camp people drank 'what is often considered (even by Northern Territory standards) an extraordinary amount of liquor' (1979: 209, 1988).[44] In the 1980s, the camps were largely violent, insular and lawless places without regular police patrols, despite the fact that residents included some non-drinkers and others whose drinking varied along a continuum from regular (moderate) to heavy (bingeing) (Collmann 1979, O'Connor 1983: 5, Jane Lloyd, pers comm).[45] Tyeweretye Club patrons who came from the south-side camps, near the club, were primarily made up of desert people (i.e. Luritja, Pitjantjatjara and Warlpiri) who had had relatively little exposure to, or experience of, alcohol (Stead 1980). They had not worked in the pastoral industry that, for some Aboriginal people, provided their (relatively controlled) introduction to alcohol. Their experience of drinking on licensed premises was confined to one or two rough, usually segregated, bars at roadside inns or in Alice Springs hotels.

---

44   Even when the club was operating, the Alice Springs police reported that they took 13,000 people a year into protective custody who were intoxicated in public, and that the extent of public drunkenness was beyond their capacity and function (Northern Territory Liquor Commission 1997: 21).

45   The Tangentyere Liquor Committee would have liked to declare the town camps as dry areas under existing Northern Territory Dry Area legislation, but this was thought to be 'too hard' because of the impossibility of policing such an arrangement (Ferguson 2003: 86). Town camps were eventually declared dry under the NTER provisions in 2007.

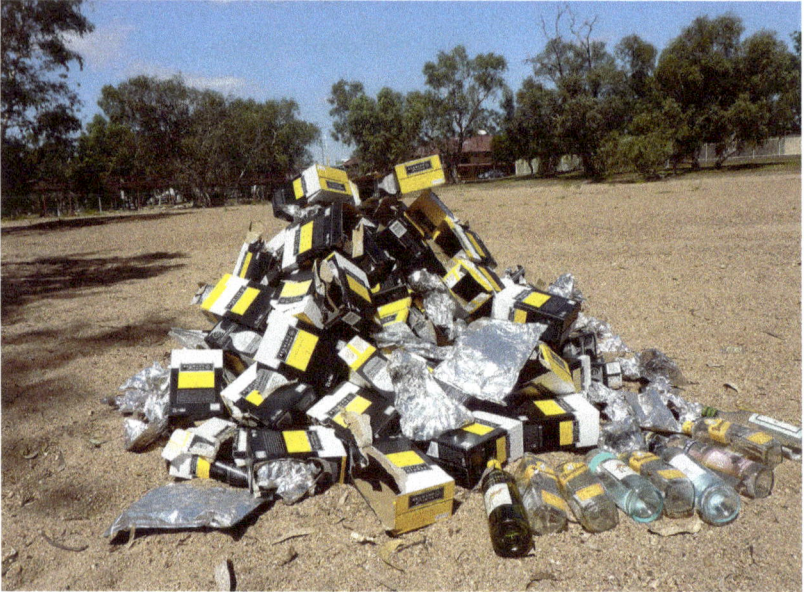

Fig. 21 Empty wine casks and liquor bottles (sold by one outlet) collected from drinking spots in the Todd River bed, 2012
Source: People's Alcohol Action Coalition, Alice Springs

The Tyeweretye Club was at a distinct disadvantage. Like all on-licences, it was unable to compete with the off-licences that provided Aboriginal people with takeaway alcohol. More specifically, it was unable to fulfil the needs of Aboriginal people who placed a high social and cultural value on the exchanges and interchanges that were made possible by takeaway alcohol. The bulk nature of takeaway alcohol (in cans, bottles or casks) makes it a *malleable* commodity, allowing it to become a form of symbolic capital through which people make and remake their social world. This dense network of sociality and exchange is essential to people's sense of self (Peterson 2013). As a fluid, liquor can be divided into different amounts and shared in different ways—from a communal cup, by the gift of a bottle, or a swig from a flagon or cask: something that is not so easily achieved when drinking at a club or bar. Local historian Dick Kimber, although he did not drink himself, used to sit with Aboriginal friends who were drinkers. He recalled:

> You'd get 20 'it makes you happy' [was what they said]. You'd make the most of what you got.[46]

---

46   Dick Kimber, pers comm, 1 August 2008.

According to Collmann (1979), liquor was a form of credit for town campers: it involved the 'entire social universe' of the town camp in which he lived. Alcohol, like other commodities, has become part of what Peterson (2013) has termed 'demand sharing'—that is, the pattern of informal sharing in which acting generously commonly takes place in response to demands. As well as being easily shared, takeaway alcohol allows for greater spatial flexibility, as drinkers can recruit and maintain their companions and co-drinkers and locate them spatially in the landscape in a manner that is not possible on licensed premises, no matter how extensive a beer garden might be (Sansom 1980, Brady 2010).

Losing the competition war

While the Tyeweretye Club tried to enact some corporate social responsibility by serving low-alcohol beer and closing for a few hours on band nights, the other, more competitive commercial outlets, ignored such niceties, commonly engaging in unscrupulous sales tactics. Some of these were exposed in 1993 when the government was forced to amend the Liquor Act to curb happy hours that lasted longer than two hours; ban the selling of 'buy-one get-one free' drinks; prevent hoteliers from offering all the liquor a person could consume for a set fee; ban drinking competitions; and prevent hotels from providing ticketing or other discounting mechanisms. All these deplorable practices had become normal in Northern Territory hotels; when they were banned, the Hoteliers Association called the new regulations 'bloody ridiculous' (*Centralian Advocate* 1993a: 3).

Meanwhile, the Tyeweretye Club's light-beer initiatives were unsuccessful and unpopular; club members did not drink it, even though it cost half the price of full-strength beer. According to the *Centralian Advocate* (18 April 1997: 3):

> The club did all the right things: it sold beer only, had entertainment at the weekends, security guards, BBQs and meat plates, grassy areas, and Aboriginal ownership. But it slowly lost money and was forced to extend trading hours and sell wines and spirits. They had argued that it was better for people to drink in a controlled area rather than in public.

Ferguson spoke in similar terms about the club's efforts to trial different opening hours:

> We tried for one year opening from 4 pm to see if we could draw people in. But no-one came. By that time, they'd have [had] a fairly good fill. We got big numbers in the early days and they stayed longer, even though the bottle shops were open, but we realised we had to have a shut-down time, or else a drunken mess around me. So about 3 pm we had a shut down. But once people left, they'd never come back.[47]

The availability of cheap takeaways, and the unashamedly profit-driven marketing strategies of nearby hotels, made the club unviable. This had been a danger from the beginning; the year the club opened, the Gapview Hotel drive-in bottle shop was selling 4 L casks of Kaiser Stuhl Riesling for $8.45, and a carton of Territory Bitter beer for $16.95 (*Centralian Advocate* 4 May 1993: 9). Customers abandoned the Tyeweretye Club en masse once the takeaway outlets opened at around midday or early afternoon. As mentioned, it was not just the lure of takeaway liquor that drew customers away; one nearby hotel put on live Aboriginal bands and set up a bar overtly designed for Aboriginal drinkers to attract on-premises sales.

The club had not become embedded in people's lives as a social and community centre—a regular drinking spot. Instead, the club became a venue for 'pre-loading'. In a reversal of the widespread practice in which young urban (non-Aboriginal) Australians engage in pre-drinking at home prior to a night out clubbing, Aboriginal drinkers used the Tyeweretye Club to whet their appetites before heading off to the takeaway outlets, after which the 'real' drinking began (Wells et al. 2009, Brady 2010).

A business or a social enterprise?

Originally, the club's proponents and management committee had hoped that it would become a community hub, providing services, training programs and rehabilitation for drinkers. There were also plans for a sporting complex on the property. According to the manager, there were even hopes that income from the club could be used to:

> Sponsor people to go to a better school or through Uni, but we never made enough to do that. Early days [we had] a turnover of $10,000 per week, then $2000. We had six pokies but didn't make anything out of them.

---

47   Bill Ferguson, pers comm.

The poker machines that KMG thought would produce $70,000 a year were hardly used. This was probably because, rather than winning cash, poker-machine players won credits that could be redeemed at the shop with vouchers. Most mainstream clubs, such as RSL clubs or sporting clubs, would not survive without the income from poker machines.[48] The Tyeweretye Club's income from food sales also dropped dramatically from 1997, because another Tangentyere Council business became the designated outlet for the exchange of food vouchers.[49]

The club's accountant described Tyeweretye as a 'mutual club', in the sense that its profits were for the benefit of members as a whole; indeed, the club's constitution stated that any profits would be applied 'in promotion of its objectives'.[50] The club was intended as a social enterprise, acting for the good of its constituents and members, rather than solely as a money-making enterprise, which is somewhat in the spirit of the community-owned, or Gothenburg-style, hotels discussed in earlier chapters. Yet, ATSIC expected the club to make enough money to repay its loan, and gave it little leeway. The accountants had optimistically predicted that the club would be self-funding, but the reality was that without ongoing outside support, it struggled to survive. Once the club was built and furnished, it received no further financial support. According to the club's accountant:

> There were no subsidies. We had to stand on our own two feet. One million to build and equip it—as good a club as you'd get anywhere. We had $200,000 left as a loan that had to be repaid over the five-year lease time at 10 per cent interest. The loan was a 'mortgage' on the five-year lease. But we only had a five-year lease and limited sales.

Running the club, and making it profitable while honouring its commitment to safe and moderate drinking, was a much more difficult proposition than had been anticipated by the sponsoring organisation, Tangentyere Council. Tangentyere had its own governance problems. Its periodic changes in direction and governance affected the club and diminished the level of both tangible and ideological support. The club's manager and principals needed more professional guidance and better

---

48   Chris McIntyre, Liquor Commission, pers comm, 8 August 2008.
49   Tangentyere Council bought a supermarket that included a liquor department, representing a reversal of its earlier policy on takeaway licences, and changing the arrangements for Tangentyere-issued food vouchers.
50   The Constitution reads: '21.2. Profits, if any, and other income of Tyeweretye shall be applied in promotion of its objectives. Dividends shall not be paid to, nor profits, income or property of Tyeweretye be distributed amongst members. 21.3. No member shall be entitled to derive any profit, benefit of advantage from Tyeweretye which is not available to every member'.

management training, but no government or non-government agency provided any follow-up support or advice, and none had the capacity to do so. The Liquor Commission dealt only with compliance issues; the government health department and the LWA program had limited practical involvement with the club. In a sense, uncertainty within government about whether the club was meant to be a business or a social enterprise (an exercise in alcohol harm reduction, or even health promotion), was a key factor in its demise.

After defaulting on its start-up loan in 2005, the club closed its doors. The club needed to generate around $100,000 per year to survive; it was driven to make the controversial application for a takeaway licence purely out of economic need—it had no interest in having such a licence beyond a financial one. A local politician who believed in the club and wanted it to survive articulated what she saw as the key question:

> The issues that have to be established by people are: do they believe that the Tyeweretye Club is a good thing, and has it delivered benefits for the community? In other words, was the situation worse in terms of the patterns of anti-social behaviour before it started. If we say yes to that, and certainly on the evidence I've been provided with I've been persuaded of that, then somehow or other we've got to ensure that the club survives. (*Centralian Advocate* 1998a: 2)

If the club had not been required by ATSIC to operate as a self-sufficient and successful business, and if it had received ongoing government support in the form of a subsidy—in recognition of its social benefit (assuming this could be demonstrated), or in anticipation of its future, long-term beneficial effect on drinking patterns—perhaps it could have survived (Christie & Young 2011).

Only one club

Several Aboriginal and non-Aboriginal commentators believed that the Tyeweretye Club failed because it was only one, instead of being one of four, as originally planned. Betty Pearce commented, bluntly, that:

> Just one club was plain stupid, better to have two or none at all! Warlpiri were always our natural enemies ... The Hermannsburg and NPY[51] mob all go there, and the town camps. Not many from Areyonga went [to the club].

---

51 NPY = in this sense refers to people from the Ngaanyatjarra, Pitjantjatjara and Yankunytjatjara lands straddling the South Australia – Northern Territory border, southwest of Alice Springs.

Why was it so important to have more than one club? While most of Alice Springs' Aboriginal residents identified as being of Arrernte ancestry, the town also had (and increasingly has) a diverse population of Indigenous people of different affiliations. As Ottosson (2014: 131) has pointed out, the town is the service hub for thousands of remote-living Aboriginal people from many different language groups: some stay for a few days, others stay for a few years, most usually live in a number of town camps. Those proposing four clubs pointed out that the town camps were largely composed of distinct Aboriginal communities based on language and ancestral connection to country or kin. The camps north of the Gap were primarily Arrernte. On the south side, near the club, there were four town camps (Little Sisters, Anthepe, Karnte and Ilparpa) and these camps produced some of the key players in the club's fortunes. The southern town camps tended to be composed of Arrernte, Luritja, Pitjantjatjara and Warlpiri people. The original idea of having four licensed clubs, each one catering to different groups, reveals something of the local complexities of Aboriginal identity politics present in Alice Springs, in which categories of people mobilise and promote their own group, affiliation or family network to differentiate themselves, associate or distance themselves from certain others. As mentioned earlier, several older Aboriginal residents disliked changes to the layout of local hotel bars that gave them fewer strategies and less 'room' to avoid certain people while drinking.

Two significant assumptions undergirded the proposal to establish four drinking clubs. First, Aboriginal people assumed that drinking would lead to trouble, inevitably bringing 'drunken-changes-for-the-worse'.[52] Second, Aboriginal people expected that this trouble could be forestalled by stage-managing the social environment. Room (2001) has observed that, given cultural foreknowledge of intoxication's role in violence, experienced drinkers will choose their drinking partners and venues carefully (MacAndrew & Edgerton 1969, Shore & Spicer 2004). As Basil Sansom (1980) has argued, grogging is inherently dangerous: to avoid trouble you drink with your own 'crew—with people you trust, your mates'. This mechanism is mentioned in several ethnographies of drinking (Sansom 1980, Brady 1988, 2010). Thus, it was believed that having different clubs to cater for different language or other groups would solve the problem of alcohol-related violence, which was endemic

---

52   Alcohol expectancy theory states that cognitions about drinking have been found to influence drinking behaviour; indeed, expectations about what will be the likely outcome of a situation have a profound effect on the actual outcome of events (see MacAndrew & Edgerton 1969, Blume et al. 2003, Shore & Spicer 2004).

in the town camps during the 1980s when the club was being planned. Rather than seeing violence in the town camps as 'normal', advocates of the four-club model rationalised such conflict as the preventable result of language groups mingling.[53] Alternatively, it could be argued that fighting facilitated by intoxication is usually about the airing of grievances that are as likely to occur within immediate kin groups. Fighting also arises from sexual jealousy; when people are drunk, even the smallest gesture can be interpreted in a particular way, leading, sometimes, to deadly violence among intimate partners (Lloyd 2014). Rather than addressing the need to change the culture of drinking, and the easy resort to violence, people sidestepped these issues and instead focused on lobbying in support of different clubs for different groups.

Having one club on the south side possibly reduced the customer base; some potential customers may have avoided drinking at the club because they did not want to mix with people from other language groups. Certainly, the customer base was nowhere near the 1,650 that had been predicted by the accountants from KMG. However, a number of knowledgeable participants in this project question this explanation for the club's demise, pointing out that, in fact, people from all language groups patronised the club and mixed together, including those from north of the Gap. The supposed distinctions between residents of the town camps seem to have been exaggerated: in any case, they have become less marked over time. It is notable that, when a sobering-up shelter[54] was being planned for Alice Springs in the mid-1980s, similar suggestions were made regarding the need for multiple facilities: people said that more than one shelter was needed to accommodate different groups. However, the manager of the relevant drug and alcohol organisation maintained that, with appropriate rules of behaviour, one shelter would suffice: it did.[55]

Four clubs may have satisfied the needs or desires of individuals who, for various reasons, were promoting their own family networks, or avoiding others, or who wished to micro-manage their choice of drinking companions to pre-empt trouble. However, multiple clubs would have faced the same ruthless competition from commercial takeaway outlets and hotels keen to attract lucrative Aboriginal clientele. If one club was not financially viable, it is highly unlikely that four clubs could have survived without substantial ongoing external support.

---

53 Several anthropologists have noted this (Sansom 1980, Shore & Spicer 2004).
54 A sobering-up shelter is an overnight non-custodial refuge for intoxicated people.
55 Carol Watson, pers comm, May 2009. The Sobering-up Shelter was opened in 1986.

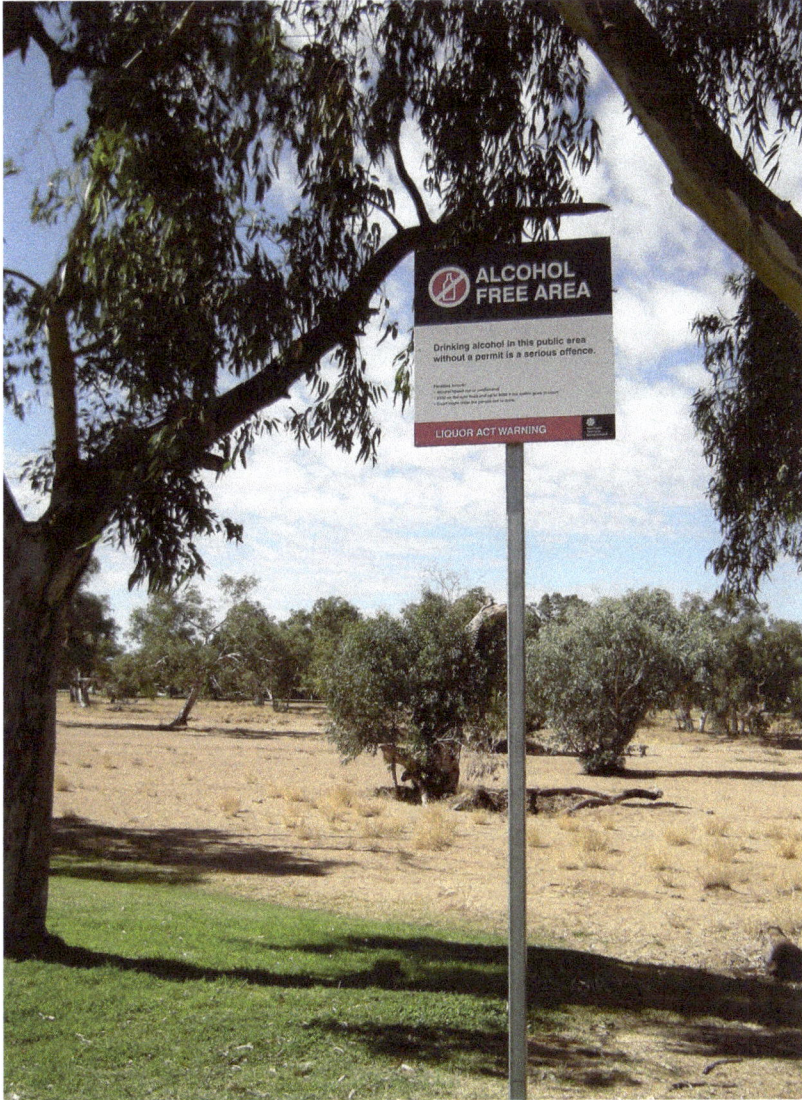

Fig. 22 Alcohol restrictions sign, Todd River, 2009
Source: M Brady

There are, naturally, differences of opinion about whether the Tyeweretye Club was, or became, a place of moderate drinking. Many of the now middle-aged and older Aboriginal musicians who played at the club talk nostalgically about the diversity of people who went there; they also talk about the fighting, and recall that the levels of drinking and drunkenness could be out of control.[56] Some of those involved with the club over the 12 years of its existence believe that it was successful, or partly successful, in modifying people's drinking behaviour:

> Bill had to really sort it out at first—it was a rough place, no way would a young woman go in there! People changed their behaviour dramatically. Half way through we started to see the change, we introduced food, had a half-time cook plus assistant, and a shop assistant … The Club tried to be an induction into community life, not just selling grog. It was living in a half way between what was 'kosher' in the town and what was 'kosher' in the bush. They learned—it was their place—rules to obey made by the club themselves [sic] 'You will behave like this. If intoxicated automatically removed from premises'. Under club rules, you were removed, [whereas] the Liquor Act [only] says not to sell any more.[57]

Supporters of the club believe they were victims of their own success: that the Tyeweretye Club did all the hard work of teaching the 'wild brumbies' how to behave on licensed premises and that other hotels reaped the benefit, stealing away their customers. Ferguson believed that the club 'worked *too* well—people were let into the Gap Hotel because they knew how to behave now!' In effect, the club was penalised for introducing its 'safe drinking' policies, for trying to create a family venue and for placing limits on its sales practices and the type of alcohol it sold. These were controls that other, more business-oriented premises, chose to ignore. Betty Pearce reflected that: '[The club] started to help with responsible drinking … but [it's] not much use now: alcohol is freely available everywhere!'[58] The Tyeweretye Club failed where other licensed outlets succeeded because it had different goals from its competitors. Given a choice between maximising profits and not selling to people for short-term profitability, the club placed its corporate social responsibility first.

After years of living in the town camps and participating in Tangentyere Council's alcohol-management efforts, the manager of the defunct club believed that the only solution to Aboriginal problem drinking was to restrict takeaway sales to a few hours, starting late in the day, with no takeaway sales on Sundays. He was convinced that this would 'result in people (who wanted to drink) being forced to drink on licensed premises in a safe and controlled environment' (Ferguson 2003: 88).

---

56   Åse Ottosson, pers comm, 30 July 2014. One local newspaper editor described the club as a 'hapless experiment in social engineering' (Chlanda 2006).
57   Gordon Fawcett (the club's accountant from 1994 to 2005), pers comm, 7 August 2008.
58   Betty Pearce, pers comm, 8 August 2008.

Notwithstanding the research evidence of aggression and violence in and around bars and the rarity of prosecutions, Ferguson is undoubtedly right in believing that drinking on licensed premises, with at least some expectation of a basic standard of comportment, is preferable to drinking in uncontrolled public spaces (Brady 2010).

Astonishingly, only four years after the Tyeweretye Club closed, the mayor of Alice Springs called for the establishment of a 'controlled drinking venue' for Aboriginal people from the town camps and bush settlements: a club (Richards 2009: 5). It is difficult to comprehend such extraordinary ignorance of the long local history of debate, research and lobbying on the subject of community-controlled drinking clubs for Aboriginal people in Alice Springs, not to mention the existence of the closed and empty Tyeweretye Club, which still stood, intact and unused, just south of the town.

6

Indigenous communities buy hotels

Among the many damaging effects of the prohibition years, the bans on Aboriginal people drinking in hotels alongside other Australians were the most mortifying. When it became financially possible for Indigenous entities to buy hotels for themselves in the 1970s and 1980s, this history of exclusion was influential in the thinking of Aboriginal organisations and government bureaucrats. Eight hotels were purchased by, or on behalf of, Aboriginal community entities over roughly a 20-year period—the first was the Finke Hotel at Finke in the Northern Territory in 1975. This was followed by purchases of the Oasis Hotel at Walgett (1983), the Transcontinental at Oodnadatta (1986), Mt Ebenezer Roadhouse (1987), Woden Town Club, Canberra (1988), the Crossing Inn, Fitzroy Crossing (1989), Daly River Hotel Motel (late 1990s) and the Wayside Inn at Timber Creek (1999). The most recent purchase of a licensed hotel was in 2014, when the Ngarluma Aboriginal Corporation and the Ngarluma Yindjibarndi Foundation, both in the Pilbara region of Western Australia, purchased the Whim Creek Hotel between Roebourne and Port Hedland.[1]

---

1   The purchase of the hotel ($1.7 million) includes an accommodation complex (*The West Australian* 2014). The new owners plan to restore and reopen the hotel and provide industry and training opportunities for local Indigenous people.

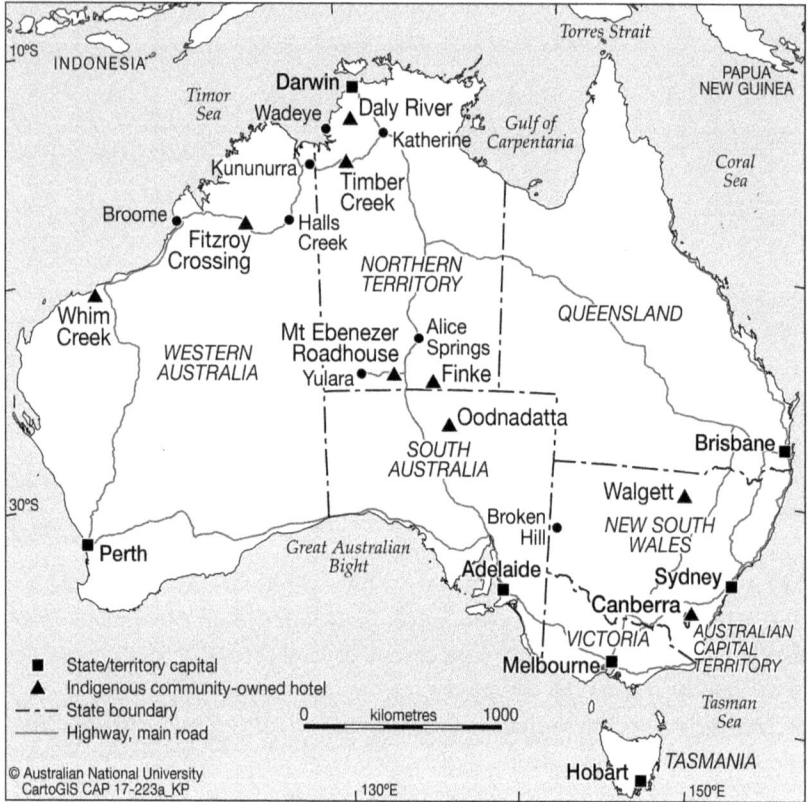

Map 2 Public hotels owned or part owned by Indigenous entities, 1975–2014

Source: CartoGIS, The Australian National University

Apart from these mostly rural, small-town pubs, in recent years, Aboriginal corporations have bought interests in several high-profile facilities that include the sale of alcohol, such as the Gagudju Lodge at Cooinda, and the Gagudju Crocodile Holiday Inn Motel, which are both in Kakadu National Park; the Dugong Beach Resort on Groote Eylandt; and the Ayers Rock Resort (Yulara) in central Australia. However, these hotels and lodges are primarily investment properties. Designed for tourists, they are focused on accommodation, and are intended neither to cater to local Aboriginal people nor to influence their drinking behaviour. By having management leaseback agreements and appointing large management companies for these properties, Indigenous associations have chosen to distance themselves from the day-to-day issues of running them; they see these enterprises as revenue raising rather than as social enterprises (Simonsen 2006).

In contrast to these investment properties, the purchase of rural public hotels by Aboriginal bodies has been largely, though not entirely, an exercise in social enterprise. A social enterprise is a market-oriented economic activity that serves a social goal, although, as Defourny and Nyssens (2010) pointed out, the definition of a social enterprise varies between countries. Social enterprises are generally defined as businesses that have social aims, such as local employment; are usually based on a commitment to build local capacity; and are answerable to their members for their social and economic effect. Defourny and Nyssens (2006: 6) suggested five criteria that, ideally, characterise a social enterprise:

1. It has an explicit aim to benefit the community and promote a sense of social responsibility locally.
2. It is an initiative of a group of citizens.
3. The decision-making power is not based on capital ownership, but the 'one member one vote' principle.
4. It has a participatory and representative structure.
5. It practices limited profit distribution, avoiding profit-maximising behaviour.

Most of the Aboriginal-owned hotels have aimed to achieve some of these criteria and have achieved varying degrees of success. As well as developmental goals, hotel purchases by Indigenous groups have been driven by a desire to manage previously uncontrolled sales of alcohol, and as an alternative to having a local hotel run by a publican estranged from the Aboriginal community (who may not care about the damage his or her product does). It has been difficult to ascertain—in retrospect, mostly— to what extent Indigenous-owned hotels have made enough profit to allow for distributions. In a departure from the 'ideal' characteristics proposed by Defourny and Nyssens, at least one Aboriginal-owned hotel has focused strongly on maximising profits. Both within and beyond the communities involved, all these hotel purchases have been controversial.

Buying hotels: A response to discrimination

While Aboriginal groups have articulated a variety of social and economic goals for buying licensed premises, one underlying motive has been to overcome the humiliation of having been refused service in public hotels. A letter to Prime Minister John Curtin in 1943 from Mr Mullins of Deniliquin epitomised this feeling:

> To the Prime Minister Mr Curtin
>
> Dear Sir
>
> Could you give me any reason why I cannot get a drink of *beer* in any Hotel especially in the town I am now living Deniliquin NSW. I have been advised to state my case to you as soon as possible. Here is my case in full. My Father is a White man and my Mother is a very light half Caste as for my colour its hard for anyone to tell its only that they know my Mother is an half caste. I have served in the AIF [Australian Imperial Force] but was discharged with bad feet. Now that my feet are good I'm willing to serve again. But Mr Curtin do you think its fair that I should be treated this way. I have just received my Enrolment Form for Home Defence so you see I'm treated like a White man in every other way still I'm not allowed to enter an Hotel. I have been on the Electoral Roll for ten years and if Probition [sic] came in I would have to vote for something that I'm not receiving. I'm not in the habit of drinking around the town and making a fool of myself but I do like my pot the same as any other man it makes you very small to be refused a drink in front of your work mates. The Police have refused me still they don't know the reason why. Mr Curtin I have one Brother a Prisoner of War in Italy as been for three yeares [sic] and another Brother in camp in Victoria so once again I will ask you do you think it is fair to me. I'm hoping you can do something in this affair.
>
> I am, Yours faithfully SA Mullins,
> 94 George St. South Deniliquin NSW.[2]

To be excluded from hotel service was a crippling social disadvantage that drove people to buy inferior types of liquor at black market prices. Writing on race relations on the north coast of New South Wales in the 1950s, Malcolm Calley (1957: 198) explained that:

---

2   Letter dated 17 February 1943. Australian Archives A461 U/300/1.

Being unable to buy alcohol in any public house is a far more serious social disability than appears at first sight … The evening 'session' in the bar is the only occasion on which members of every stratum of the community meet on a footing of equality, to gossip, to conduct business and often to arrange and issue invitations to … social gatherings, sports meetings, functions … In any small country town the hotel is the hub around which the life of the district revolves.

At around the same time, Jeremy Beckett (1958: 249) observed, succinctly, that the hotel was a 'visible expression' of Aboriginal people's peculiar, underprivileged status. The pub was the locus of power in small towns. As Ann McGrath (1993: 109) noted:

To enter [the pub] freely was a constant reminder of inequality. Only via the patronage of white men (or exempted men, if they dared risk it) could they obtain liquor. Removal of restrictions promised a status alongside white men. Access to alcohol meant access to power.

There was also the anomalous (and ridiculous) situation in which an Aboriginal person could legally drink in a hotel in one state and not in another. An Aboriginal taxi driver told Elizabeth Eggleston (1976: 218) that it was marvellous to be free to go into the pub in Darwin, but that when he was back in his home state of Western Australia, his status changed. Once drinking rights were gained, sitting down and drinking in a hotel was seen as recognition of equality and *civil* rights: for people living in the camps and shanty conditions of most town reserves—tin shacks and mud floors—the hotels were warm, dry and comfortable (Kamien 1978, Chesterman 2005). The granting of drinking rights did not eliminate all discrimination: for example, Indigenous ex-servicemen were still refused membership of RSL clubs. This was something that the Student Action for Aborigines' (SAFA) 'Freedom Riders' campaigned against in New South Wales in the 1960s (Curthoys 2002).[3] An Aboriginal man may have fought in the war or been fully employed in the post-war years, but he would still be refused service. Those who received service were often served in segregated areas of hotels via a side door. Even if they held exemption certificates, which, in most states, provided legal exemption from the provisions of the Aborigines Act, Aboriginal people

---

3   Organised by students from the University of Sydney, the Freedom Ride toured country towns in northern New South Wales in February 1965; they picketed and campaigned against discrimination and segregation in swimming pools, rural hotels and RSL clubs.

of mixed descent could still be refused service in hotels because white patrons would refuse to drink with them.[4] Dress requirements were also used to keep Aboriginal people out.

The patent unfairness of this situation was captured in the experiences of Aboriginal activist and politician Charles Perkins, whose personal history was marked by several alcohol-related incidents; however, he was not a drinker himself. In the 1950s, at a time when Perkins was becoming a significant sportsperson (a footballer and a cricketer), he recalled being refused service of a soft drink in a Port Adelaide pub. The barman served him, grudgingly, through a side window while Perkins's white cricket teammates drank inside (Perkins 1975: 56, Read 2001: 54–5). The humiliation of this incident lasted a lifetime. Perkins's experiences as a member of the Freedom Ride in 1965 confirmed that Aboriginal people in outback New South Wales were experiencing similar humiliations.[5] He observed that:

> They were not allowed in any of the hotels and they had to get their beer and were sold cheap plonk through the back windows at three times the price, through sly-grogging operations. (Perkins 1975: 76)

The Freedom Riders demonstrated outside hotels that discriminated against Aboriginal people; in doing so, they saw their role as 'liberating' hotels and clubs from the colour bar. Perkins described the Freedom Ride as a new idea and a new way of promoting a rapid change in racial attitudes in Australia: 'I felt I might have been lacking courage in the face of this kind of prejudice', he explained, '[so] I decided … to try and beat the system' (56).

One of the New South Wales towns targeted by the Freedom Ride was Walgett. After World War II, the town had initially welcomed back its Aboriginal servicemen at the RSL club; subsequently, they were banned from drinking there. The Freedom Riders arrived at Walgett 20 years later to find that publicans and the RSL were still discriminating against Aboriginal people; the Oasis Hotel had a sign on the door of the bar lounge that stated 'Aborigines admitted only by invertation' [sic]. The Freedom Riders, mostly students from the University of Sydney, picketed

---

4   As mentioned in Chapter 3, these Acts were a complex mix of exemption and citizenship, with varying preconditions and criteria in each state (Chesterman 2005).
5   Charles Perkins was president of SAFA; the Freedom Riders took their inspiration from the Reverend Martin Luther King.

the Walgett RSL club and were confronted by a crowd of angry white townspeople: heated debate and heckling ensued. Later that night, as they left the town, a local grazier's son driving a Dodge truck forced the students' bus to swerve off the road (Curthoys 2002). Aboriginal locals found the protest confronting: Ted Fields, a local Aboriginal man, recalled that discussing contentious issues, such as alcohol consumption and other sensitive racial issues, in public 'scared the life out of us' (Zagar 2000: 116). However, in the wake of the protest, *New Dawn* magazine[6] reported that the Freedom Ride had brought about big changes in towns like Walgett and Moree: at the Oasis Hotel, Aboriginal and white people could be seen having a drink together, 'purely out of friendship' (*New Dawn* 1971: 1). Perkins continued his activism on his return to Sydney, staging a 'drink-in' at the Burlington Hotel in Haymarket. He and a group of Aboriginal men and some Freedom Riders met for a drink there as an act of defiance. Their photograph was printed in the *Sydney Morning Herald*.[7]

Considering this history of overt and covert discrimination against Indigenous people, it is hardly surprising that, with the advent of self-determination policies and emphasis on employment and training, when government support became available, communities started talking about buying pubs themselves. It was believed that owning their own outlets would enable Indigenous groups to tackle racist practices, provide appropriate amenities and welcome Indigenous customers. As it turned out, Perkins was to play a pivotal role in this endeavour. After serving as deputy secretary of the DAA, he became inaugural chair of the ADC in 1980;[8] he held this part-time position for four years before becoming an acting commissioner. From March 1984 to November 1988, he was secretary of the DAA. Undoubtedly influential, Perkins's personal history and optimism drove his support for the purchase of hotels and clubs.

Evidently, Perkins and other bureaucrats did not perceive any moral hazards in Aboriginal ownership of hotels. Owing to the deregulation trends of the 1980s, alcohol was already becoming more freely available in Australia. The thinking behind Aboriginal ownership was that these sales might as well be in Aboriginal hands, as this would remove the risk of racial discrimination at the point of sale, and enable an Aboriginal

6 *New Dawn* was published by the New South Wales Aborigines Welfare Board.
7 *Sydney Morning Herald* 30 March 1965.
8 The ADC had nine other commissioners, including Gatjil Djerrkura, deputy chairman, and Lois O'Donoghue, who later became chairperson of ATSIC.

entity to reap the financial rewards, rather than an outsider. There was a strongly held view that Aboriginal drinking problems were historically determined—that they derived from past prohibition policies, and from past and present experiences of racism and discrimination in hotels and clubs. Surely, if Aboriginal people themselves owned the premises, this would help to prevent a kind of reactive alcohol abuse?

The idea of Aboriginal people buying into a hotel had been raised in 1971, by Prime Minister John Gorton, who proposed that the Yirrkala Aboriginal community in northeast Arnhem Land buy a share in the new Walkabout Hotel in Nhulunbuy, a mining town on the Gove Peninsula.[9] However, given that the Yirrkala community had repeatedly, vociferously and unsuccessfully *opposed* the granting of a licence to the Walkabout Hotel, the CAA was 'disgusted' by the suggestion. Interpreted charitably, one could argue that perhaps the prime minister believed that owning a share would confer some control over sales to Yirrkala people.

Case studies

The Finke Hotel, Finke, Northern Territory

The first purchase of a licensed hotel by an Aboriginal group was in 1975 at Finke in the Northern Territory. It was the only hotel in town. A siding on the railway line linking central Australia to the south, Finke had a small population that included several Torres Strait Islander railway employees as well as other gangers and Aboriginal people. The local pastoralists all drank at the Finke Hotel. Uniting Church worker, Margaret Bain, recalled the effect of excluding Aboriginal men:

> Many [Aboriginal] men from Finke were stockmen. When the muster was over, they'd be turned off—and the white men who'd been working with them, they'd go into the hotel and drink and the boss would go into the hotel, and the Aboriginal workers weren't allowed in.[10] They [Aboriginal men] thought that what men were doing had a kind of religious significance. It was like a ceremony, part of the cattle business. They could join in everything, except for that last part of the ceremony. They felt inferior, juvenile, if you know what I mean. They had done the ceremony

9   B Dexter, pers comm, 2005.
10   Although Aboriginal people were not allowed to drink at the hotel, one or two local people were employed there as domestics; they received £3 a week plus food and clothing.

all the way until the 'king hit'. They would have had a relationship [with another stockman] and all of a sudden that was chopped off. [After the law was changed] it was *significant* when they were allowed [to drink]— it was more than an invitation—it was 'be one of us' sort of thing.[11]

Jim Downing, another Uniting Church worker, agreed with Bain that when Aboriginal drinking rights came in 'there was a push from people who thought that now they were citizens they *should* drink—people started to drink like the pastoralists did. [There were] tremendous brawls and injuries'.[12] The Finke Hotel held a 24-hour licence and sold flagons of cheap wine. Heavy drinking among the Aboriginal population undermined work practices, and relations between Aboriginal people and police were said to be worsening in the township, where the only consistent employment was provided by a housing parts factory.

Change came with the innovative Whitlam Labor Government in 1972: the policy of self-determination was introduced and the DAA was established, with Perkins appointed assistant secretary. According to Bain, the idea to buy the Finke Hotel, which had been on the market for some time, came from two local Aboriginal men[13] and Northern Territory politician Bernie Kilgariff.[14] The 'driving force' behind the purchase seems to have been Kilgariff. He recalled how the two 'old men' asked him for a yarn about the hotel:

> 'That man at the hotel is a bad bugger, he is killing our people. We want to buy that hotel.' They said: 'you gotta go and get that money from that government man' [Senator] Cavanagh. I knew him from South Australia. I went to see him and told him about the Aputula mob: 'They want to buy this hotel', He said, 'you're kidding'. 'No, they want to bring it under control.' He said, 'all right you can have that money but you've got to be part of the board—when it all goes broke I'll have you to blame'.[15]

---

11   M Bain, pers comm, 2004. Bain had visited Finke regularly with the supply truck that drove across from Ernabella Mission to collect supplies arriving by train; she eventually lived at Finke.

12   J Downing, pers comm, 2004.

13   One was Toby Ginger, a Pitjantjatjara man.

14   Kilgariff founded the CLP and became the first Speaker of the Legislative Assembly and Member for Alice Springs, later a Senator. Bill Ferguson described him as the 'driving force' behind the purchase of the Finke Hotel. Ferguson later became the manager of the Tyeweretye Club, Alice Springs (see Chapter 5) (pers comm, 6 August 2008).

15   Bernie Kilgariff, interview, Alice Springs, 8 August 2008.

Letters were written to arrange the funds. Jim Cavanagh, Minister for Aboriginal Affairs, agreed to the purchase: this was before the advent of the ADC.[16] With a federal grant of $30,000, a holding deposit of $1,000 raised from the community's own funds and Kilgariff's support, the Aputula Social Club bought the Finke Hotel. Senator Cavanagh hoped that owning the pub would help Aboriginal elders at Finke to control the drinking problem, and also improve race relations in the town. He thought the plan had a 'strong chance of achieving its goals providing certain strict conditions attached to the grant were met'.[17] It is important to point out that this purchase took place in the period before Aboriginal groups and liquor licensing authorities began to negotiate in earnest about alcohol restrictions: subsequently, certain conditions of sale were either written into the licences held by individual premises or were informally agreed to by licensees. Arrangements such as these, which usually target takeaway sales, were not common prior to the 1980s.[18] For the Aboriginal community at Finke, buying the hotel was the only solution to the problem of unconstrained sales. Downing believed that, in the case of Finke, most aspirations for ownership cohered around the control over sales:

> People said if they bought the pub, then they could control it. Bernie Kilgariff helped. It was the people's idea to buy the pub there so they bought it, and said we won't sell takeaway, we won't sell takeaway to our blokes. The fellas would go off at lunchtime, so they restricted it to evenings only; it worked up to a point.

It was unusual enough for the *Daily Telegraph* in Sydney to run a story on the hotel's Aboriginal buyers, headlined 'Blacks will buy the only pub in town':

> If you're clean and decently dressed you'll be welcome to a beer at the Finke Hotel, no matter what the color of your skin. The pub is the only watering hole in Finke, a tiny railway settlement about 321 km south of Alice Springs ... The elder of the Aboriginal community saw the purchase of the hotel as a means of regulating ... drinking. (*Daily Telegraph* 1975)

---

16   It is unclear whether Charles Perkins was involved in the Finke Hotel decision, although later he fully supported Aboriginal purchases of hotels. His relationship with Jim Cavanagh was fraught (Australian Dictionary of Biography 2007).

17   DAA (1975). Media release, JC/178, 1 May.

18   At the time, the Northern Territory had a Licensing Court presided over by a Licensing Magistrate. The Northern Territory Liquor Commission was established in 1979, along with a new Liquor Act that gave the Commission many flexible powers. In South Australia, the first restricted licence was issued in March 1981 to a hotel at Marla Bore in the far north of the state: at the request of the Aboriginal community, the sale of takeaway liquor is prohibited, except to lodgers or bona fide travellers.

A non-Aboriginal man from Alice Springs was hired as the manager, and a hotel management board, with eight Aboriginal community members, four non-Aboriginal members and two members of the Legislative Assembly of the Northern Territory, was established. The board's first act was to ban off-premises sales of wine and spirits, resulting, reportedly, in a decline in hotel profits and a rise in store profits (Downing 1976: 1147). Four years later, the intensity of violence and the disruption of sleep and work had diminished, and any troublemakers were 'disciplined' by the Aboriginal council.

Significantly, there had been no reference to the hotel becoming a source of locally generated funds or jobs once it was Aboriginal owned. Kilgariff recalled that there were no Aboriginal drinkers *in* the pub itself (in the early days at least); consequently, it appears that the purchase of the hotel was not associated with a campaign to teach 'civilised' drinking on premises. In 1979, Superintendent Symons of the South Australian police claimed that, although there was still intoxication and fighting at Finke (despite Aboriginal ownership of the hotel), the community was more settled; he used the Finke Hotel to support his argument in favour of extending the sale of beer at the Yalata community canteen.[19] A local resident of Finke, Torres Strait Islander Harold Matasia, remembered things differently: there was too much fighting and 'kids crying' when the people owned the pub, he claimed.[20]

In the long run, the Finke Hotel did not survive. When, in 1980, the railway line (the Ghan) linking Finke to the outside world was rerouted, and the road to another source of alcohol (at Kulgera) was improved, the manager of the Finke Hotel decided to let his stocks run down. The community raised no objections and the hotel eventually closed. The original stone building was renovated and is now the Shire office.

The Oasis, Walgett, New South Wales

In 1983, nearly two decades after the Freedom Riders' confrontation at Walgett, the ADC, with Perkins as chair, acquired the Oasis Hotel for around $450,000. The hotel was leased to Gamilarai Ltd, an Aboriginal community company instituted for the purpose of managing the hotel.

---

19 HD Symons, South Australian Police to BJ Powell, Regional Director, DAA, Adelaide, 19 March 1979, DAA files, South Australia.
20 D Nash, pers comm, 2009.

Accounting firm Coopers and Lybrand recommended that the ADC purchase the nearby Imperial Hotel instead, as it had better trading results: also, its relationship with Tooheys Brewery meant that staff would be trained by brewery-sponsored supervisors (Commonwealth of Australia 1989a: 21). However, owning the Imperial Hotel lacked the symbolic value of owning the Oasis; it is difficult not to assume that sweet, symbolic justice, motivated the purchase.

The ADC's stated purpose in buying the Oasis was to provide employment and training for 12 Aboriginal staff and to enhance social and economic development (Commonwealth of Australia 1989a). There was vague talk of controlling sales, but this seemed an illogical rationale to some local Aboriginal people. Echoing the early arguments of temperance advocates against the establishment of community or 'Gothenburg-style' hotels, one Aboriginal town councillor in Walgett commented that he could not 'understand why they'd want to buy a hotel in Walgett … if you're going to try and resolve the alcohol problem you wouldn't go and buy a pub!'[21]

Almost from the outset, there were problems of governance and management at the Oasis Hotel, with sales either not charged or undercharged, cash receipts not going into the till and stock being removed from the premises. There were eight different (non-Aboriginal) managers over a five-year period and the hotel lost around $10,000 per month. The Commonwealth Audit Office found that Aboriginal directors had interfered in the day-to-day running of the hotel—to the point of harassment of managers; had paid themselves unauthorised sitting fees; and had breached their statutory duties by failing to lodge company tax returns. The Audit Office rebuked the ADC, commenting that public funds of around $1 million dollars could have been spent 'more carefully and productively' (Commonwealth of Australia 1989a: 23). The Oasis Hotel continued to require financial assistance until it was sold to non-Aboriginal interests.

The Transcontinental, Oodnadatta, South Australia

In 1986, the ADC was involved in another hotel purchase, this time at Oodnadatta in South Australia. Like Finke, Oodnadatta was an outback railway town that had provided limited employment for Aboriginal

---

21   ABC Radio National, AM, transcript, 13 January 2000.

people until it was bypassed by the railway in 1981. The town had a small population of between 100 and 200, more than half of which was Indigenous. Buying the hotel was the initiative of George and Maude Tongerie, a local Aboriginal couple who were qualified welfare workers. When the Department of Community Welfare withdrew from the town, George Tongerie became the community adviser, setting up a self-help program of 'outstanding enterprise' (Mattingly 1988: 212).[22] The Tongeries (both non-drinkers) conceived taking over the Transcontinental Hotel as an alcohol-control measure—a solution to the upsetting number of alcohol-related deaths in the town. The purchase seemed 'all in God's plan', according to George Tongerie:

> Well, Charlie Perkins was at a meeting at Port Augusta. But we didn't know that. And we were at a meeting at the other end of the same building. And anyway, we came out of the meeting and bumped into Charlie Perkins, and of course we said, 'Charlie, we don't know what to do! [about the drinking]. They haven't given us any funding, we haven't got anything there we can start with … the only thing we can do is buy the hotel to have control', and he said 'well, how much do you want to buy the pub?' and I told him, and he got his secretary to go and get his briefcase … He was secretary of the ADC. He's like us, he was brought up in the camp, like us. So we bought the pub, we set up a board of directors, and Maude and I are still on it.[23]

Perkins was an acting commissioner at the ADC at the time and secretary of the DAA.[24] Whatever the truth of the matter, it is clear that the Tongeries *believed* that Perkins was the person who made the purchase happen. The Oodnadatta Aboriginal Housing Society, which had been a driving force behind local social improvements, was renamed Dunjiba Community Council; it became the owner of the hotel on behalf of the community. With the backing of the community, Dunjiba also bought the licensed general store and post office, the railway station and several houses. The ADC Annual Report does not give details of the cost of the hotel, merely noting that it was 'funded'.

---

22 George Tongerie (1925–2013) was brought up at Colebrook Home, which moved from Oodnadatta to Quorn. He knew Charles Perkins from their time together with the Aboriginal Progress Association in Adelaide in the 1960s.
23 George Tongerie, interview, 11 March 2008.
24 Shirley McPherson was Chair of the ADC at the time of the Transcontinental Hotel purchase.

George Tongerie and other senior community members at Oodnadatta saw owning the hotel as a means of controlling sales, especially the sale of fortified wine (port) that came in 2 L glass flagons. With its high alcohol content and sweet taste, port was the (troublesome) drink of choice for many Aboriginal drinkers. Maude Tongerie recalled that the drinkers 'were having flagons for breakfast'. A local doctor reported that alcohol-related injuries and trauma were common causes of visits to the Oodnadatta hospital (Johnston 1991). Once it owned the hotel and the general store, the first action of the Dunjiba Community Council was to get rid of the flagons that were being sold from the store in the hours before the hotel opened for on-premises drinking. The council staged a spectacular and symbolic act of destruction:

> The first job—we had to get someone to dig a hole, a great big pit. We brought out all the plonk from the store. The boys lined them all out and guess what they were doing all day, for half a day? Shooting them down this big hole! The damage—the 'red ned'—all down the big hole!

After this, both the hotel and the store were restricted to selling a maximum of two bottles of beer per person per day over the counter, and the premises were closed at 8 pm. It was agreed that wine and spirits would be available to non-Aboriginal patrons of the hotel dining room only. No formal training or advice was provided to the Aboriginal board on alcohol policy, governance matters or hotel management—'we just used common sense', Maude Tongerie explained. She recalled that they actively encouraged people to eat before drinking alcohol: 'I said, if you're going to have your drinkies, have your *mai*, have your *mai*'.[25] She also advised patrons to have a rest and a shower before going for a drink; however, apart from this, there is little evidence of any conscious attempt at teaching moderation. Instead, Maude and George led by example:

> We were the only two non-drinkers [at first]. It was only down the line that we got more non-drinkers on there, because once we went there and we were their auntie and uncle drinking lemonade and cold water.

Two years after buying the hotel, the Dunjiba Community Council applied to declare the areas in town where the children played 'alcohol free' (*Adelaide Advertiser* 1988: 4). These early attempts at harm reduction were accompanied by welfare strategies and other initiatives, such as arranging for people to have better access to second-hand clothes, and

---

25   *Mai* = food from plants or food generally, or 'whitefella' food.

providing curtains for their houses to give people a psychological 'lift'. The extent to which these strategies worked can be seen in the report of the Royal Commission into Aboriginal Deaths in Custody (Langton et al. 1991), which noted that the Aboriginal community at Oodnadatta had moved from relative dependence with no land and no economic base in the 1950s, to a position in which they owned business enterprises and 40 houses and had a strong community council.[26] The store and the hotel both employed Aboriginal people, even though they were managed by non-Aboriginal people. Although there have been no formal evaluations of the effect of Aboriginal ownership of the Transcontinental Hotel, the restrictions were judged successful by observers who commented on Aboriginal people's improved health and drinking habits (Shaw & Gibson 1988: 170, Mattingly 1988: 212).

The purchase of the Transcontinental Hotel owes more to George and Maude Tongerie's temperance leanings, and fortuitous connection with Charles Perkins, than any considered government strategy to regulate alcohol sales or support Aboriginal self-determination. George Tongerie knew Perkins from their time together in the Aboriginal Progress Association in Adelaide in the 1960s. George was an ex-serviceman, Justice of the Peace and Member of the Order of Australia: he was celebrated enough that when he died in 2013, the Premier of South Australia attended his memorial service. Maude was a non-drinker who, while not being an official member of the WCTU in South Australia, was clearly known to them, as she features in a WCTU publication celebrating Aboriginal women pathfinders who served their communities (Beeson 1980: 61); she was also a Member of the Order of Australia.

Woden Town Club, Canberra, Australian Capital Territory

In 1988, the ADC guaranteed loans for the development of a licensed Aboriginal club in Canberra, the Woden Town Club—a controversial decision enabling returns not only from alcohol but also from poker machines.[27] Several government offices, including the DAA, were located in Woden, and the club was designed to attract Indigenous public servants

---

26   Comments made by Commissioner Elliott Johnston (1991).
27   I have included the Woden Town Club in this discussion of hotels as it differs from other Aboriginal social clubs that are primarily within discrete, remote Aboriginal communities.

from around the country who lived in Canberra. Perkins supported the development of the club and became its president, thus fulfilling his long-held desire for a club for Aboriginal people. Aware that there were numerous clubs for different ethnic groups in Australian cities (e.g. Croatian clubs, Italian clubs, Greek clubs), Perkins had long wanted a similar-style club for Aboriginal people.[28]

The ADC approved a grant of $286,300 to the Aboriginal Corporation for Sporting and Recreational Activities, and a loan of $100,000 for refurbishment and renovation of the club premises. Established in the windowless basement of Bonner House, a building owned by the ADC, the club opened in June 1988. The premises soon ran into serious financial difficulty, incurring losses of $10,000 a month. Subsequently, the club, and Perkins himself, became enmeshed in controversy over the role of the ADC in the purchase of poker machines for the premises (Christie & Young 2011).[29] The Minister for Aboriginal Affairs, Gerry Hand, asked for an audit and an investigation into the ADC's role in the purchases of the Woden Town Club and the Oasis Hotel in Walgett. As a result, Perkins's actions were subjected to intense scrutiny by the Senate Estimates Committee and the Audit Office.

Characteristically, the Audit Office was more interested in the viability of these enterprises than their social benefits; it found that the ADC had not satisfied itself that the Aboriginal owners were capable of engaging in the enterprise, as required by the *Aboriginal Development Commission Act 1980* (Commonwealth of Australia 1989a, 1989b). At the Senate Estimates Committee hearing, CLP Senator Grant Tambling (Northern Territory) was particularly unrelenting in his pursuit of Perkins, suggesting that it was irresponsible to have used 'taxpayers' money' to start the Woden Town Club when so many other clubs were failing. Perkins replied, with asperity, that 'Blacks are taxpayers as well, which some people tend to forget'. Further, he argued that the club had only just opened, that it usually took around two years for such a venue to get on its feet, and that the original grant had been spent on renovations because the previous owner had left the place in a 'shambles'. Teething problems were only to be expected. Another senator's question, about who the club was for, gave Perkins an opportunity to explain the club's purpose:

28 See *Fire Talker,* a documentary about Perkins's life by Ivan Sen (2008).
29 The club acquired 47 poker machines, something that would raise eyebrows today in view of current concerns about the damage caused by Aboriginal people's use of poker machines.

It is a club for Aboriginal people and their friends. Everybody is welcome down there. You have two other clubs near there which compete for clientele, and that is natural enough … There is not one Aboriginal club in Australia. We want to start one because we think it is important for Aboriginal people to have some facility where they can go, where they know there are standards set, in terms of dress and behaviour, by Aboriginal people, by the board.[30]

Unconvinced, the Audit Office criticised the ADC for funding projects that placed 'undue' emphasis on employment opportunities and on creating social facilities for Aboriginal people, rather than focusing on business activities. As Perkins explained, the club was intended, at least partly, as a venue for inculcating moderation and standards of social behaviour. However, the Audit Office did not attach importance to these social goals. The Woden Town Club went into liquidation and closed after six months, making it impossible to observe its social impact, either beneficial or detrimental (Christie & Young 2011). Unlike the 'Aboriginal' hotels in rural communities such as Oodnadatta or Finke, and the community-based licensed social clubs in discrete remote communities in the Northern Territory or Queensland, the Woden Town Club lacked a local community of interest that could mobilise to support the project.[31]

Mt Ebenezer Roadhouse, Northern Territory

In 1987, the Pitjantjatjara-speaking community of Imanpa in the Northern Territory bought Mt Ebenezer Roadhouse on the Lasseter Highway. The highway took tourist traffic from the Stuart Highway south of Alice Springs to the motels and resorts at Uluru. The Imanpa community made the purchase with no assistance from the ADC.

Imanpa was a new community, formed when local pastoralists, the Kunoths, offered to excise a living area for Pitjantjatjara-speaking people from their station; they chose an area away from the highway and roadhouse in the hope of dismantling a drinking camp that had developed there. The roadhouse had a monopoly on sales of alcohol

---

30   Perkins was omitting the 'clubs' located on remote communities in the Northern Territory and the taverns in Queensland communities in saying that there was not one Aboriginal club in Australia, parlinfo.aph.gov.au/parlInfo/search/display/display.w3p;query=Id:committees%2Festimate%2Fecomd881026a_ece.out%2F0025.

31   After this episode, Perkins was dismissed from his DAA position by Gerry Hand, but was later exonerated of any wrongdoing.

to Aboriginal people in the region. By 1980, Aboriginal drinking had become sufficiently problematic for the Liquor Commission to persuade the licensee to suspend takeaway sales. At one stage, the Aboriginal community considered establishing a licensed club at Imanpa, as a way of counteracting the sale of beer from the roadhouse, and they asked the Liquor Commission for advice on setting one up. Their request was not answered, and the community lost interest. Instead, in 1987, the community bought the Mt Ebenezer Roadhouse by raising funds for a deposit through profits from the store at Imanpa, and via contributions from a community 'chuck-in' system (Tangentyere Council 1991: 97–8). The store had been established with help from Uniting Church advisers; its purpose was to pay for the community's essential services and maintenance. Imanpa's financial integrity qualified it for a bank loan of $500,000. This was paid to the community's company, Lisanote Pty Ltd, which became the owner of the roadhouse. The people of Imanpa were proud of managing this without any government support.

The aims of the purchase were threefold: to help Imanpa people secure an economic base; to raise funds for the purchase of a nearby cattle station; and to reduce the harm from alcohol sales (Pitjantjatjara Council 1990: 35–9): in other words, a mixture of economic and social goals. Once the community owned the premises, new rules were put in place; the non-Aboriginal manager was directed to de-emphasise liquor sales and to focus on catering to tour buses by improving the décor, providing food and selling locally made Aboriginal artefacts. Lisanote's additional liquor restrictions included a six-can takeaway limit for Imanpa people, restricting alcohol sales to the late afternoon and stopping all sales on request during ceremonies or community festivities. Ownership of the premises gave community members the freedom to introduce a harm-reduction strategy that, while unusual, was culturally appropriate; a list of names of non-drinkers who had *asked the licensee to prevent them from buying alcohol* was posted so that they could not be pressured to buy alcoholic beverages for their drinking relatives (Pitjantjatjara Council 1990: 39). This request represented a peculiarly Aboriginal form of social control, in which individuals externalise authority—by giving it to an individual or a regulation—to take the socially awkward step of refusing requests (Brady 2004: 116). It is unlikely that any ordinary hotel or roadhouse that was not community owned would agree to implement such a policy.

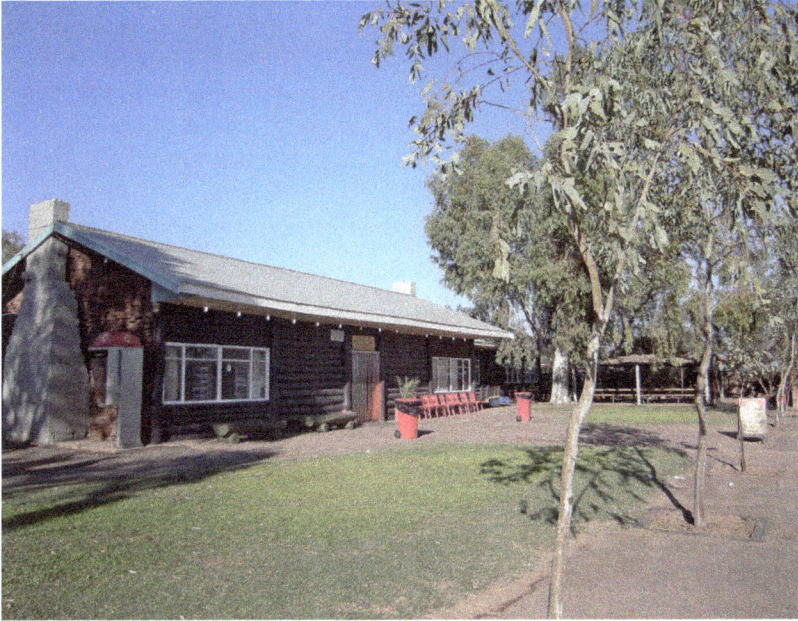

Fig. 23 Mt Ebenezer Roadhouse, Lasseter Highway, 2009
Source: M Brady

Unknowingly, the Imanpa community's priorities—to de-emphasise liquor sales and to improve sales of food—echoed the ideals of the Gothenburg system of alcohol control. However, these locally created social-control initiatives were soon undermined by the liberal sales practices of two competing roadhouses. In 1988, a roadhouse at Curtin Springs to the west, changed its previous, more restrained practice, and began selling greater volumes of takeaway beer to local Aboriginal people. In 1989, Erldunda Roadhouse, located to the east of Imanpa, applied for a takeaway licence. In a vain attempt to keep the region relatively 'dry', the Imanpa community and the Pitjantjatjara Council objected to Erldunda's application. However, given that the Imanpa community owned a similar outlet at Mt Ebenezer, its objection was complicated to argue and difficult to sustain. The Northern Territory Liquor Commission was not sympathetic. It noted, derisively, that the community had 'its own liquor outlet'; that out of 40 adult males, only two were non-drinkers; and that most of the drinkers had severe alcohol problems. Disagreeing that the addition of a takeaway licence at Erldunda would attract Aboriginal people, the Liquor Commission granted Erldunda an unconditional takeaway licence (Rae 1989). Alcohol-related injuries to Imanpa people increased following the end of the virtual monopoly that Mt Ebenezer had enjoyed. The uncontrolled sales of takeaway beer along the Lasseter Highway precipitated a long campaign for sales restrictions led by the NPY Women's Council (Lyon 1991, d'Abbs et al. 1999, Brady 2005: 132). The Women's Council eventually succeeded in prompting an inquiry by the Race Discrimination Commissioner into non-discriminatory mechanisms for restricting alcohol sales to residents of Aboriginal communities in the region. The Women's Council eventually persuaded the roadhouse at Curtin Springs to try various restriction regimes (Race Discrimination Commissioner 1995).

Imanpa faced many problems in the 1990s, not all related to alcohol consumption or ownership of the Mt Ebenezer Roadhouse. For example, there were governance and accountability problems related to debts accruing from the purchase of a cattle station; community indifference regarding governance; stealing from the community store; and problems with staff. The community board continued to instruct the roadhouse manager to implement alcohol-management regimes; however, at least one manager expressed frustration that he did not have the freedom to apply any of his previous experience of running a licensed club in an Aboriginal community—he was 'just the publican' with no power. By May 2009,[32] a four-can limit of full-strength takeaway beer was in place, and the arrangement worked well; a community member managed the list of names of ineligible drinkers as well as a list of those who were banned for bad behaviour. For such an arrangement to work, the keeper of the lists has to be tough and consistent: inevitably, they had to deal with either close kin or long-term companions. Imanpa was fortunate in having competent leaders, including several women, who were prepared to involve themselves in these roles. The community council also put in place a number of other limitations. For example, it was decided that Aboriginal people should not use the roadhouse dining room and should consume their beer allowance away from the roadhouse—partly to prevent them importuning tourists for more beer. Another limitation put in place by the Aboriginal council was that alcohol could not be supplied to residents of the Anangu Pitjantjatjara Yankunytjatjara lands. These limitations undoubtedly affected the profitability of the enterprise.

32   The author made a field visit to Mt Ebenezer in 2009; further information and background was provided by Norman Steele, Glendle Schrader and Matthew Ellem of Wana Ungkunytja, and Richard Preece.

By the late 2000s, Mt Ebenezer Roadhouse was not trading well, and was using all surplus funds to clear a large debt that had accrued over several years. As well as having difficulty creating the economic base that people had hoped for originally, the roadhouse suffered from the Global Financial Crisis, which resulted in a change in the type of tourists it attracted. After 2008, there were fewer international visitors, and more Australian 'grey nomads' who tended to cater for themselves. In March 2012, the roadhouse became insolvent and closed. It reopened in October 2013. In conjunction with the Ngaanyatjarra Council, the Imanpa community decided to try a new arrangement in which it still owned the land and the roadhouse buildings, but was no longer involved in the business itself. The business was leased to a branch of the Ngaanyatjarra Council (Indervon), which employed managers and took over the liquor licence.[33]

The aim was (and is) to use the lease money to pay off old debts; once the business becomes viable again, it will be returned to community ownership. Ngaanyatjarra Council is an Aboriginal organisation concerned with the wellbeing of Aboriginal people. This means that, although the Imanpa community no longer has a direct role in running the roadhouse, the present managers still act in the interests of Aboriginal people. By mutual agreement with the community, they stopped selling takeaway alcohol as a separate item. To be eligible to buy four cans of beer, all customers (including those on tour buses) must first purchase hot food to be consumed on the premises. Owning the roadhouse has not been easy, and the expected financial rewards have not been forthcoming; however, as has been the case in several other instances, Aboriginal ownership has enabled a measure of local control over alcohol sales. The roadhouse artefacts shop and gallery cuts out unscrupulous traders, and gives Aboriginal craftspeople a fair return for their work.

Another instance of a community attempting to constrain a troublesome outlet by buying it was at Daly River, where, in the late 1970s, two Aboriginal communities, Peppimenarti and Daly River, had objected to the renewal of the liquor licence at the Daly River Hotel Motel. They argued that any licence in the area should be under Aboriginal control to regulate consumption. When the hotel was offered for sale, the Peppimenarti community applied for funds so that an Aboriginal association could purchase the facility as part of a tourism venture (Stanley

---

33 Indervon Petroleum Pty Ltd, is the fuel distribution arm of the Ngaanyatjarra Council (L Hewson, Manager, pers comm, 2014).

1985: 34). Their offer failed. In the late 1990s, the Nauiyu Nambiyu Aboriginal Corporation at Daly River purchased the Daly River Roadside Inn and caravan park.[34]

The Wayside Inn, Timber Creek, Northern Territory

In 1999, Aboriginal organisations bought into two licensed hotels at Timber Creek, a small remote township on the Victoria Highway between Katherine and Kununurra in the Northern Territory: the Wayside Inn and the Timber Creek Hotel. The township of Timber Creek lies between the East Kimberley of Western Australia and the Victoria River District of the Northern Territory, two regions popular with tourists. Timber Creek is also in the heart of pastoral country. Hence, hotel customers were often ringers, stockmen and cattle-truck drivers, as well as tourists and local Aboriginal people.

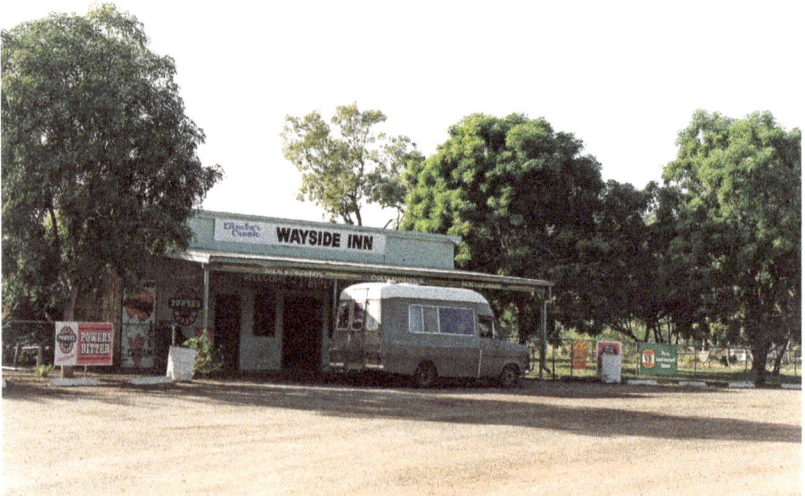

Fig. 24 The Wayside Inn, Timber Creek, 1991
Source: M Brady

The Timber Creek Hotel, which grew out of an original outback store known as Fogarty's, had a single air-conditioned front bar, a restaurant and a convenience store. Next door was the Wayside Inn, a licensed

---

34   At Fitzroy Crossing in Western Australia, the Aboriginal communities of the Fitzroy Valley purchased the Crossing Inn in 1988–89; this case is discussed in the next chapter.

roadhouse with a beer garden, petrol bowsers, tourist camp and small supermarket. The Wayside Inn was licensed to cater 24 hours a day to long-distance travellers. Its extended opening hours, limited restrictions, cheap grog and outdoor facilities where smoking was permitted made it popular with Aboriginal drinkers.

Two organisations representing Aboriginal communities in and around Timber Creek, the Ngaliwurru-Wuli Association and Gunamu Aboriginal Corporation, entered into a joint venture with the non-Aboriginal couple who owned both the Timber Creek Hotel and the Wayside Inn. The Aboriginal entities took a 50 per cent share in the Timber Creek Hotel and took over full ownership of the Wayside Inn, with the licence being issued to the Timber Creek Wayside Inn Joint Venture Pty Ltd. In what the Licensing Commission (2008) later referred to as an 'unusual' joint venture, two ostensibly competing, and adjoining, hotels were owned or part owned by the same Aboriginal entity, and were managed by the original owners and joint-venture partners. This complex arrangement was further complicated by the involvement of the two Aboriginal organisations, one of which (Gunamu Aboriginal Corporation) owned the title for the land on which the Wayside Inn stood,[35] while the other was responsible for management.

In previous years, the owner of the Timber Creek Hotel, Mr Fogarty, after consultation with the local community, had limited takeaway sales to six cans of beer, banned sales of wine and spirits to Aboriginal people and prohibited 'book up' (selling on credit). These initiatives had cost Fogarty 25 per cent of his sales (Legislative Assembly of the Northern Territory 1991: 151). Nevertheless, both outlets were lucrative. The gross profit from a small number of poker machines alone earned the Wayside Inn $133,000 (Northern Territory Department of Justice 2009: 119–26). In purchasing the Wayside Inn, the Aboriginal community entered into a business arrangement; additionally, it sought to use the opportunity to deal with binge drinking. The Inn's new owners barred unruly customers and experimented with alcohol-management strategies, such as restricting troublemakers to light beer for a certain period, as determined by a 'tribunal' led by an Aboriginal policewoman (who was also a member of the main landowning family) (*Weekend Australian* 2000: 1–2). New rules proscribed abuse of staff, fighting, refusing to leave the premises, bringing

---

35   The Indigenous Land Corporation transferred title for the 2 ha of land to Gunamu Aboriginal Corporation in July 1999 when the joint venture commenced.

weapons into the town, spitting, theft, humbugging, supplying to barred persons, bad debts, damage to property and disturbing the peace. The Inn was closed for ceremonies and funerals, as directed by the traditional owners (Bartlett & Duncan 2000: 229). It is difficult to know whether these interventions made a difference, because Aboriginal people drank at both hotels, which were virtually side-by-side.

The Wayside Inn had to repay a substantial loan, which meant that there was pressure on the manager to make money. It is unclear whether there were any profits remaining after expenses had been paid that could have been distributed for the benefit of local people, or upkeep of the property. The property, which was under attack from white ants (i.e. termites), did not get the maintenance it required.

In 2009, the original 10-year joint venture came to an end, and the traditional owners decided they wanted to own the Wayside Inn independently. The Ngaliwurru-Wuli Association announced on its website that it planned to take over management of the supermarket, tourist camp and adjoining Wayside Inn. However, according to the Licensing Commission, the previous licensee (i.e. the joint venture) had failed to transfer the licence to any new entity before it dissolved, and had also failed to submit redevelopment plans for the building itself. One or both Aboriginal organisations were responsible for material alterations, renovations and redevelopments, which (for licensed premises) required the agreement of the Liquor Commission. Licensing inspectors and lawyers repeatedly tried and failed to resolve these issues (Northern Territory Licensing Commission 2010a). Meanwhile, white ants, which are endemic in the Northern Territory, continued to eat the Wayside Inn, transforming what was already a complex situation into a disastrous one. A decision was made by Ngaliwurru-Wuli to pull down the dilapidated building and restart the business in another form.

The situation descended into farce. The building was demolished but Ngaliwurru-Wuli failed to obtain building permissions or a properly qualified project manager; a new concrete slab poured at the site of the demolished pub turned out to be non-compliant and unusable. No one, including the Licensing Commission, knew who held the licence of the (non-existent, white-ant consumed) hotel. Without informing or consulting with its lawyer, Ngaliwurru-Wuli decided to relinquish the liquor licence; in July 2010, in a fax to the Licensing Commission, it announced that the board did *not* wish to continue with the transfer of the licence.[36] On these instructions, in September 2010, the Licensing Commission cancelled the gaming machine and liquor licences of the Wayside Inn under a section of the Liquor Act that states that cancellation can occur if the premises have not been used for the sale of alcohol for a period of 90 days.[37] Why Ngaliwurru-Wuli surrendered its valuable liquor licence rather than organise an interim arrangement for alcohol sales, or transfer the licence to another entity, is unknown. There is no annual fee for a liquor licence, which means there was no financial disincentive for the organisation to have the licence suspended rather than cancelled. The decision appeared illogical to both Aboriginal and non-Aboriginal observers, not least because a 24-hour liquor licence is worth a considerable sum. An Aboriginal community member who had been positive about the extra controls made possible by local ownership, was taken aback at the demise of the licence:

> I don't know why the licence got sent back! We had restrictions in our own way because we [were] the licence holder. We say 'don't serve to particular people'; if [there were] domestics, leader would come up and say 'you are banned from the pub'. It was really good. Now if you want to not serve people it's complicated. [After a death] people would ask 'you mob shut down while we grieve, one or two days?' It happened quite often. I don't understand why Ngaliwurru gave it back … We got bad advice from legals and I know the community wanted the development because the building was falling apart, we wanted to make a more welcoming 24-hour licence. At the time when [joint-venture partner] and his family had it, the building was run down. The directors said we're not renewing the agreement in 2009 because of this. We got a floor plan drawn up, concrete etc. I told [Ngaliwurru-Wuli director] 'We can keep licence on hold until we build a new setup'. But the CEO they had, gave bad advice and let the licence go. I was in Darwin when this happened. They didn't get any advice. I was not called to give evidence at the cancelling hearing.[38]

The disappearance of the Wayside Inn deprived the travelling public of the four basic services that such licensees are required to deliver 24 hours a day (food, accommodation, fuel and hospitality). Wayside inns are still

---

36 The President of the Ngaliwurru-Wuli Association sent a fax to the Liquor Commission on 22 July 2010 to this effect (Northern Territory Liquor Commission 2010b: 3).

37 The Timber Creek Wayside Inn Joint Venture Pty Ltd was finally deregistered by ASIC in 2011 (ASIC Gazette A064/11, 5 August 2011).

38 Brady fieldnotes, 12 August 2014.

important in the outback because of the lack of population centres and service points, even if their need has diminished in recent years (Racing, Gaming and Licensing Division 2003).

Only one source of alcohol remained in the township, the Timber Creek Hotel, which had an indoor bar with minimal features (e.g. a pool table), and restrictions on takeaway times and types of alcohol.[39] Drinkers could no longer move to an alternative drinking place with longer opening hours and a beer garden, as had happened in the past. However, despite having no involvement in the ownership of the hotel, the community was able to negotiate restrictions and other arrangements with the licensee, such as closing the bar to Aboriginal people when ceremonies or funerals were on. The hotel manager agreed to maintain an incident register and a banned person register (Northern Territory Licensing Commission 2010b). As it turned out, it was not necessary for Aboriginal people to *own* the premises to negotiate alcohol controls. However, such controls were only possible because the community had a longstanding relationship with the licensee; there are no guarantees that the controls would survive a change of licensee.

While some local Timber Creek people resented the hotel for making money out of 'us blackfellas' 'who buy all year round' (unlike seasonal tourists), other Aboriginal community members were ambivalent. One spoke about the original purchase of the Wayside Inn:

> We wanted to buy it to reduce alcohol intake but it created more problems, people drank more. [We] wanted to get a business to make money—and alcohol makes more money. Now we want to buy a block and make an art and craft centre, sandwiches and coffee, make a facility we can use to have meetings in.

Although the Wayside Inn has gone, an Aboriginal association, Gunamu Aboriginal Corporation, owns the businesses on the site—the Wirib[40] tourism park, caravans, fuel pumps and a store—and has sought professional advice on management and finance. Plans have been drawn up for a new supermarket on the site, but there is to be no liquor licence there. All that remains of the Wayside Inn is a concrete slab, on which the hotel's original coolroom has been cemented as a memento; a mural above it depicts the dingo dreaming, painted by the grandson of a senior traditional owner.

---

39 Prices for takeaways are extremely high; for example, $80.50 for a carton of 24 cans of full-strength beer and $20.50 for a sixpack (as at August 2014).

40 *Wirib* = 'dingo', 'a significant local dreaming'.

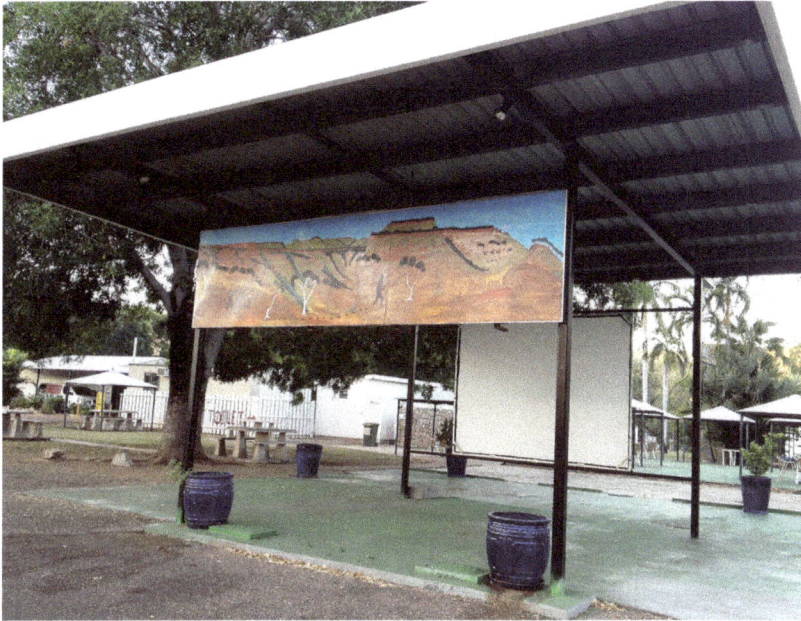

Fig. 25 Remains of the Wayside Inn, Timber Creek, 2014
Source: M Brady

The Indigenous community hotels: Hopes and outcomes

Most of the hotels discussed here were purchased during the 1980s, a decade when serious alcohol problems were becoming evident in the Indigenous population (cf. Hunter 1993), as shown in Table 2. Aboriginal people and government officials had anticipated that Aboriginal people would exert control over alcohol consumption, but this did not always develop. Funding agencies, such as the ADC, as well as the Australian Government, promoted self-management, self-determination and economic and social development for Indigenous people. These goals at times contradicted the motivations that led Aboriginal people and organisations to seek licences to sell alcohol, such as a desire for social improvement and economic development; to prove that Aboriginal people were capable of running economically viable enterprises; to provide employment and training; to enable Aboriginal people to socialise, set their own standards and learn to moderate drinking behaviours; and to gain a degree of control over their own lives.

Table 2 Public hotels purchased by Indigenous groups, 1975–2014

Year	Licensed premises	Aboriginal organisation	Sponsorship	Stated aims
1975–80	Finke Hotel, Northern Territory	Aputula Social Club	Federal Minister for Aboriginal Affairs, Jim Cavanagh	Control the drinking problem; improve race relations
1983–?	Oasis Hotel, Walgett, New South Wales	Gamilarai Ltd – Barwon Aboriginal Community Ltd	ADC; Charles Perkins ($428,211)	Commercial venture, training, control of sales
1986	Transcontinental Hotel, Oodnadatta, South Australia	Dunjiba Community Council	ADC; Charles Perkins	Control sales of fortified wine
1987	Mt Ebenezer Roadside Inn, Northern Territory	Imanpa Community (Lisanote Pty Ltd)	Bank loan ($500,000)	Gain secure economic base, accumulate assets, control supply of alcohol
1988–88	Woden Town Club, Canberra, Australian Capital Territory	Aboriginal Corporation for Sporting and Recreational Activities	ADC guaranteed loan; Charles Perkins ($386,300)	Create an Aboriginal social environment; set standards of dress and behaviour
1988	The Crossing Inn and Fitzroy River Lodge, Western Australia	Leedal Pty Ltd (40% ownership)	ADC loan	A development project; reduce harm from takeaway alcohol
c. 1998	Daly River Hotel Motel, Daly River, Northern Territory	Nauiyu Council	Not known	Regulate drinking, tourist enterprise, have Aboriginal control of outlets
1999–2010	Wayside Inn, Timber Creek, Northern Territory	Ngaliwurru-Wuli Association and TC Hotel Wayside Inn Joint Venture Pty Ltd	Indigenous Land Corporation	Commercial venture; greater control over sales
2014	Whim Creek Hotel, Pilbara, Western Australia	Ngarluma Aboriginal Corporation and Ngarluma Yindjibarndi Foundation	$1.7 million	Promoting Indigenous tourism, employ local Indigenous as chefs, barmen and tourist operators

Source: Author's data

Social improvement and economic development

Indigenous and non-Indigenous community-hotel enterprises had their philosophical origins in sometimes idealised notions of social improvement and self-help, as described in Chapter 2. In the Barossa and the Riverland regions of South Australia, where notions of self-sufficiency were deeply embedded in Lutheran communities and agricultural cooperatives, community ownership of the local hotel was seen as an integral part of fundraising for the betterment of the town. Many, if not all, of the non–Indigenous run South Australian hotels seem to have achieved this goal; they distributed substantial sums to local community and educational activities, town parks and gardens, and charities and sports associations. However, an obvious influence on their profitability, and thus their ability to be generous to local causes, was the size of the population base. Towns such as Ceduna, Nuriootpa, Loxton and Renmark—whose community hotels raise enough revenue to make substantial financial donations to local organisations and facilities—have resident populations ranging from 3,000 to 7,500 people, and these numbers are boosted by tourists and other travellers. By contrast, several of the Indigenous-owned hotels were in towns with very small resident populations. Timber Creek and Imanpa – Mt Ebenezer have resident populations of around 250. Even though both locations are supported by substantial through traffic and visitors, much of their customer base is seasonal and can be affected by economic downturns. As a result, they made minimal (if any) distributions of revenue for the benefit of their communities, and Mt Ebenezer Roadhouse became bankrupt.

Despite the aspirations for social improvement and job creation that accompanied Indigenous purchases, none of the hotels profiled here provided much Aboriginal employment. It was their considered decision *not* to employ local Aboriginal people in direct sales of alcohol, and not one had an Aboriginal manager. Aboriginal people tended to be employed as groundsmen, gardeners and cleaners, rather than front of house staff.[41] Indeed, as employers of local people, Indigenous community-owned hotels compare woefully with their non-Indigenous counterparts. The Loxton Hotel in the Riverland, for example, employs 85 local people; the Nuriootpa Vine Inn, a community-owned hotel in the Barossa Valley, has a staff of 120. As well as having bigger populations, these non-

---

41   At the Crossing Inn in the Kimberley, backpackers work behind the bar.

Indigenous premises are located in relatively rich tourist towns, operate substantial accommodation and restaurant facilities, and have a work-ready local population from which to draw their workers. The Oasis Hotel in Walgett was said (optimistically) to have been purchased to provide hospitality training and employment for local Aboriginal people. This failed to eventuate because the training program was poorly planned and implemented, and neither the ADC nor the hotel license holders, took any responsibility for it: no trainee learned how to tap a keg or run a cellar and no Aboriginal person was enabled to engage in business to the point of self-management and self-sufficiency (Commonwealth of Australia 1989a, 1989b).

The goal of controlling sales

In 2001, Justice Tony Fitzgerald identified control over alcohol supply as a major priority for Indigenous communities: it was the major determinant of Indigenous submissions to the licensing authorities regarding nearby liquor outlets (Fitzgerald 2001, Brady 2004). However, there are impediments to any community group—especially an Indigenous group—attempting to regulate sales from 'normal', commercially run premises: the legislation is complex, the criteria for objections are narrow[42] and the procedures involved are often protracted (Bourbon et al. 1999). Licensees vigorously contest any attempt to 'unfairly' limit their trade (Pitjantjatjara Council 1990: 18). Some licensees have started petitions objecting to community moves to change sales practices (Wright 1997, Brady et al. 2003: 67) and some have argued (ironically, in view of their history) that they could not impose certain restrictions on sales because these would be racially discriminatory (Lyon 1991, Race Discrimination Commissioner 1995).[43] In their access to licensing authorities, Aboriginal groups and licensees are not equal. Not all Aboriginal groups can afford legal representation to present their case, and many lack the resources to

---

42   For example, harm minimisation has only been an explicit objective of the South Australian Liquor Licensing Act since 1997 (Bourbon et al. 1999: 13, Brady et al. 2003). In 2014, a CLP Government announced that it would abolish the Northern Territory Licensing Commission (to save 'red tape') and hearings (thus reducing the opportunity for community objections) (Vangopoulos 2014).

43   Actions that would otherwise be unlawful can be exempted if they constitute a 'special measure'. However, there is a dilemma; normally, special measures treat a disadvantaged group advantageously but, in the case of alcohol restrictions, they treat the disadvantaged group *disadvantageously*—that is, by restricting a person's rights to purchase 'goods'. The dilemma is addressed by the fact that the restrictions confer a group or collective right (Calma 2004).

present supporting evidence for their submissions.[44] Conversely, liquor industry lobby groups support licensees; have contact with ministers, policy advisers, policy writers and the liquor licensing authorities themselves (Secker 1993); and tend to be antagonistic to Indigenous and government harm-reduction initiatives.[45] In view of these factors, it is understandable that some Indigenous groups have found it easier to become licensees themselves than to object to the practices of other licensees.

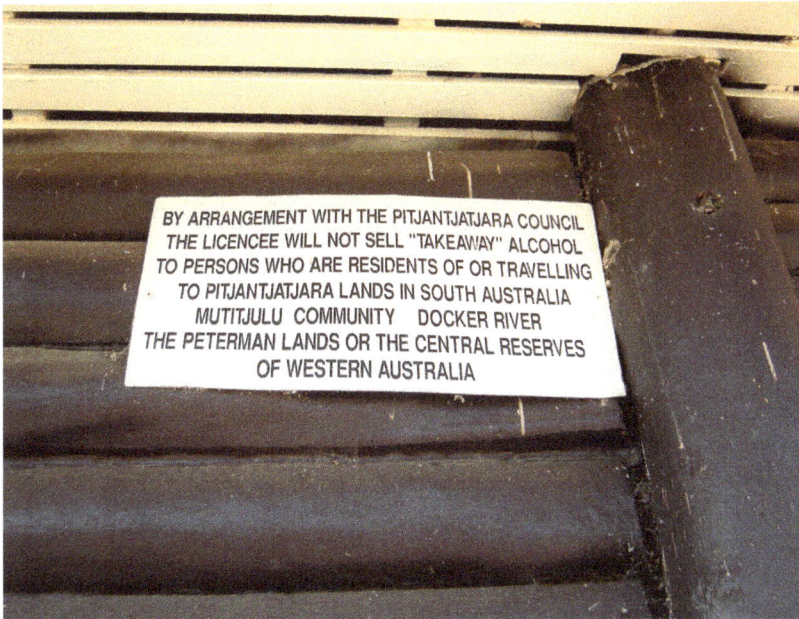

Fig. 26 Notice at Mt Ebenezer Roadhouse, 2009
Source: M Brady

---

44   In its submission to the Sessional Committee on the Use and Abuse of Alcohol by the Community in the Northern Territory in 1990, the Pitjantjatjara Council wrote that while it had been successful (before the South Australian licensing court) in obtaining changes to licence conditions reflecting community desires, in the Northern Territory, it had had to rely on a mix of formal and informal arrangements, some of which were not noted on the liquor licence concerned 'depending on the proclivities of the licensee and the prevailing philosophy of the Liquor Commission at the time' (Pitjantjatjara Council 1990: 16).
45   For example, the Australian Hotels Association. Other liquor industry groups, such as the Brewers Association and Distilled Spirits Industry Council, have also objected to National Health and Medical Research Council drinking guidelines, and to health warning labels on alcohol containers (Ford 1988: 5, *ABC News* 2004, 2007a, Stark 2008: 7).

All the case studies discussed in this chapter followed similar patterns: after taking control of the hotel, the community group limited trading (Saggers & Gray 1998). The hotels at Finke, Oodnadatta, Mt Ebenezer, Daly River and Timber Creek were purchased to 'control the drinking problem' or 'reduce harm'. At Mt Ebenezer Roadhouse, a sign on the outside wall of the premises explained some of the background to the community-instigated controls over sales: 'By arrangement with the Pitjantjatjara Council, the licencee [sic] will not sell "takeaway" alcohol to persons who are residents of or travelling to Pitjantjatjara lands in South Australia'. These publicly displayed notices were needed to quell disputes with disappointed drinkers and to clarify for naive tourists—who might otherwise be persuaded to buy beer for Aboriginal people—that the rules were put in place by the Aboriginal community. Some of these rules might appear authoritarian to outside observers; however, decisions about what is acceptable and unacceptable that are made by Aboriginal owners or communities represent a more legitimate form of authority than those made by (possibly racist or unsympathetic) non-Aboriginal licensees.

Vague plans to moderate drinking

Some government advisers and many Aboriginal people who advocated for licensed clubs mentioned wanting to teach Aboriginal customers moderate and 'civilised' drinking patterns—as an alternative to explosive binge drinking. This was never a *defining* rationale behind the purchase of hotels by Indigenous associations: rather it was a vague hope, occasionally voiced. Once owned by Indigenous groups, hotel enterprises paid more attention to controlling sales than changing drinking *behaviour*. In fact, it is difficult to find any examples of Indigenous-owned hotels introducing behavioural change programs *for on-premises drinking*, although some attempted to implement harm-reduction measures, such as providing good quality food and diversionary activities that might have contributed to minimising the demand for alcohol. Examples of what could have been done include the 'Sober Bob', or designated driver, programs that police sometimes run in hotels; providing sober drivers with free non-alcoholic drinks; installing a breathalyser machine so that customers can see how rapidly their alcohol levels can rise; demonstrating the effects of intoxication on perception by showing people 'drink goggles'.[46] In some

---

46   Drink goggles = goggles used in health education, which can be worn to simulate alcohol impairment.

instances, such as the Finke Hotel (in its early years) and Mt Ebenezer, local Aboriginal community members were actively *discouraged* from drinking on premises, which meant that no attempt was being made to use the premises as a venue for cultural change in drinking. As will be discussed in the next chapter, at Fitzroy Crossing, Aboriginal drinkers were at liberty to buy takeaway beer from their community-owned hotel and consume it off premises, in an adjacent park; this went on for many years. Most Aboriginal customers followed this practice: only a minority of Aboriginal customers drank in the hotel. When takeaway sales were finally banned in 2007, these unrestrained outdoor drinkers were forced, under protest, to drink on premises. In an ironic reversal of the civil rights struggle to repeal drinking bans and to force licensees to accept Aboriginal people into their pubs, many of the outdoor drinkers of Fitzroy Crossing objected to having to drink in their own hotel.

Rather than trying to re-educate drinkers or engage with customers about reducing the harm caused by heavy drinking, Aboriginal community-owned premises have relied on a plethora of signage—what might be called 'arms-length instruction'. There seem to be more signs in Aboriginal-owned hotels, and in the social clubs in remote communities, than in other licensed premises. Dress requirement signs once kept Aboriginal people out of hotels: now they are prominent in Indigenous-owned premises— 'No singlets. No thongs. Sleeved and collared shirts only after 6.00 pm'. Numerous signs deal with proscribed behaviours: 'No spitting in the garden bar or you will be banned from the Inn for 3 months'; 'If you hit a staff member the pub will close immediately'. There are signs explaining the (often elaborate) barring rules: life bans, barring until further notice, barring for different periods of time—'drunk and refusing to leave: 1 to 7 days; aggressive arguing: 1 to 7 days; humbugging: 1 week'. It is difficult to know how strictly some of these are applied. There are also signs about who is allowed where: 'Children most welcome in lounge'; 'When you are allowed back in the pub, you will only be allowed back in for 3 hrs (12 noon to 3 pm) for the first week'; 'No open drinks to leave the bar'.[47]

---

47 Signs seen at Indigenous-owned hotels at Fitzroy Crossing and Oodnadatta.

The challenges inherent in community ownership

There is little evidence that Indigenous community-owned hotels have become truly social enterprises. Most have struggled to achieve the basic aims of benefiting the community, promoting a sense of social responsibility and having a workable participatory structure (Defourny & Nyssens 2006). Most have also struggled financially, except for one hotel, which is economically viable but whose profit-maximising behaviour makes it atypical of social enterprise. This case is discussed in the next chapter, together with an analysis of the complex reasons underlying developments in this instance.

Before buying a hotel, a community group should, ideally, engage in long-running consultation and should be prepared for a polarising and bitter debate (Lang 1994: 223). It must then form a proprietary company, organise business plans and obtain loans, set up management structures, arrange community representation and decide on policies. Such an organisation and the hotel itself must be compliant with the features of the relevant state or territory's Liquor Act. This is just the beginning: there is much more to running a hotel than this. The case of the Wayside Inn at Timber Creek illustrates how Indigenous organisations (which are often small, unskilled and isolated) and the communities they represent are sometimes badly advised about the legal structure and joint partnership arrangements for their purchase: the Wayside Inn closed, at least in part, because government, quasi-government and non-government bureaucracies with the potential to provide competent advice and ongoing guidance failed to do so.

The Australian Hotels Association, a peak organisation that represents the interests of its hotel members, does not provide Indigenous-owned hotels with any special help or advice on governance or management matters. It offers its members general assistance on industrial issues, such as policy documents on responsible service and the hiring and firing of staff.[48] State licensing authorities restrict themselves to providing random checks on staff, weights and measures, infrastructure (i.e. exits and toilets) and compliance issues (i.e. serving underage and intoxicated drinkers); they have no capacity to assist community hotels (either Indigenous or

---

48   Information provided by the Australian Hotels Association, South Australia.

non-Indigenous) with governance issues and appear to have no interest in taking on this responsibility. It is unfortunate that licensing authorities (or other agencies) do not offer such help, for Indigenous community-owned hotels are subject to many of the same challenges and difficulties as their non-Indigenous counterparts in South Australia, but they have fewer resources to deal with them. Exacerbated by living in small, interwoven, rural or remote communities, these challenges include staffing and governance issues and the pressures of remaining financially viable.

Indigenous-owned hotels find it difficult to recruit and retain competent staff, including managers, because of the isolation, remoteness and particular stresses of dealing with alcohol sales and Indigenous people—an issue fraught with historical, social and cultural sensitivities.[49] The manager's job is more complex in an Indigenous-owned entity, for he or she must liaise with a board that is usually made up of community members who have no special training or experience in the hospitality industry, may not be fully literate and may themselves have ambivalent attitudes towards drinking. Board members are usually untrained in governance matters; research into Indigenous organisational management has highlighted the need for boards *and* managers to have adequate governance training and guidance (Mantziaris & Martin 2000, Brady 2002, Sharma 2005). At times, boards misconstrue the boundaries of their role and that of the manager, as was the case at the Oasis Hotel at Walgett where there was no articulated 'separation of powers' between the manager and the directors. Arguably, a manager needs to be able to operate independently of his or her community board. A manager should have the authority to caution staff who break the rules—for example, by giving free drinks to relatives—and to bar customers from service. However, in an Indigenous context, these powers carry advantages and disadvantages that vary greatly and depend on the qualities of the manager. Managers inexperienced in Indigenous contexts need to be monitored by board members and pulled into line if necessary.

Another difficulty peculiar to community-owned premises rests on the misinterpretation of what 'community ownership' means. This confusion was manifest at Walgett; some Aboriginal directors initially believed that their ownership of the Oasis Hotel gave them the right to make free use

49   In one case, a newly appointed manager at Mt Ebenezer Roadhouse claimed he had been threatened by a community member with a spear and had jumped out of a window to escape, 'running for his life' (Phelan 2012).

209

of the hotel's stock (Commonwealth of Australia 1989a: 21). It seems that non-Indigenous residents of Ceduna had the same idea when the community bought the hotel there in 1949: some thought the drinks would be free (Larkins & Howard 1973). Local staff at Indigenous and non-Indigenous premises are sometimes pressured to give special privileges or free drinks to their friends and relatives. Several of the South Australian community hotel managers dealt with this by having daily stocktakes and spot checks. Indigenous hotels have attempted to avoid or circumvent some of this pressure by hiring non-Indigenous workers—'neutral' people from beyond the community—or by displaying signs that prohibit unwanted behaviours. Nevertheless, if might have been useful had the Indigenous hotels and their governing boards or corporations known of the existence of the non-Indigenous community-owned hotels in South Australia; perhaps both groups could have benefited from networking and exchanges of experiences and strategies? Indigenous-owned hotels have struggled with numerous dilemmas: keeping turnover high, repaying loans, keeping customers happy and distributing profits, while simultaneously maintaining some social responsibility to minimise alcohol-related harms among their local population.

7

The Indigenous purchase
of the Crossing Inn

In 1989, at a time of upheaval in the Australian government's management of Aboriginal affairs, community groups at Fitzroy Crossing formed a company and, with an ADC loan, bought shares in several enterprises. These included a supermarket, shops, a caravan park and Fitzroy Crossing's only licensed hotel and source of takeaway alcohol, the Crossing Inn. While there was widespread support for the purchase of the supermarket and caravan park, buying into the Crossing Inn was controversial from the beginning. Local people hoped that as a development project, the purchases would improve their social and economic circumstances, and that owning the hotel would encourage people to drink on the premises (rather than off premises) and adopt a less damaging drinking style. Nearly 20 years later, several official inquiries found—and a good deal of public opinion agreed—that neither of these goals had been achieved.

The history of the Crossing Inn

The Crossing Inn has been part of the lives of the pastoral workers of the Fitzroy Valley in the Kimberley region of Western Australia since the 1890s. Joe Blythe, the first pastoralist in the region, established Brooking Springs station in 1888, and built his homestead where the Crossing Inn now stands. The settlement of Fitzroy Crossing takes its name from the place where travellers once forded the Fitzroy River. Blythe's rough shanty homestead originally served as a hotel and store, and his son held the first official 'wayside house' licence in 1897. Amid the 'crazed' drinking style of the frontier, the pub undoubtedly did well (Pedersen & Woorunmurra 2007: 85, Hawke 2014). Today, Fitzroy Crossing has a settled population of approximately 1,500, and a mobile population of around 4,500 living in 45 discrete communities within a 200 km radius. The town lies in the southeast corner of Bunaba country, between Broome in the west and Halls Creek in the east; however, the region itself lies at the intersection of several traditional groupings of people who speak different languages: some from the Kimberley cultural bloc, others from the Western Desert region (Kolig 2000). In this instance, as in many others, the pub was part of the colonialist project: it aided the conquest of new areas. Pubs on the frontier provided accommodation and grog to new settlers as they pushed inland (hence the notion of the 'wayside house'), and introduced alcohol and drinking to those who had been displaced (Kirkby 1997: 28).

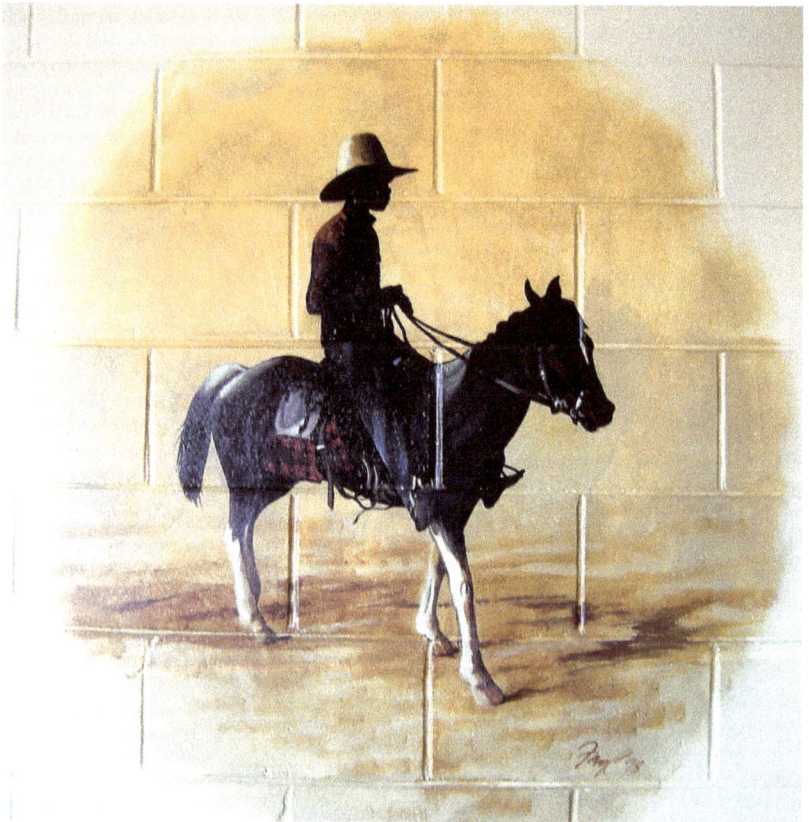

Fig. 27 Mural in Salem Shelter, Halls Creek
Source: M Brady

Apart from its drinking, the Kimberley region is noted for the violence of its frontier history. During the 'era of stockwhip and rifle', Aboriginal groups were violently displaced by pastoralists: it was colonisation in its harshest form (Kolig 2000: 14). There were massacres of Aboriginal people by police and pastoralists, outright warfare and strong resistance by Aboriginal people, both passive and active, exemplified in the exploits of Aboriginal warriors such as Jandamarra (Marshall 1988, Pedersen & Woorunmurra 2007, Hawke 2014). The arrival of the Catholic Church in the region in 1934 (at Rockhole Station and Balgo Hills), and the United Aborigines Mission (UAM) in the 1940s, provided Aboriginal people some protection from the excesses of the frontier (McDonald 2001: 56–7). In 1952, the UAM took over from the Department of Native Affairs' Depot at Fitzroy Crossing, running a children's home and distributing rations. The children's parents were largely working on the cattle stations of the Fitzroy Valley. This was the fertile land of Nyikina, Bunuba and Gooniyandi traditional owners, and the people had become part of the labour force of the cattle industry, joined later by the Walmajarri and Wangkatjunka groups who moved into the stations from the desert regions.

In 1965, the embryonic town of Fitzroy Crossing was isolated and remote; it consisted of a police station and residence, a post office and residence, an Australian Inland Mission nursing post, the UAM mission and the hotel, which was at the end of a track near the river. Ten Aboriginal people were employed at the hotel, with the men earning between £1 and £3 per week, and the women from £1 to £2 10s. At the time, the basic wage was £15 19s (Hawke 2014: 27–8). These Aboriginal workers lived near the hotel at a camp that lacked any amenities, was littered with tins and bottles, and where pigs and dogs roamed freely. The hotel's publican agitated for the removal of the camp and disclaimed any responsibility for it. According to Steve Hawke, it was the Licensing Court that suggested the creation of a proper native reserve to accommodate the Aboriginal people living there. The equal wages case for Aboriginal pastoral workers was in the offing, and the camp's population began to increase once the surrounding properties started evicting Aboriginal workers and their families; some people walked off the stations voluntarily. The evictions and mass unemployment that spread to the Western Australian pastoral industry followed the requirement for station-owners in the Northern Territory to pay Aboriginal workers award wages. It meant that the population of Fitzroy Crossing exploded during the late 1960s and early 1970s. The UAM 'packed people in' (Hawke 2014: 165), and different mobs from pastoral stations began to set up their own squatter camps in and around Fitzroy Crossing, such as the people who walked off Noonkanbah in 1971.[1] This, together with the expectations of political change following the 1967 Referendum and the abolition of the last alcohol restrictions in Western Australia in 1971, made it a dramatic period of turmoil and transition (Oscar & Pedersen 2011: 89–90, Thorburn 2011). Not all Fitzroy Valley Aboriginal people were in favour of these changes at the time, or in retrospect: some believed that drinking rights 'ruined everything' and that equal wages did 'a lot of damage' (Marshall 1988: 23, 30).

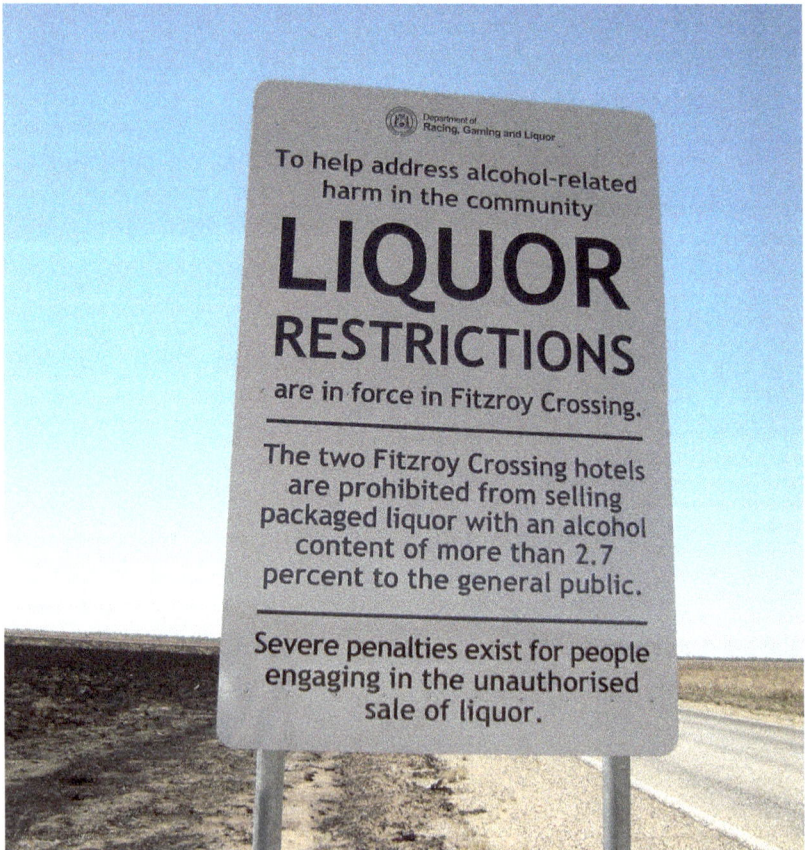

Fig. 28 Liquor restrictions sign, Fitzroy Crossing, 2009
Source: M Brady

---

1   These camps eventually became the different communities (or neighbourhoods) in and around Fitzroy Crossing. The Go Go Station mob became Bayulu; the Christmas Creek mob became Wangkatjunka; the residents of old Mission camp became Junjuwa community; the Noonkanbah mob from Loanbung became Kadjina and Yungngora; and the Fig Tree Camp people were incorporated as Kurnangki community (Hawke 2014: 196).

Selling grog

According to a local observer in the 1970s, young and old Aboriginal people imitated the drinking behaviour of their white peers in style and quantity, which is to say that Aboriginal men were no heavier drinkers than 'respectable' white men in the north of Western Australia (Kolig 1974: 51). The Crossing Inn was happy to supply them all. While talking about his life to Paul Marshall (1988: 76), Jock Shandley, a Walmajarri man and Fitzroy Valley drover, told of buying takeaways from the Crossing Inn:

> I used to be a drinker myself. After Aborigines were given citizenship rights, we used to go in to the Fitzroy Crossing pub and tell Dick Fellon that we wanted rum or whiskey or whatever. He'd say, 'Yeah, come into the store'. He'd give us as many bottles as we wanted. He had to make his money I suppose, and he must have made a lot of money out of us. I used to drink all that stuff back then, but I began to realize what it does to you. That's when I stopped drinking.

The sale of copious quantities of canned beer from the Crossing Inn resulted in what locals described as 'Fitzroy snow'; from the air, you could look down on shady trees and see, glinting in the sun, a carpet of white cans surrounding them where seated drinkers had chucked their empties. Moderate alcohol consumption was a style of drinking that never gained a foothold on the northern 'frontier', nor in Fitzroy Crossing. Hawke (2014: 190) has written about the ferment of new ideas, hope and activism in the town in the 1970s that ran alongside an orgy of self-destruction, as rampant drinking and alcoholism quickly became a feature of life in the fringe camps. According to Shandley (cited in Marshall 1988), the grog was too strong and it led people away from the old rules. In 1974, anthropologist Erich Kolig (1974) described the drinking problem at Fitzroy Crossing as 'acute'; he reported that senior Lawmen—who, at the time, were attempting to revive traditional punishments—organised a roster of 'prestigious men' to patrol the public bar at the Crossing Inn, to remove drunken people and seclude them in bush camps (46).[2]

Oscar and Pedersen (2011: 92) noted that during these years, the non-Aboriginal owners of the Crossing Inn ignored the social and health consequences of their desire to make money. A study of morbidity rates at

---

2   According to Kolig (1974: 49), Aboriginal elders believed that the Western judicial system and the use of jail was 'too soft' by comparison with Aboriginal Law. However, he was pessimistic about whether the traditional *kerygma* (mythology, dreaming) would provide any solutions to people who were 'sodden' with grog—a situation, he said, which had no sacred precedent.

Fitzroy Crossing between 1978 and 1983 found that violence and alcohol were the most common causes of hospital attendance for both men and women (Holman & Quadros 1986: 31). By the 1980s, the hospital records showed that between 75 per cent and 85 per cent of fatal injuries incurred at Fitzroy Crossing were alcohol related (Moizo 1991: 184). An anthropologist who made fieldwork visits there, Bernard Moizo, described the situation at various times between 1980 and 1987. At the Crossing Inn in 1980, there were three bars: the lounge bar, the garden bar and the 'Blackfellow' bar. No bare feet were allowed in the first two and, as Aboriginal people were, for the most part, the only ones with bare feet, they congregated in the 'Blackfellow' bar, or went bush with their takeaways. Moizo explained:

> The 'Blackfellow' or 'Aboriginal' bar was a large dark room with high concrete walls that separated it from the garden bar. There were no lights, no tables, no chairs, only two wooden benches. A huge grid, welded at the top of the bar on one end and fixed at the ceiling on the other end, symbolised quite clearly the racial relations within the pub. Aborigines handed the money through the square holes of the grid and were handed back glasses of beer … I was struck by the atmosphere. Between twenty and thirty Aboriginal, [sic] men and women, most of them drunk, were shouting, arguing, swearing or fighting each other. The noise was amplified by the size of the room and the concrete walls. The ambience was pathetic, but it got worse when the iron curtain dropped down on the bar and the police walked in … In the garden bar things were different: a few non-Aboriginals would enjoy their beer under the cool shade of centenarian trees. Here there was no shortage of tables, chairs or bar stools. Inside, in the air conditioned lounge bar … a few customers emptied their stubbies … Patrons in the garden and lounge bar were probably as drunk as were the Aborigines, but they were quiet and enjoyed their drinks in a pleasant ambience. (51–2)

Five years later, it was increasingly common to see young Aboriginal people in the more salubrious lounge or garden bars, but these drinkers were people holding regular jobs or who had been to Perth for schooling. On Friday nights, there were cheaper prices ('happy hour') in the garden bar where most of the non-Aboriginal population drank, but not in the Aboriginal bar, which was often closed on Friday nights.[3] The clientele

---

3   Moizo (1991: 68, note 5) documented one occasion when around 40 Aboriginal people walked into the garden bar to protest about the unfairness of this and to demand 'their' bar be reopened on Fridays with 'happy hour' prices.

of the Aboriginal bar had dropped off, as more drinkers made the switch to takeaway alcohol. Once a taxi service became available in 1984, they used the pub as a bottle shop:

> They called a taxi, were driven to the pub, bought a carton of beer and were dropped off in one of the many drinking spots in the bush around town. This presented some definite advantages. Firstly, one could choose with whom one would drink. Secondly it was easier to flee into the bush when the police arrived or when a fight was about to start. (56)

The advent of the taxi service, and the increasing availability of private vehicles, meant that grog could more easily be carted in larger volumes to a variety of drinking places, including those far away from the pub and town. Prior to this, open-air drinking with takeaway beer had taken place anywhere and everywhere, most often under trees close to the pub or, to avoid trouble when walking home, close to home communities. An Aboriginal man, 'Patrick', explained this practice to Moizo:

> You see us Bunaba … we drink here, right under that big fig tree. Number one place this one … we are next to that hotel, when you want more grog you just go there and get some. Look behind, well there is that creek, if you need one good cool bath to sober you up a bit this is the place now … I know that track all the way [home], even dead drunk I can go back home. (178)

Moizo mapped the spatial distribution of drinking spots, most of which were established in the late 1970s. These revealed the tendency for members of the same kin and language groups to choose to drink together. Despite, or perhaps because of this, disputes and arguments among drinkers frequently degenerated into violent fights, triggered by a drunken lack of control in speech, heedless mention of secret Law matters or jealousy. By mid-1988, the drinking was so problematic that local women formed an action group called Women Against Alcohol (WAA). The group was led by Topsy Chestnut, an influential Gooniyandi woman involved in community development work (cf. Hawke 2014).[4] The WAA aimed to raise local awareness of problem drinking and alcohol-related domestic violence. Clinical research showed a high prevalence of alcohol-related problems among Aboriginal drinkers in the region (including

---

4   It is worth noting here that 1988 was also the year in which Aboriginal women in several other regions began to mobilise against alcohol-related troubles—in the Northern Territory at Wadeye, the Tiwi Islands and at Curtin Springs in the Pitjantjatjara lands.

Fitzroy Crossing), with two-thirds scoring two or more on the CAGE[5] questionnaire, which is sensitive in detecting 'excessive drinking' (Hall et al. 1993: 1095, Hunter 1993). Three-quarters of this sample identified alcohol use as a major community concern in the Kimberley. In view of the amount of alcohol being consumed, this is not surprising; Hall and colleagues (1993) found that median consumption over a drinking occasion or day was approximately 10 standard drinks per person (i.e. 104.5 g of pure alcohol).[6]

Non-Aboriginal people monopolised most jobs in the town, which circulated among them without being advertised; they also dominating the local enterprises and businesses. The publican, for example, owned the supermarket, the caravan park and the shopping complex. Between 1985 and 1987, four Aboriginal people were employed at the pub for weekly rubbish collection. The low level of Aboriginal employment, their exclusion from participating in, and benefiting from, local enterprises, together with increasing problems associated with alcohol from the Crossing Inn, created growing dissatisfaction and a mood for change. The ADC, which was established to assist Aboriginal people to engage in business enterprises (among other aims), gave people an opportunity to buy into local businesses and to change things at Fitzroy Crossing.

The proposal to buy the Crossing Inn and other businesses

In 1988, the owner and licensee of the Crossing Inn, Jack Sandford, placed the business on the market, together with other holdings owned by his family over several decades: the supermarket, shops and a caravan park. Alerted to this impending sale, the ADC had the Sandford holdings valued; subsequently, the ADC (and its successors) became a significant player in the future of these Fitzroy Crossing enterprises. The ADC engaged Bill Arthur, a social scientist at the Aboriginal Economic Research Unit in Perth, to investigate the feasibility of purchasing the businesses for the Aboriginal communities of the region. Arthur's terms of reference included explaining to Aboriginal people the implications of the

---

5   CAGE is an acronym for the four questions that make up the questionnaire.
6   At the time, the National Health and Medical Research Council definition of a 'harmful' amount of alcohol was more than 60 g a day for males (Hall et al. 1993: 1096).

purchases, documenting Aboriginal support or objections, and putting forward ideas for a Trust structure and options for ownership and control of the enterprises.

Arthur's observation, that the issues were 'complex and new', was an understatement. As was the case with other Aboriginal hotel purchases, Aboriginal people at Fitzroy Crossing had limited educational backgrounds and little, if any, experience of planning or running such an enterprise; they were also completely unaware of the existence of mainstream community-owned hotels in South Australia, from whom guidance could have been sought. At most, some Aboriginal people at Fitzroy Crossing had experience running cattle stations; however, some of these had not been commercially successful.[7]

Arthur's (1988) Interim Report pointed to a difference of opinion within the Aboriginal community about buying into the hotel. Although they supported community ownership of the supermarket, caravan park and shops unconditionally, people were guarded about the purchase of a share in the Crossing Inn. Arthur reported that 'directly negative statements only apply to the hotel … and people are uncomfortable about it at this stage'.[8] Those who were most uncomfortable were older men (although only two older men had stated categorically that the community should *not* be involved with the hotel) and women. The supporters of the hotel purchase were mostly younger adults who appreciated the potential for commercial development, including Patrick Green, a Bunaba man, who was to have an ongoing role in the businesses. The supporters of the idea perceived its potential: capturing the hotel's profits would give local people the opportunity to purchase other enterprises, which would make them less reliant on government. Arthur (1989a) wrote:

> The bottom line for them appears to be that if they don't own [these enterprises] then someone else will, and that by owning them they will stop the money flowing out of Fitzroy Crossing. (executive summary)

Arthur (1988) soon discovered another difficulty: that different players— the ADC and various Aboriginal community interests—held different perspectives on the *purpose* of the purchases. There was the ADC view, which saw the purchases in a commercial light; a local view, which saw

---

7   However, in 1991, ATSIC acquired Leopold Downs Station for the Bunaba people, a large and very productive cattle station with a river frontage (Thorburn 2011: 108).

8   Arthur's (1988) Interim Report was not paginated.

the purchases as a way to address a social problem; and another local view that saw the purchases as a means of generating both commercial and social benefits.

According to Arthur, local expectations that owning the hotel would alleviate excess drinking took precedence over commercial discussions of both the hotel and the supermarket. Despite these differing—divergent—aims, *someone* was going to buy the hotel and sell alcohol to the Aboriginal population (so the thinking went), in which case, it might as well be locally owned, enabling some measure of control over sales: the obvious ethical dilemma of profiting from the sale of a substance that was so patently damaging to so many Aboriginal people, notwithstanding. The problem, from the perspective of various Aboriginal community members, was the packaged nature of the deal: presumably the hotel could not be excised. To overcome the potential conflict between commercial success and negative social consequences, the Aboriginal community hoped to find directors of the company and managers of the facility who had 'special' qualities, not just commercial qualifications or experience in running businesses. As Arthur (1989a) explained:

> People do not see the project in simply commercial terms. They see it as a development project and as a means of improving their social and economic circumstances through participation. Therefore to own the hotel as assets in which they have no involvement, has little or no attraction.

It seems that the majority of mature-age Aboriginal people ultimately were persuaded that owning the hotel would 'relieve the alcohol problem'. Their main concern was over the sale of bulk takeaway liquor from the Crossing Inn. It was suggested that, once they owned the hotel, takeaway sales could be restricted or prohibited to encourage people to drink inside the hotel:

> In the old days the pub was open from 6 am. He [the owner] didn't care about our people. Wanting to buy in was wanting to control liquor sales and [we] didn't want them to wake up with a beer early morning. Let them have food in their guts first.[9]

Somewhat drily, Arthur (1989a) explained that: 'It is not that there is simply heavy drinking but that there is a certain style of drinking with features which I suggest were not envisaged by the Liquor Act' (10). Apart

---

9   Patrick Green, pers comm, 16 August 2012.

from curbing sales of takeaways, during these preliminary consultations, local Aboriginal people suggested a few other harm-reduction strategies that, it was thought, could be put in place once they owned the Crossing Inn. These included introducing by-laws to restrict the amount of takeaway alcohol that could be purchased using taxis; upgrading on-premises drinking areas to make the atmosphere more 'civilised'; introducing more hotel entertainment to encourage social drinking; using the profits to mount alcohol-education programs; and hiring 'certain Aboriginal staff'—that is, people with particular qualities who would be able to effectively control on-premises drinking.[10]

In view of subsequent events, it is significant that from the outset, takeaway sales were identified as a key problem and that there was a plan to restrict (or even stop) such sales. The loss of revenue presented another major dilemma, as Arthur (1989a) reported:

> People can see that if drinking is limited then profits may be reduced and the project may not be able to repay the loan. Their concern here is that *they would be blamed* for the resulting lack of commercial success. I suggest that this issue represents something of a dilemma for people. (11, emphasis added)

Arthur's observation implied that, under pressure from the Australian Audit Office and a tough new approach by the minister, the ADC had made its financial support dependent on the project's commercial viability. This worried some people. Buying the Sandford holdings package was not a decision taken lightly by the Aboriginal people of Fitzroy Crossing. Eighteen months of consultations and meetings enabled people to air their views and debate the issues: it took that long for them to agree on a final structure for the company and the governance of the enterprises.

Leedal, governance and the sharing of benefits

In March 1987, Leedal Pty Ltd was incorporated as an investment company—not an Aboriginal corporation; the Fitzroy Crossing Trust was created at the same time, with Leedal as Trustee. Each of the Trust's six beneficiary communities had different shareholdings within the Trust, which acquired a 50 per cent interest in the Crossing Inn, the supermarket

---

10   In retrospect, this seems an unduly optimistic aim. With intimate knowledge of the close kinship networks within Fitzroy Crossing, how was it possible for people to believe that Aboriginal staff—regardless of how well chosen they were—would be able to 'control bar sales'?

and caravan park using a $1 million loan, and an additional grant from the ADC. Several non-Indigenous people with liquor industry experience bought shares in the businesses as joint-venture partners with Leedal. One was the developer, joint-venture partner and manager of the Fitzroy River Lodge (Coppin 2006: 10). Three other non-Indigenous joint-venture partners were well-known identities in Kimberley towns (such as Broome, Halls Creek and Kununurra) where they owned high-profile and lucrative alcohol-oriented enterprises, including bars, liquor stores, hotels and tourist facilities.

The beneficiaries of the Fitzroy Trust were (and are) the Junjuwa, Marra Worra Worra,[11] Yiyili, Kadjina, Bayulu and Kurnangki communities. Following Arthur's suggestion, Junjuwa Community Inc., as the representative of the majority of local traditional owners, held the major stake: 40 out of 100 ordinary shares.[12] The remaining shares were divided between the five other communities: 12 shares each.[13] Regarding the allocation of benefits, Arthur (1989a) explained that:

> Beneficial ownership will extend to all communities of the Fitzroy Valley. Representatives of the communities will meet to discuss allocation of benefits. The spirit of this arrangement will be that Junjuwa (and finally the Bunupa of Junjuwa, being the traditional land group) will have the greatest and final say regarding all matters including allocation of benefits. Junjuwa can be seen as the principal (but not exclusive) beneficial owner. (i)

Leedal's (2014) board comprised a nominated representative from each of the six beneficiary communities. The ADC insisted that a legal adviser and an accountant or financial adviser be appointed to the board as well.[14] Learning from the financial collapse of the Woden Town Club in late 1988, and incompetent management of the Oasis Hotel at Walgett,[15] and mindful of enquiries into its conduct, the ADC was anxious to protect its investment and to ensure that professional advice was available to

---

11   Marra Worra Worra is not a community; it is an Aboriginal corporation and multipurpose resource centre designed to service decentralised communities. It is the oldest and largest Aboriginal resource agency in the Kimberley. It grew out of regular meetings about development programs held in the late 1970s by leaders of seven communities in the Valley (Sullivan 1996, Hawke 2014: 198).
12   Thorburn (2011: 111) reported that Junjuwa Community Inc. contributed $100,000 to Leedal's investments: the existence of this original contribution provokes ongoing discussion about how much the organisation should 'earn' from Leedal.
13   Current Company Extract for Leedal Pty Ltd, ASIC database 2012.
14   Since approximately 2000, there has also been a 'chief operations officer' for Leedal.
15   Woden Town Club and the Oasis Hotel in Walgett had been purchased with ADC loans (see Chapter 6).

the Trust. As in other licensed hotels owned by Aboriginal community interests, the manager was (and still is) a non-Indigenous person. Staff working in the bar were also non-Indigenous; Aboriginal barmen were tried initially, but the peer-group pressure was found to be 'too hard' for them.[16]

The ADC (1990: 19) announced the deal in its 1989–90 Annual Report:

> In February 1990, the Minister for Aboriginal Affairs, Mr Gerry Hand, officially opened the Region's most important enterprise project for the year, at Fitzroy Crossing. The purchase of the town's supermarket, caravan park and a half-share in the hotel and motel facilities in Fitzroy Crossing was undertaken on behalf of some twenty-five Aboriginal groups in the Fitzroy Valley. These enterprises are managed by a Trust Company whose board operates the ventures for the Aboriginal people.

It was anticipated that after repayment of the loan, the 'benefits' (i.e. financial benefits) of owning the hotel and other businesses would be substantial enough for distribution between several Aboriginal groups in the region. Indeed, there were discussions about how widely these should be shared out. Consultant Bill Arthur presented people with two options to consider. First, profits could be banked annually; communities could apply for loans or grants that would be decided upon by some kind of representative group. Alternatively, the annual profits could be shared out equally among the groups (meaning that each share would be rather small). To diminish the tensions that were likely to result from these arrangements, Arthur suggested that 40 per cent of the benefits be reserved for Junjuwa community, in recognition of the significant landowning status of Bunaba people. While two other language groups lived in the Junjuwa community, Junjuwa was where the most influential Bunaba people resided in 1989. It was thought that the financial benefits accruing from the hotel and other businesses could be used to support smaller communities that were short of resources, or to set up other ventures. Clearly, the Aboriginal people of Fitzroy Crossing believed that owning a 50 per cent share in the hotel would enable them to stimulate 'social development' through employment and training, as well as to improve the alcohol problem (Arthur 1989a).

---

16 Fieldnotes dated 21 June 1993, supplied by Bill Arthur. According to a Leedal spokesperson (interviewed in 2012), backpackers were the 'backbone' of the workforce at the Crossing Inn. Employing non-Indigenous bar staff is common practice in other Aboriginal-owned premises too.

In an attempt to give the structure a more social and community focus, and to enable community views to be made known to management (a suggestion made by Arthur after his earlier consultations), a Management Liaison Group (MLG) was established. The MLG sat between the board of directors and the Aboriginal communities in and around Fitzroy Crossing. The MLG, which had an open membership, was intended to represent the wider community, not just one faction; it was expected to have an understanding of the social problems of the hotel and be interested in improving the social and economic situation of the people (Arthur 1989a: 7).

Initially, Leedal owned less than a 50 per cent share in the Crossing Inn, and the Tarunda supermarket, Fitzroy shopping centre and caravan park outright. In 1989, the Fitzroy River Lodge, an extensive tourism accommodation facility that included a restaurant and bar, was built a short distance from the town. The Fitzroy Crossing Trust bought a share in that too.[17] As one Leedal director stated:

> In the past people would come in, set up a business and charge what they liked … now you do business in Fitzroy Crossing with Leedal or you don't do business at all … now we are big enough to say you either work with us or we will run you out. (Walker 1995: 5)

Evidently, Leedal soon developed an appetite for such investments. Enabled by further loans and grants, the Trust continued to acquire new properties and to increase its share in existing ones, including the Crossing Inn and the Fitzroy River Lodge.[18] In corporate terms, following its inception, Leedal accumulated capital and grew its asset base, ostensibly to generate revenue for the communities it represented (Coppin 2006: 7). However, despite owning millions of dollars in assets with profits of

---

17   Fitzroy River Lodge has 40 motel units, 30 safari tents, 90 caravan sites, coach and camping facilities, pool, tennis courts and golf course. There are no takeaway facilities, only an on-premises licence.

18   For example, in 2001, the Trust bought a 42.5 per cent interest in Fitzroy Lodge, with the help of a $1 million grant from ATSIC and a $1 million loan from IBA. The purchase of Fitzroy Lodge brought into existence a joint-venture partnership between Leedal, Mapigan Pty Ltd, and IBA's holding companies, Fitzroy Inn Investments Pty Ltd and Fitzroy Lodge Investments Pty Ltd (Irving 2007: 6). Mapigan was a proprietary company, with Wayne Bowen (the licensee of the Crossing Inn) as the sole director and secretary (Irving 2007: 30). In 2006, the Trust borrowed a further $750,000 from IBA to acquire further interests in the Fitzroy Lodge and the Crossing Inn; by 2007, Leedal owned a 70 per cent interest in the two joint-venture businesses, IBA held a 26.43 per cent interest and Mapigan held the remaining 3.57 per cent interest (Irving 2007: 31, Hope 2008: 114–15). Apart from the Crossing Inn and the Fitzroy Lodge, in 2007 Leedal owned seven other commercial interests in Fitzroy Crossing.

around $1 million a year, Leedal's pursuit of these corporate goals occurred at the expense of the community; rather than distributing profits to its six 'beneficiary' communities, it donated relatively insignificant amounts, from time to time, to various community activities.

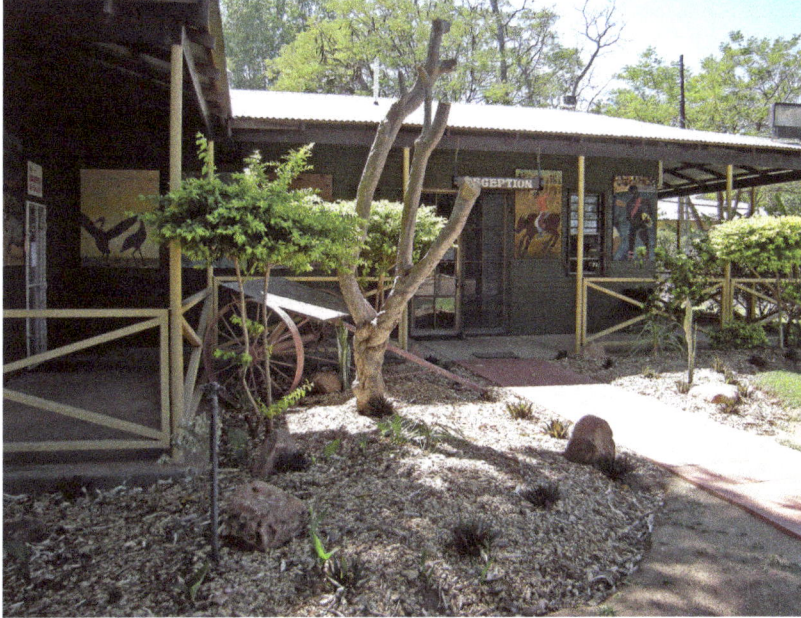

Fig. 29 The Crossing Inn reception, Fitzroy Crossing
Source: M Brady

The trajectory of alcohol-related harm 1989–2007

There is no doubt that, once it was partly owned by Aboriginal interests, the Crossing Inn implemented some harm-reduction measures. Soon after the purchase by Leedal—whose constitution obliged it to monitor alcohol consumption in the Fitzroy Valley (Leedal 2014: 5)—the Crossing Inn banned on- and off-premises sales of fortified wine (port) and sales of flagons. Subsequently, the hotel voluntarily reduced its hours of opening, banned sales of 4 L, then 2 L, casks of wine, and discounted mid-strength beer (Hope 2008: 123). However, owning only *half* of the business meant that Leedal had to negotiate any changes with its commercially driven joint-venture partners (one of whom was the nominee of the Crossing

Inn). In 1996, community leaders persuaded Leedal and the hotel's joint-venture partners to run a trial in which the sale of packaged alcohol was restricted until after 12 noon, as morning drinking was disrupting community employment projects. Although the trial was successful, the policy was discontinued due to disagreements among the partners. Restrictions, such as selling only light beer, or delaying takeaway sales until noon, were put in place in the football season and during funerals and other community events at the request of the community, and these interventions were reported positively to this author in 1998 (Brady 2005: 150). Nevertheless, the mere existence of the Crossing Inn, with its bars and particularly its off-premises sales, and its location as the only outlet for alcohol sales between Derby (260 km to the west) and Halls Creek (300 km to the east), constituted an irresistible attraction to a captive clientele. Financially, the hotel—and Leedal—made the most out of this monopoly.

In 1994, five years after the original part purchase of the Crossing Inn by Aboriginal interests, Fitzroy Crossing was described (along with Halls Creek) as having the highest drunkenness arrest figures in Western Australia (Midford et al. 1994: 5). Drinking in the Valley was said to be an 'unmanaged epidemic' involving a 'tide of poison' in which violence had become normalised (Oscar & Pedersen 2011: 92). Clearly, the hotel was *not* monitoring or slowing down alcohol consumption. During pay weeks, the area around the premises was populated by drunken staggering people, as described by a senior medical officer, Dr J Rowland:

> There would be little fires lit in the bushes and people surrounding those fires, drunk and drinking, and people wandering around and bodies scattered in various poses all around ... many stuporous bodies on the ground ... people that are waving, drunk, bottles and rocks, all approach the ambulance and you don't feel very safe ... 'Which of these bodies lying around is the unconscious one we need to assess?' (cited in Hope 2008: 109)

Opposite the Crossing Inn was a poorly lit area known to all as 'Billabong Park' where drinkers consumed the takeaway alcohol bought at the hotel. At least one rape and one murder took place there. It was so dangerous that even the police were unwilling to enter. Late in 2006, by agreement between the police and the Shire (which owned the land), the area was closed. This action did not stop alcohol-related brawls and assaults; instead, the violence moved to people's homes, making policing even more difficult.

By 2007, the annual consumption of pure alcohol in Fitzroy Crossing was estimated to be 27 L per person, equating to 35 cans of beer per week for every person in town (Dr John Boulton, cited in Fitzpatrick et al. 2015b). As the Crossing Inn was the only source of packaged alcohol in town, and with takeaway sales far outweighing on-premises sales at the Crossing Inn and the Fitzroy River Lodge, the Crossing Inn was the source of the majority of those 35 cans per person, per week. According to evidence given later at a coronial inquest, the Crossing Inn's licensee reported that alcohol sales in the 2006–07 financial year totalled $4 million (Strutt 2007b). By the time this calculation was made, Leedal had increased its equity in the Crossing Inn, giving the Aboriginal company majority (70 per cent) ownership.[19]

Aboriginal people of the Kimberley were suffering a complex social and health crisis; alcohol abuse was both a cause and a result of many of the problems (Western Australian Department of Health 2009). This crisis became evident in several ways—primarily through the high number of alcohol-related deaths and prevalence of fetal alcohol spectrum disorder (FASD). Between 2000 and 2007, there were 22 deaths of Aboriginal people in the Fitzroy Crossing region that required coronial investigation and that were believed to be linked with alcohol abuse. In one year alone, 2006, there were eight self-harm deaths. Drinking in pregnancy was also common. Out of a sample of 122 women in the Fitzroy Valley who gave birth between 2002 and 2003, one-quarter reported alcohol-related injuries and one in seven needed an alcohol-related hospital admission. Using the AUDIT C assessment tool, 60 of these women were found to drink alcohol at risky or high-risk levels during their pregnancies; 55 of these consumed seven or more standard drinks on a typical drinking day (Fitzpatrick et al. 2015b: 332).[20] The researchers considered that these calculations were probably underestimations, and noted that such levels of alcohol consumption were generally associated with high rates of FASD.

Aboriginal people, particularly those at Fitzroy Crossing, were gradually becoming aware of the existence of FASD. Many suspected that it was present among the community's children. Around half the students at the local primary–secondary school were reported to have 'learning difficulties' associated with FASD or with other social and environmental

19 In late 2006, Leedal acquired a further 27.14 per cent equity in the Crossing Inn from IBA, which still owned a 16 per cent partnership share in the Inn (IBA 2007: 135).
20 AUDIT = Alcohol Use Disorders Identification Test.

challenges (Irving 2007: 36). When assessments were conducted a few years later, 13 out of 108 children were found to have FASD or partial FASD, giving a prevalence of 120 per 1000, which is among the highest FASD prevalence in the world (Fitzpatrick et al. 2015a: 454). Of the children with FASD, 69 per cent had microcephaly, 85 per cent had weight deficiency and all had central nervous system damage, commonly showing as attention deficit hyperactivity disorder.

With all the drinking going on in town, the women's refuge was kept busy: 96 women sought refuge there over a six-month period in 2006, with one woman attending on 24 separate occasions in less than a year. Over a six-month period, 85 per cent of all trauma patients admitted to the local hospital/clinic were intoxicated (Irving 2007: 33, 39). These very high rates of alcohol-related harm began to provoke deep concern in the community, and local people, particularly women, started to mobilise to do something about them. Aware of these rumblings of discontent about alcohol consumption, the Crossing Inn voluntarily changed some of the rules about takeaway sales in late 2006 or early 2007. The hotel's licensee, presumably in consultation with Leedal, decided that packaged alcohol would no longer be sold to people walking into its takeaway shop—it would only be sold to people *driving in* with a vehicle. After this relatively minor adjustment, Leedal resisted further efforts to negotiate a voluntary accord to restrict sales of alcohol (Oscar & Pedersen 2011: 94).[21] One participant reported at the time:

> There are some self-imposed restrictions. We're saying the current restrictions are not working to their full potential. There's been the closure of Billabong Park across the road from the takeaway … they used to go over there. Then the licensee upgraded it, but the downside was uncontrollable, there were rapes etc., it was very difficult to police. The Shire, whose land it is, said it was a breach. It was closed down but the purchase of alcohol continued. They had a ruling that you have to be in a vehicle to purchase but alcohol was being transported back into communities. There was a collapse of senior leadership in the communities and the same with the community in town, not functioning at all.[22]

---

21 Leedal stated in 2007 that since buying the hotel in 1989, sales had declined by 29 per cent because of self-imposed restrictions (Taylor 2007).
22 Brady fieldnotes, 14 August 2007.

The mobilisation of the community

A tipping point was reached between December 2006 and December 2007, when the growing alarm expressed by community members and service providers within and beyond Fitzroy Crossing triggered a cascade of events. After a spate of alcohol-related suicides and other deaths at Fitzroy Crossing, in December 2006, the Kimberley Aboriginal Law and Culture Centre (KALACC)[23] wrote to the state coroner, insisting that a coronial inquest was needed 'to jolt the systems of government, and *some elements within the local community*, into an appropriate level of response' (Hope 2008: 2, emphasis added). Their request was supported by local MLA, Tom Stephens. The following July, a bush meeting of women from the four language groups of the Fitzroy Valley agreed to campaign for a 12-month moratorium on takeaway sales, citing unacceptably high levels of violence, assault, rape, suicide, incarceration, FASD, child abuse and neglect, and the low life expectancy and quality of life associated with harmful alcohol use.[24] They resolved to confront Leedal and to approach the director of Liquor Licensing. The plan caused uproar: its proponents were confronted with accusations, threats and coercion.[25] One of the proponents was Topsy Chestnut, who had been the chair of the WAA group in 1988. The July women's meeting came up with three aspirations: to restrict full-strength alcohol, to invest in the needs of men and boys and to turn the police around to a more community-based policing style. Further community meetings were held in Fitzroy Crossing across all language groups at which people expressed concern about the levels of drinking, the deaths and the suicides. Senior women made a presentation to the senior men of KALACC outlining the damage alcohol was doing to the communities and seeking their support: 'We want to bring about a future where we have respect for our culture, respect for our leaders, and safety for our children and families', the women declared. At the end of July, the chair of KALACC, statesman John Watson, issued a press release supporting the moratorium.[26] In the following weeks, *The West Australian*,

---

23   KALACC is a peak body supporting the Law, culture and languages of 30 Aboriginal groups in the region.
24   These effects were listed in an Outline of Marninwarntikura Draft Submission to the Director of Liquor Licensing, 24 August 2007 (in the author's possession). Senior paediatrician in the Kimberly Dr John Boulton also publicly called for urgent action on alcohol abuse (*ABC News* 2007b). The bush meeting was organised by the Marninwarntikura Women's Resource Centre.
25   The stressful nature of this period is captured in interviews with protagonists in the film *Yajilarra* (Hogan 2009).
26   *Kimberley men resolve to support Fitzroy Crossing women* (2007). Media release, 31 July.

the national press and the ABC ran a flood of stories on the proposed takeaway ban. The media focused on the fact that the Crossing Inn was Aboriginal owned, with one front-page story describing the hotel as the Aboriginal pub 'that poisons its own' (*West Australian* 22 July 2007).

The director of Liquor Licensing gave the communities six weeks to find locally agreed solutions, after which he intended to commence formal proceedings under Western Australia's Liquor Control Act (Department of Racing, Gaming and Liquor 2008). Fortunately for everyone involved, by this time, the director had greater flexibility in decision-making, and could place less emphasis on purely 'legal' factors in decisions; this was as a result of the abolition of the previous Western Australian Liquor Licensing Court in May 2007. Prior to this, one Licensing Court judge had ruled that it was not within his power, or the Act itself, to restrict the sale of alcohol to promote public health (National Drug Research Institute 2007: 136).

There were last-ditch proposals by Leedal and its partners in the two licensed premises for additional self-imposed restrictions, such as having no alcohol sales on Sundays and Mondays. These were considered 'weak' by the women's group, as these days were already known to be slow sales days when there was little cash around. Even though the restriction would not affect the Fitzroy River Lodge,[27] its general manager circulated a petition during the six-week discussion period, urging customers to be 'calm and patient' and to write letters to the director of Liquor Licensing protesting against the proposed moratorium on takeaway sales:

> Please be advised that the licensees of both the Fitzroy River Lodge and the Crossing Inn Hotel are doing what they can to resolve the issue to the satisfaction of all members of the community … [You can] visit the Lodge and sign the current petition opposing a total ban on takeaway alcohol!

By this time, many different players were involved in an increasingly fractious, polarised and public debate. *The West Australian* and other media continued to print articles on alcohol-related problems and the role of Leedal. The bad publicity made IBA and its responsible federal minister increasingly uncomfortable. IBA, which had inherited the ADC's financial interests in Leedal, owned a 26 per cent interest in the Crossing Inn (down from 43 per cent in 2006). At the prompting of

---

27   The Fitzroy River Lodge (by this time 70 per cent owned by Leedal) already held a restricted licence that allowed residents only to consume alcohol in their rooms.

the Minister for Employment and Workplace Relations, Joe Hockey, IBA ordered a review of the hotel's sales practices and restrictions, and of the social and economic effect of the Crossing Inn and Fitzroy Lodge. IBA's review added to the quarrelsome atmosphere. On one side were those who supported the proposed moratorium on takeaway sales and the interrogation of Leedal's conduct. They included the original lobbyists for the takeaway ban (i.e. prominent Aboriginal women and senior Aboriginal men); the commissioner of police; the local member for Central Kimberley-Pilbara, Tom Stephens; the director of Liquor Licensing; and Aboriginal spokesperson Lionel Quartermaine, formerly a deputy chair of ATSIC. Arguing that there was nothing worse than 'our own people' living off the misery and illness of others', Quartermaine called for the Australian Securities and Investments Commission, rather than IBA, to investigate Leedal (Strutt 2007a). The other side included Leedal spokespeople who argued that banning takeaway alcohol would be a removal of Aboriginal people's rights, and those aligned with them who asserted that the review of Leedal was 'racist' (*ABC News* 2007c). Leedal fought tenaciously against what became an unstoppable flow of events (Oscar & Pedersen 2011: 92). An article published on the front page of *The West Australian* on 25 August 2007, headlined 'Grog hurts quarter of Kimberley under-fives', highlighted alcohol's damaging effect on babies; this made it politically impossible to oppose the restrictions.[28] From 1 October 2007, the sale of packaged liquor was restricted.[29] Perth barrister, George Irving, reviewed Leedal's practices as requested by IBA.[30] Meanwhile, the state coroner conducted an inquiry into multiple drug- and alcohol-related deaths.

The inquest

One week after takeaway restrictions were imposed, Coroner Alistair Hope arrived in Fitzroy Crossing to conduct hearings as part of an inquest into 22 Aboriginal deaths (including suicides) in the Kimberley that were

---

28 Dr John Boulton, pers comm, 18 July 2016. The article in *The West Australian* was by Jessica Strutt.

29 The director of Liquor Licensing imposed restrictions (initially for six months) from 1 October 2007 on the sale of all packaged liquor exceeding 2.7 per cent ethanol to anyone other than a lodger at either of the two licensed outlets in Fitzroy Crossing (the Crossing Inn and the Fitzroy River Lodge).

30 IBA proposed a review team consisting of its chairman, a staff member and Perth barrister, George Irving. However, Irving was concerned at the perceived bias in this approach, and the terms of the review were adjusted so that he alone would consult broadly and report back to IBA, who would in turn report to the minister. The review was announced on 25 July 2007.

associated with either alcohol or cannabis (Hope 2008). The abuse of alcohol was identified by all witnesses as a major cause of child neglect, domestic violence, assaults, threatening behaviour and abject poverty: noisy drinking and fighting kept hundreds of people awake at night— every night. The respected epidemiologist, Professor Fiona Stanley, gave evidence about alcohol's association with damage to the fetus. During the hearings, it became clear that the Crossing Inn was gravely implicated in many of the deaths. Two intoxicated male pedestrians were found to have been killed by drunk drivers on two separate occasions while walking away from the hotel, one being run over *twice*. Two individuals had drowned trying to cross the flooded Fitzroy River: one was trying to reach the Crossing Inn, the other was leaving the hotel. A man had died of a heart attack while drinking in Billabong Park opposite the takeaway outlet at the Crossing Inn. Others had committed suicide after consuming extraordinary amounts of alcohol bought at the hotel.

Of the 22 Kimberley deaths investigated by the coroner, most were caused by self-harm. The coroner was particularly concerned about a cluster of eight suicide deaths in 2006[31] in the Fitzroy Crossing region.[32] Most of these individuals had consumed copious amounts of alcohol; in 11 cases, the blood alcohol levels were over 0.2 per cent, which is extremely high (see Table 3). It is worth noting that a person with a blood alcohol concentration of between 0.200 and 0.300 may be disoriented, anxious, aggressive and violent, have poor coordination and trouble breathing. A blood alcohol reading of 0.318 (the highest noted in Table 3) indicates probable stupor; an individual so affected would have little comprehension of where they were—any higher and they would risk death from respiratory arrest (Brady et al. 2005). Blood alcohol concentrations as high as these provide irrefutable evidence that drinkers were able to access and consume extraordinary amounts of alcohol.[33]

---

31 In 2006 alone, there were 21 Aboriginal deaths from self-harm across the Kimberley region.
32 The total population of the Fitzroy Crossing region was about 3500.
33 It is, of course, illegal to continue to sell alcohol (for on- or off-premises consumption) to a person who is already intoxicated.

Table 3 Alcohol-related deaths at Fitzroy Crossing investigated by the
Western Australian coroner, 2007

Individual	Age	Date of death	Place of death	Blood alcohol level	Cause of death
1	56	13/03/2000	Fitzroy River	–	Drowned trying to reach the Crossing Inn
2	21	15/04/2000	Fitzroy River	–	Drowned in river after drinking at the Crossing Inn
3	35	26/05/2000	F. Crossing	0.318%	Run over (by drunk driver) Sandford Rd
4	17	14/02/2002	F. Crossing	0.226%	Hanging
5	57	28/01/2004	F. Crossing	0.140%	Multiple injuries, run over by two different drunk drivers near the Crossing Inn
6	29	18/11/2005	F. Crossing	0.238%	Hanging after attending the Crossing Inn
7	11	07/10/2005	F. Crossing, Perth hospital	–	Hypoxia (intentional or unintentional hanging)
8	52	12/01/2006	Billabong Pk, F. Crossing	0.189%	Ischaemic heart/coronary arteriosclerosis, died while drinking
9	33	16/04/2006	F. Crossing	0.236%	Hanging
10	40	10/10/2006	F. Crossing	0.157%	Hanging after attending the Crossing Inn
11	23	26/10/2006	F. Crossing	0%	Hanging
12	24	30/11/2006	F. Crossing	0.171%	Hanging
13	24	26/12/2006	F. Crossing	0.180%	Hanging

Source: Compiled from Hope (2008)

The coroner's inquiry and subsequent report ranged over many aspects
of Aboriginal life in the Fitzroy Valley[34] and drew critical attention to the
role played by the Crossing Inn. It was a matter of concern, Hope (2008:
108) observed:

> That evidence at the inquest revealed that most of the alcohol purchased
> by [the] deceased persons … was supplied by the Crossing Inn Hotel,
> a hotel part-owned throughout the relevant period by Aboriginal people

---

34   Apart from alcohol and cannabis use, the coroner's report dealt with the social context
surrounding the deaths, including government services to Fitzroy Crossing, housing, education,
school attendance, mental health, the role of the police and the hospital.

through a Trust, The Fitzroy Crossing Trust, the trustee of which is a private company, Leedal Pty Ltd (Leedal), which had originally been incorporated through the instigation of the Aboriginal Development Council [sic], a Commonwealth Government organisation.

Hope found that Leedal's self-imposed restrictions had *not* been successful. He was dismissive of Leedal's claim to be selling alcohol responsibly and was unimpressed when the hotel's licensee claimed that the new takeaway sales ban was 'ill-conceived' and 'incorrectly implemented', since objective evidence clearly showed the measures to have been extremely effective (103, 123). Reminding Leedal that the original purpose of owning an interest in the Crossing Inn had been to correct local alcohol-related problems, Hope asked why the organisation had not supported the takeaway ban. More damaging was his focus on Leedal's failure to substantially benefit the community over its 18 years of operation. Instead of helping Aboriginal people in Fitzroy Crossing and surrounds, Hope pointed out that Leedal had harmed them, while making millions of dollars in profits and acquiring assets. The residents of the 'beneficiary communities' had received no distributions or dividends from Leedal's profits; nor had they 'escaped the damaging effects of alcohol abuse':

> It is not surprising that members of the community beneficiaries are extremely concerned that there have been considerable social and economic and health costs which have resulted from the sale of alcohol, particularly from the Crossing Inn Hotel, but that community members have seen little or no benefits. (120)

Three of the deceased persons took their own lives in the community that was the largest shareholder in Leedal (and which therefore held a substantial interest in the Crossing Inn). In observing this tragic irony, Hope (2008: 124) suggested that Leedal should consider its credibility and 'not act in a way which would be seen by the local community as being motivated by self-interest'. His words reprised the insights of nineteenth-century temperance campaigners, one of whom wrote:

> The secret of most of the mischief now worked by the [liquor] trade is that the monopoly of the sale of liquor is connected with private interests … The brewer, the distiller, the publican, the shareholder, are all deeply interested in promoting the sale of liquor. (Wilson 1894: 7)

The aftermath

These events—the inquest, the attention of the director of Liquor Licensing, the investigations into FASD by prominent medical professionals and the intense public scrutiny—combined to provoke a series of outcomes and responses from government and associated agencies, the management of the Crossing Inn and Leedal itself.

Government responses

The Western Australian Government was quick to respond to the coroner's findings. It announced that a new alcohol and drug treatment service would be established in Fitzroy Crossing (Department of Indigenous Affairs 2008), and authorised the state's Drug and Alcohol Office to fund research on the effect of the restrictions. Produced by researchers at Notre Dame University, the first six-monthly monitoring report in March 2008 showed an overall reduction in harm: less violence, fewer police and emergency department callouts, fewer alcohol-related crimes and an increase in school attendance. After 12 months, the local emergency department reported a 36 per cent reduction in monthly presentations and reductions in the severity of injuries (Henderson-Yates et al. 2008, Akesson 2009).

The federal government also responded with alacrity. The public scrutiny of Leedal and its activities reflected negatively on IBA, which still owned a share in the Crossing Inn, and on Hockey as the responsible minister. Before Irving's review was completed, Hockey instructed IBA to sell its share of the Crossing Inn, retaining only its interests in the Fitzroy River Lodge and other investments (Barrass 2007: 6).[35] On 9 August 2007, ABC's *Message Stick* reported that, as a result of the Australian government's 'new stance on alcohol in Aboriginal communities', in connection with the imminent 'Emergency Intervention' in the Northern Territory,[36] as well

---

35 The chronology of events is as follows: on 23 July 2007, Joe Hockey demanded that IBA conduct an investigation into the social and economic effects of the Crossing Inn. On 25 July, IBA approached Irving to conduct the investigation, with a short turnaround of 10 days. The terms of reference were reviewed and released on 2 August. On 8 August, Hockey instructed IBA's board to sell its share in the pub 'after he became aware of the damage the hotel was doing to the community' (Barrass 2007: 6). At the time, Irving had not completed his report: he was still at Fitzroy Crossing. Irving's report is dated 13 September 2007.
36 This 'new stance' on alcohol is a reference to the tightening of liquor regulations affecting Indigenous communities, which accompanied the NTER (the 'Intervention') announced in September 2007.

as unfavourable media attention, IBA had offered to sell its share in the Crossing Inn to the other joint-venture partners. The sale was finalised some months later. Significantly, the Crossing Inn was not included in the IBA's map of 'principal investment sites' in its Annual Report for 2007–08 (IBA 2008: 22). However, it was not until the following year's Annual Report that IBA reported its divestment of the Crossing Inn (IBA 2009: 29). No attention was drawn to the fact that IBA gave Leedal a grant through its Economic Development Initiative that enabled Leedal to buy out IBA's share. Since the funds were categorised as a grant rather than a loan, they were quite separate from IBA's investment program (IBA 2009: 68).

Not everyone supported IBA's withdrawal from the Crossing Inn. Tom Stephens wanted IBA to stay involved and to stick to the original business plan, which was to ban the sale of takeaway grog (Barrass 2007). Irving (2007) also recommended that IBA should stay involved. On the basis of his government-sponsored investigation of the Crossing Inn, he advised the agency to provide mentoring, training and support to the community beneficiaries and Leedal, until Leedal could be 'transferred to an appropriate governance structure, comprised of the community beneficiaries' (47). Mentoring, training and support were clearly required; however, they would not be provided by IBA.

Changes at the Crossing Inn

Leedal's principals complained that they had been 'slandered', but they had in fact been shamed. Even the United Kingdom's *Independent* newspaper featured a story describing the strange irony of the fact that the Crossing Inn and the Fitzroy River Lodge were owned by 'the very people whom those businesses are "poisoning" ' (Marks 2007). The directors of Leedal and the management of the Crossing Inn were forced to make changes: beginning in 2008, the hotel implemented several harm-reduction strategies that, arguably, should have been in place long before. As one community member stated:

> It was easy for them before. They sold takeaways and said goodbye. It's only since the restrictions came in that the hotel's been forced to take responsibility, and [ask] the police for help.[37]

---

37   Brady fieldnotes, 4 August 2009.

The ban on takeaway sales had an immediate effect on the Crossing Inn. In the three months before the restrictions, takeaway sales from the hotel had totalled 8,500 L of pure alcohol; in the three months following, they were down to 949 L of pure alcohol.[38] The hotel also experienced a surge in the number of Aboriginal people drinking *on the premises*. Extra security and staff had to be engaged. There was a 44 per cent increase in the amount of pure alcohol (by volume) purchased for consumption on the premises (from 819 L in July–September 2007, to 1,180 L in October–December 2007). Overall, the restrictions had a direct and immediate effect on the volume and type of alcohol sold: the amount of pure alcohol sold from the Crossing Inn reduced by 77 per cent.

In March 2008, in a letter to the researchers from Notre Dame University who were evaluating the effectiveness of the restrictions, the Crossing Inn's manager revealed the challenges of trying to bring rapid change to entrenched drinking styles:

The bars at the Crossing Inn took a dramatic change from having nearly nobody in [them] after 1.00 pm to having … between 100 to 150 in the bars from 10.00 am till 10.00 pm most days. The ban has forced them to seek full strength beer in the bars. From my experiences from working in the bar I am well aware that this is not what they enjoy doing … they have always chosen to take their alcohol way [sic] to drink. Whether it be at home with friends and family or under their favourite tree … After the first week of the ban it was pretty obvious that they were not accustomed to drinking in the bars for a long period of time as opposed to drinking at home … I had to come up with some sort of strategy to slow them down and try to help them drink responsibly and to give them some sort of break during trading hours. So it was decided to try the following, open the bar from 12.00 noon and then close from 3.00 pm till 5.00 pm to give them a breather … but … they just caught a taxi out to the Fitzroy River Lodge for the next 2 or 3 hours … Quite often we are forced to close early. This of course has had a huge effect on our regular contractors and locals that used to drink at the Inn because now they just don't. These [Aboriginal] people are being forced to drink in an environment that they are not used to and don't want … A lot of these people do not realise that they are not allowed to be drunk on [licensed] premises as a lot of them have not drunk in the bars and have only done so since this most irresponsible decision was handed down forcing them into the bars. (Henderson-Yates et al. 2008, appendix VIII: 109)

---

38 These takeaway sales would include sales of low-alcohol beer, and sales of full-strength beer made to lodgers at the Crossing Inn. Data from the Western Australian Drug and Alcohol Office, August 2009.

Usually only the haunt of tourists, the Fitzroy River Lodge reported large numbers of Aboriginal patrons drinking at their bar. Both the Crossing Inn and the Fitzroy Lodge were chaotic, inundated with uncontrolled drinkers who, it was reported:

> Did not understand the strict bar regulations that applied. When refused service because of drunken behaviour and non-observance of other bar regulations, they became aggressive to staff and with each other. At the same time personal fights would develop between family members. (Henderson-Yates et al. 2008: 33)

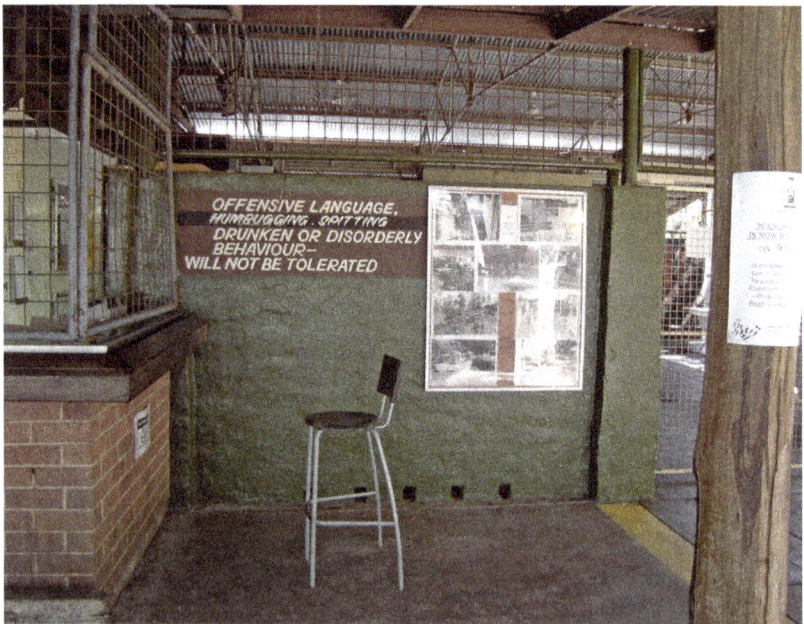

Fig. 30 Signage at the Crossing Inn
Source: M Brady

As a result, signs were installed behind the bar about the behaviours expected of customers on the premises (e.g. 'no spitting, no humbug'), and the Crossing Inn displayed responsible service of alcohol posters.[39] The manager began to sit on a local alcohol and other drug management committee established by the Western Australia Drug and Alcohol Office, which was dedicated to reducing alcohol-related harm in the community. With so much attention now focused on the effects of alcohol on unborn

---

39   These were reported in the Leedal *Newsletter* 2008, November (3).

children, the Crossing Inn agreed to have plastic beer glasses printed with FASD warning messages on them; the Fitzroy River Lodge refused to use them, arguing that it was a tourist facility.[40] The Crossing Inn started to provide hot food over the bar and lunches and afternoon teas in the gallery during the tourist season. Pamphlets were printed for members of the public explaining what the liquor restrictions were and why they had been imposed; new road signs were erected outside the town announcing the restrictions.

In the wake of the restriction on takeaway sales, there was a slight decrease in takings at the Tarunda supermarket (part of Leedal's holdings), which suggested that some Fitzroy Crossing residents were travelling away from home to purchase alcohol *and* food. It was still possible to buy sly grog in Fitzroy Crossing. Nevertheless, following a six-month review, the director of Liquor Licensing extended the restriction on the sale of takeaway liquor indefinitely (Department of Racing, Gaming and Liquor 2008, Oscar & Pedersen 2011). He declared that the restriction, which was subject to regular review, was in the *public interest*:

> Negative impacts, and inconvenience experienced by those residents who wished to purchase full strength packaged liquor for takeaway, did not outweigh the social and health benefits that had been experienced by the broader community since October 2007. (Department of Racing, Gaming and Liquor 2008: 23)

Damage control at Leedal

The public exposure of Leedal's failings provoked it to improve its image by publishing a quarterly newsletter. Commencing in 2008, the newsletter featured (mostly) laudatory stories about its contributions to the community, business awards and appointments to its board, and an opinion column written by the chairman. That year, Leedal also implemented a strategic management plan to ensure that its directors had 'a clear understanding of all major business decisions before voting on them'. The aim was to 'develop the economic base of Fitzroy Crossing and to assist Indigenous community members who want to develop their own businesses'. A publicity pamphlet—'All about Leedal'—presented the names and qualifications of the company's bankers, auditors and legal advisers. Leedal also made several new professional appointments to its

---

40 Such an argument implies that FASD is not a problem for the general population: it is.

board, including a lawyer from a respected Perth law firm, and a new financial adviser. An earlier legal adviser had been found to be corrupt,[41] and the original financial adviser had reportedly been responsible for Leedal's commercial strategy of redirecting profits to loan repayments and new investments, rather than the community.

Irving's review had found that, instead of instituting an orderly mechanism for the distribution of profits to beneficiaries, Leedal had gifted negligible sums of money—apparently at whim—to various clubs, organisations, school projects and individuals not directly associated with the shareholding communities (Irving 2007: 44–5). The issue was treated critically by the media[42] and reiterated by Hope (2008: 120–1), who pointed out that Leedal had no plan in place that 'would involve some distribution of that income in the relatively near future'. The coroner urged the Department of Indigenous Affairs to intervene; however, neither it nor the Drug and Alcohol Office had any authority over Leedal (Department of Indigenous Affairs 2008: 23).

Stung by these revelations, in 2010, Leedal announced that it was providing $250,000 to create a new charitable fund: Yapawarnti Fund Inc.[43] Directed by representatives from Leedal's six 'beneficiaries' (Junjuwa, Kurnangki, Marra Worra Worra, Kadjina, Bayulu and Yiyili), Yapawarnti's purpose was to support Fitzroy Valley's youth. Funding applications were to be assessed by the Yapawarnti board, the makeup of which was similar to Leedal itself: it included the directors of Leedal and the same chairman. The formation of this charitable association was Leedal's first (belated) attempt to share some of its profits in an orderly way with the communities that had made it rich—profits that included those derived from the sale of alcohol at the 'community' hotel.

---

41 The ADC had insisted from the beginning that there be a qualified lawyer and an accountant appointed as directors of Leedal. Unfortunately, the chosen lawyer was later struck off the roll of legal practitioners, after having been found guilty of embezzling money belonging to the Australian Paralympic Committee; he narrowly avoided jail (ABIX 2007).

42 There were headlines including 'ASIC must investigate profits from Fitzroy pub', *The West* 26 July 2007; 'Minister wants probe of Fitzroy pub profits', *The West* 10 August 2007; 'Leedal at centre of Fitzroy funds row', *The West* 1 March 2008.

43 The Yapawarnti Fund was Incorporated under the *Associations Incorporation Act, 1987* (WA) ('Investing in our children', *Leedal Newsletter* 7 August 2010).

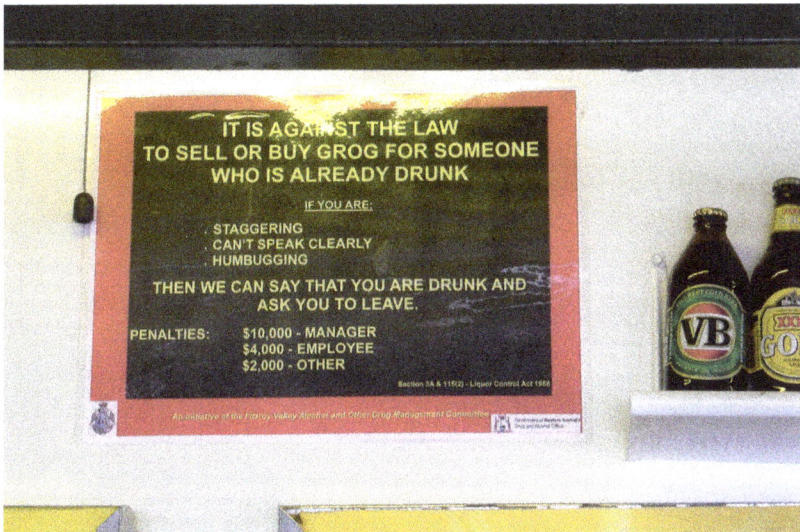

Fig. 31 Rules of behaviour at the Crossing Inn bar
Source: M Brady

Analysing what happened in Fitzroy Crossing

Unlike other Indigenous-owned hotels, the project to buy the Crossing Inn and other businesses was carefully planned, with consultations carried out by a locally known researcher who worked with relevant communities and interest groups. Local residents genuinely hoped for improvements to drinking behaviour as a result of their partnership in the purchase. Of all the hotels purchased by Indigenous associations since the 1970s, the Crossing Inn purchase underwent the most thorough preliminary planning. Yet, the hotel came to be responsible for damaging sales of alcohol to the communities it was supposed to benefit most. Irving (2007), in his report to Minister Hockey and IBA, stated that the Fitzroy project had been successful and disastrous at the same time. He explained succinctly:

> If success is measured by corporate growth then the Fitzroy Project, through Leedal, provides an outstanding example of social and economic development. Leedal is now the largest and most successful commercial enterprise in Fitzroy Crossing … [However,] if success is measured in terms of community involvement in and ownership of the outcome of a project, or in terms of improvements to the community's wellbeing, then the Fitzroy Project must be judged as having failed the community it set out to benefit. (5, 6)

There are a number of interlocking explanations for what went so wrong: Leedal and its funders placed profits before people; governments, caught up in a period of upheaval in Aboriginal affairs policy, failed in their oversight; and the 'beneficiary community'—the Aboriginal communities of Fitzroy Crossing and surrounds—was neither willing nor able to intervene in the direction pursued by Leedal.

Putting profits before people

With community ownership enacted through representation on Leedal's board, it would not have been difficult to amend the Crossing Inn's licence to end the sale of takeaway alcohol. An approach to the liquor licensing authority in Western Australia, demonstrating community support and a plan to negotiate with local Aboriginal service providers in health and legal aid, would have sufficed. At the time, in the late 1980s and early 1990s, negotiations such as these were beginning to happen in parts of central and southern Australia (Gray et al. 1995, Brady et al. 2003, National Drug Research Institute 2007).

An informed observer of long experience, Stephens (cited in Barrass 2007: 6), blamed 'IBA and its joint venture partners' for diverting the project to the new goals of asset acquisition and rapid loan repayment. He reflected that:

> A key feature of the initial business case upon which the joint venture was established involved a strategy that was widely endorsed within the local community and supported by me, involving an end to the sale of takeaway alcohol … Instead, IBA and its joint venture partners have effectively put in place an alternative business strategy that has seen aggressive sales of takeaway alcohol underpinning these excessive profits and returns, allowing the joint venture partners to pay back their loans and cover their borrowings at a rate much faster than ever originally planned. This reneging has compounded the human misery within Fitzroy Crossing and significantly contributed to the alcohol-related deaths and suicides within this community.

The focus on commercial rather than social goals for the Crossing Inn had commenced with community consultations, which revealed fears that, should the hotel and other enterprises not be a commercial success, Aboriginal people would be 'blamed' (Arthur 1989a: 11). When Leedal initially devoted considerable effort to repaying its $1 million loan from the ADC, it was presumably responding to such pressure. Leedal decided that its guiding principles were to develop an economic base in the region, which is understandable. The joint-venture partners encouraged this emphasis on profitability. Leedal originally owned less than half the shares in the businesses. The other partners in the original joint venture were part of the liquor industry; they were hardly likely to be sympathetic to public health strategies and ideas about harm reduction or social wellbeing. They were well-known Western Australian entrepreneurs who owned regional tourism and hospitality businesses in the Kimberley and elsewhere; their association with the business of selling liquor pointed Leedal in a particular direction. The less experienced Aboriginal board members, drawn from local communities, may have wished to take the business in a different direction, but their voices were not as strong. One early board member recalled:

> We had no training when we started as directors of the company, no idea. We were making decisions about the business that were ill-informed. We relied on [name] and others [non-Aboriginal board members] to supply that information about the industry.[44]

However, there is more to the story. The loan to the ADC was paid off relatively quickly. By the turn of the twenty-first century, the company was wealthy. Leedal acquired other assets and increased its equity in the Crossing Inn, strengthening its position. Why was Leedal persistently unwilling to keep faith with the original spirit of the purchase—to reduce alcohol harms, regardless of profits? Why did it not curtail off-premises sales for the benefit of the community? Leedal claimed to own assets worth more than $10 million, held in trust for the six beneficiary communities.[45] Right from the beginning, Leedal had diversified its investments; it owned shops, a supermarket, the hotel, a tourist lodge and a caravan park. With such a diversified portfolio, Leedal could have lost some revenue from alcohol sales at the hotel without negatively affecting its overall financial security.[46] However, when members of a state committee of inquiry into alcohol-treatment services asked Leedal where its profits went, the chairman answered that after loan repayments, the priority was to 'build the assets'. Leedal's operations manager replied more fully:

---

44 Brady fieldnotes, KP, interview, 2009.
45 'All about Leedal' (2009) [Pamphlet].
46 By 1992–93, three to four years after its part purchase by Leedal, the Crossing Inn's alcohol sales were estimated to be at least $3 million and the Tarunda supermarket was not far behind with sales of $2.2 million (Smith 2006: 263).

Regarding where the funds go, I want to emphasise that 10 years ago when I started here, the company owed more than $1 million in a loan. Where does the money go? The Leedal Pty Ltd is a trust for the Fitzroy Trust. Obviously the funds stay within that trust. As mentioned ... each of the beneficiaries or communities that own the company have a director from each of those beneficiaries. We have four meetings a year—one every quarter—when funds or profits are available we put it to the board to decide what to do and it goes back to the communities and discusses it with council or community members to acquire a bigger percentage of what they had. This is where we have got to own 100 per cent of the Crossing Inn. When I first started here it was 42 per cent. In 10 years we acquired 10 per cent of that. This was 42 per cent as well, Patrick, am I correct. Now it is 70 per cent. (Subcommittee of the Education and Health Standing Committee 2010: 5–6, cf. Education and Health Standing Committee 2011)

It is not surprising that the operations manager's testimony gloried in Leedal's commercial success. Many accolades from the business and mining sector have been heaped upon the company and its directors, including the West Kimberley Small Business Award in 2013, the Rhinehart Development of Northern Regional WA Award in 2014, and the Horizon Power Leadership and Development Award in 2015.[47] However, rewarding this version of 'success' begs the question of whether an Indigenous business—more so, perhaps, than any other type of business—should be seeking to incorporate *social* benefits (or harms) as valid indicators of good (or less good) performance, or as part of their 'normal' commercial aspirations? (Arthur 1999).[48] In a discussion about welfare and enterprise, one commentator observed:

While from one perspective the drive to accumulate may be seen as a corruption of the original intent to alleviate the effects of Aboriginal unemployment and social dislocation, from the point of view of the Indigenous business leaders who run them, it may be seen as a normal commercial aspiration to retain profits for expanded operations. (Smith 2006: 264)

---

47 It should be noted that in the same year that Leedal's businesses won several awards, June Oscar, who was one of several leaders responsible for the ban on takeaway sales, was made a member of the Order of Australia in recognition of her work campaigning against alcohol-related harm—an accolade that was reported in the *Leedal Newsletter* (12 July 2013).

48 Another decision that could, arguably, be interpreted as being harmful to the physical wellbeing of local people occurred when Leedal awarded the franchise to operate a shop within its Tarunda Supermarket complex to a fast-food fried chicken outlet, rather than selecting a more healthy (although possibly less profitable) option. 'Rosie's Chicken' is a small takeaway franchise designed to compete with McDonald's and KFC.

Welcome to Fitzroy Crossing

Fitzroy Crossing is located on the bank of the Fitzroy River in the heart of the Kimberley region and is a great place for travelers to stop when heading either west, east or somewhere in between. It is a small town, but it has some big "Must See" attractions.

- Geikie Gorge National Park is just 18km north east of the town via a sealed road. Boat tours are available as well as walking trails which allow you to see all the beauty of the Gorge.
- Take a walk along the river via the Old Concrete Crossing.
- Visit the Crossing Inn which is the oldest pub in the Kimberley and has some great artwork around the outside of the building and has a good collection of local art on display in the art gallery.
- Mimbi Caves are an untouched cave system not far from the town, and you can enjoy a tour through them led buy the traditional Aboriginal owners.

Enjoy Alcohol Responsibly

In an effort to address some of the alcohol related harm members of the Fitzroy Crossing community lobbied for a restriction on the sale of takeaway alcohol.

The community has been successful in their pursuit of alcohol restrictions and the following information is provided to help you enjoy your visit to the unique and spectacular part of the country.

The liquor restriction in Fitzroy Crossing relates to:

The sale of packaged liquor, exceeding a concentration of ethanol in liquor of 2.7 per cent at 20°c, is prohibited to any person, other than a lodger (as defined in section 3 of the Liquor Control Act 1988).

In practical terms this means you can only buy light beer as takeaway in Fitzroy Crossing.

What can you do?

✓ You can bring alcohol into town that you have purchased elsewhere for your own personal consumption (be aware that throughout WA it is against the law for persons of any age to drink in public, such as in the street or park).

✓ You can go to the Crossing Inn or the Fitzroy River Lodge and enjoy a full bar service.

✓ You can purchase takeaway light beer from the Crossing Inn.

✓ If you are staying at the Fitzroy River Lodge in a hotel room, cave you can purchase takeaway alcohol to have in your room (See Lodge staff for conditions).

✓ If you are staying at the Crossing Inn in a hotel room you can purchase takeaway alcohol to have in your room (See Crossing Inn staff for conditions).

What can't you do?

✗ If you are staying in a caravan park, you are not able to purchase takeaway alcohol other than light beer from the Crossing Inn.

✗ If you bring alcohol with you, you cannot sell it to others in Fitzroy Crossing.

These conditions are in place to protect the health and wellbeing of everyone living in the Fitzroy Valley as well as those visiting this wonderful part of the world. Your compliance with these conditions, while being a legal requirement, is also greatly appreciated by the community.

What You Need To Know About Alcohol Restrictions In Fitzroy Crossing

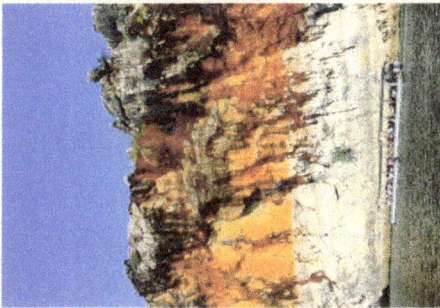

Department of
RACING GAMING AND LIQUOR

Fig. 32 Flyer explaining the liquor restriction in Fitzroy Crossing to members of the public

Source: Department of Racing Gaming & Liquor and WA Police

Failing to act for the community good

Many—probably the majority—of Fitzroy Crossing people had agreed to the community's purchase of equity in the Crossing Inn, believing that it would put an end to sales of takeaway alcohol and lead to on-premises, sociable drinking. The underlying hope was that the culture of explosive, binge drinking, would change. This did not happen, even though Leedal's growing equity in the Crossing Inn gave it greater power over the other partners.

The other way that Leedal was supposed to act for the community good was in returning money to community shareholders. This practice would usually distinguish classic community-owned hotels from typical commercial premises: it was what made the idea of community hotels so appealing to local citizens in South Australian towns in the late nineteenth and early twentieth centuries. However, Leedal failed to quarantine profits that could be distributed for the community's benefit. Profits from all its entities (including the hotel) were *reinvested*, and millions of dollars worth of assets were consolidated, while it made ad hoc and negligible donations to various local causes. When asked where the communities' funds had gone, Leedal's operations manager replied, disingenuously, that the board had 'believed that if we gave cash to communities … [it would] end up back down at the pub' (Subcommittee of the Education and Health Subcommittee 2010: 5–6). It is unlikely that anyone ever seriously suggested that Leedal's profits should be distributed in the form of cash payouts to communities. That these can be disastrous was well documented in several instances some years ago; communities that manage compensation or royalty payments have long since devised numerous sensible alternatives to cash payouts (Altman & Smith 1994, 1999).[49]

Leedal's failure to be receptive to the wishes of the community—its shareholders—raises an important question: how is 'community' defined and how are its wishes ascertained? By 2006–07, one expression of community wishes was the groundswell of concern over alcohol-related harms emanating from communities in and around Fitzroy Crossing (i.e. Leedal's member communities) that were backed up by reports from

---

49   Although, in previous years, mining royalties, compensation and other similar payouts have been paid in cash, these days, royalty and other distributions to Aboriginal communities are more likely to be allocated to community purpose projects (cf. the Central Land Council's website), www. clc.org.au/frequently-asked-questions/cat/clc.

visiting health professionals. Far from responding sympathetically to these genuine rumblings of alarm, Leedal consistently and vociferously opposed the suggestion of a six-month moratorium on takeaway sales.[50] Even more extraordinarily, once the trial restriction imposed by the director of Liquor Licensing was over, Leedal argued against its continuation, despite clear evidence of its positive effect. Highlighting the perversity of Leedal's stance, Coroner Hope (2008: 122) reminded the public that the original purpose of the acquisition of equity in the Crossing Inn had been to 'correct local alcohol problems'. At least one Leedal board member left over this issue: 'the crunch came when women called for restrictions and the board wouldn't support it. I resigned'.[51]

Leedal's opposition to the takeaway ban was evident in its self-published quarterly newsletter and in the submissions it made to every relevant state or federal government inquiry, senate committee or other investigation (Leedal 2009, 2013, 2014, Subcommittee of the Education and Health Subcommittee 2010). In these commentaries, Leedal labelled the restriction on takeaways 'prohibition': for example, the policy 'in many ways reflects "Prohibition"' (Leedal 2014: 7). In reality, the restrictions were merely a ban on the sale of packaged alcohol containing more than 2.7 per cent alcohol content, not a ban on *all* alcohol consumption. Nevertheless, Leedal's use of the term 'prohibition' was significant, for it allowed Leedal to draw a lesson from Prohibition in the United States in the 1920s—namely, that prohibition was a disaster that masked underlying problems (Leedal 2009, 2014: 2).[52] Leedal (2014) also cited a controversial American sociologist, David Hanson, who is critical of the prevailing view of clinicians on the effects of alcohol consumption on health.[53] Confronted with the positive evaluation of the takeaway ban produced by Notre Dame University, Leedal's chairman claimed that the study was inadequate. He refused to accept the view expressed by politicians and others that the alcohol bans had improved conditions

---

50   This was proposed by June Oscar, Emily Carter, the women's group and the senior men of the KALCC.

51   NP, interview, 4 August 2009.

52   Leedal correctly pointed out that prohibition can be accompanied by an increase in illicit alcohol production. However, they failed to cite the World Health Organization, which found that during Prohibition in the United States, mortality from cirrhosis declined by around 50 per cent. They also ignored a wealth of international evidence on the efficacy of liquor sales controls in reducing harm (Edwards et al. 1995, Cook 2007).

53   David Hanson promotes the idea that alcohol improves cognitive functioning and is good for health; he argues that the public health approach endorsing alcohol restrictions is a puritanical and moralistic temperance movement in disguise.

and that children were eating and sleeping better.[54] Leedal's submissions to various inquires sought to direct attention away from alcohol-control measures and towards individual responsibility, alcohol education and the need for medical treatment and care for those with alcohol-use disorders. In other words, they sought to blame the consumer. In doing so, Leedal deployed the same argument the alcohol industry has relied on for decades (Burnham 1993, International Center for Alcohol Policies 2004, Sellman 2010, Leedal 2014).

By denying how serious the situation was in the past, and by publicly condemning the restriction on takeaways, Leedal was up against a strong body of community and expert opinion that perceived an overall improvement in life at Fitzroy Crossing. The awkwardness of Leedal's position, in which it both failed to act for the good of its own community and continued to deny its role in alcohol-related problems, was captured in questioning at a state Standing Committee in 2011:

> Mr PB Watson (Committee member): Most people think that alcohol is a problem in the community. But you have got Aboriginal groups owning the places that sell liquor. Is that a problem? Is that an embarrassment to the communities, when their biggest problem is alcohol, but the people who are selling it are the communities themselves? Is that an issue to you?
>
> Patrick Green (Leedal chairman): It is perceived as a problem. But 20-odd years ago we bought it so that we could curb the drinking problem.
>
> Mr Watson: Has it worked?
>
> Patrick Green: I would like to think that we were able to help the community in having access to alcohol on certain days and restricting it on others. (Subcommittee of the Education and Health Standing Committee 2010: 5–6, cf. Education and Health Standing Committee 2011)

Service providers at Fitzroy Crossing today deal with a community that is significantly different to the one that existed prior to the restriction on takeaways. Before the restrictions were in place, the town experienced

54 Following the introduction of restrictions in 2007, there were regular spikes in the count of alcohol-related injuries, continued alcohol runs to buy takeaway supplies elsewhere and some increases in emergency department presentations to the Fitzroy Crossing hospital. However, in 2011, a thorough and evidence-based Standing Committee report noted that *overall* there had been reductions in ambulance call-outs and presentations of domestic violence cases, and a decrease in overall alcohol-related trauma. Contrary to claims that up to 400 people had moved from Fitzroy Crossing into Broome to drink, a headcount found only 35 Fitzroy Crossing residents there (Education and Health Standing Committee 2011: 22).

almost constant late-night parties and disturbances that particularly affected children (Akesson 2009). While there are lingering problems, such as illegal sales of alcohol and increased movements of people to buy grog (Akesson 2009; Kinnane et al. 2009), no one ever claimed that stopping off-premises sales would solve all the alcohol problems; to the contrary, advocates of the takeaway ban had anticipated such effects.

Problematic local politics

What prevented the Leedal board members nominated by the six beneficiary communities from insisting on ending sales of packaged alcohol? There appears to have been no concerted effort to put community pressure on the board, despite overt dissatisfaction with Leedal's direction. Two prominent Aboriginal people resigned from the board in 1995 and, as mentioned previously, another board member resigned in protest when Leedal declined to support moves to trial a ban on takeaways in 2007. A former board member said simply, 'it started off good, but greed got to them'. Another former board member recalled feeling increasingly unhappy with Leedal's direction:

> I got really unhappy about Board's direction, and it wouldn't engage with the community. I thought I could make a difference. [It] wouldn't engage with the community … The original idea was to control corrupt and irresponsible service [of alcohol] but when aligned with [joint partner name], the focus was on making money, it lost its community focus. I became disillusioned with everything.

Unlike other community-owned pubs, both Indigenous and non-Indigenous, the Crossing Inn had no governing board of its own. The hotel has always been one branch of an extensive portfolio of businesses belonging to a proprietary company. The Leedal board governed the entire portfolio. However, overseeing shops and a caravan park is not the same as overseeing a hotel, especially one servicing a vulnerable community: the issues are manifestly different. In this respect, the Crossing Inn is unlike a Gothenberg-style hotel. Each of the Gothenberg-style hotels of rural South Australia, as well as numerous Aboriginal-owned licensed premises, such as the Finke Hotel, the Transcontinental Hotel and Mt Ebenezer Roadhouse, had boards whose sole responsibility was the hotel. Indeed, one of the principles underlying the cooperative ideal of community hotels was the election of local people to the hotel board, as this gave residents the opportunity to hear directly from the hotel manager about the status and conduct of the hotel, and contribute to hotel policies. The absence of a hotel board undermined the capacity of local people to question the hotel's direction, effectively cocooning it from criticism.

A further explanation for the lack of action by community members, or Leedal board members, lies in the nature of people's affiliations and allegiances to different organisations and residence groups in the region, and the fact that people in key positions are related to one another (Thorburn 2011). Individuals may have been concerned about the direction taken by Leedal, but they were unable to change it. Several of Leedal's 'beneficial community' shareholders were corporations registered in their own right under the Office of the Registrar of Indigenous Corporations (ORIC)—a registration and monitoring body with considerable regulatory powers of intervention. In principle, this provided shareholders with some leverage, as they had the authority to seek assistance from ORIC. However, ORIC's powers to compel compliance with corporate law would not have had any effect on Leedal's policy on alcohol sales, which was within the law. Disputes over the composition of Leedal's board and the community bodies represented on it have further complicated matters.[55] Some prominent individuals have fulfilled multiple (and sometimes overlapping) roles and have retained these positions for extended periods. While this provides stability, it also contributes to conformity in (and domination of) an organisation's direction.[56] For example, the chairman of Leedal has been a director since 1991. The longest serving Leedal board member, he is also a company director of two of Leedal's beneficiary organisations[57] and chairman of the charitable fund set up by Leedal in 2010. In a small, close-knit and historically embedded population such as Fitzroy Crossing, these features of community representation are perhaps inevitable, even if they are not desirable. Rightly or wrongly, the perception in the local community was that 'no-one had input into Leedal'.

---

55 For example, Junjuwa, the major shareholder, was restructured. Although the community of Junjuwa still exists, in 2000 its administrative and economic arm was incorporated under a new name: Bunaba Inc.

56 A professional observer familiar with Leedal's business structure observed, drily, that the word 'plutocracy' comes to mind in this context.

57 These are Bunaba Inc. (previously known as Junjuwa Aboriginal Corporation), and Marra Worra Worra Aboriginal Corporation, both 'beneficiary organisations' of Leedal.

The original plan for consultation and governance had included an MLG, which was supposed to serve as a conduit between the communities and the business management arm of Leedal. This group was intended to have the *social* interests of the communities at heart; however, for reasons unknown, it lasted only a few years and folded in 1991. When the campaign for a trial ban on sales of packaged alcohol finally gathered momentum in 2007, it polarised opinion in the town, pitting family members and organisations against each other. If the MLG had still been in existence, perhaps these fractious relationships could have been improved?

In his early planning reports, Bill Arthur emphasised that the purchase of the Crossing Inn and other businesses was perceived by community members as a *community development* project. Anthropologist Patrick Sullivan has questioned whether an Aboriginal community organisation should ever become the controller of large businesses, suggesting that, as new projects are spawned in the name of the community, 'the possibility of effective community control recedes' (Sullivan 1996: 97). Community development theory has taught us that communities are not always homogeneous; that community leaders do not always act in the best interests of their people; and that government and community workers do not always share the same goals for development (Foster 1982, Rifkin 1986, cf. Purtill 2017). In the case of Leedal and the Crossing Inn, these lessons seem pertinent.

Who was responsible?

Three agents can be held responsible the Crossing Inn's failure to restrain or arrest damaging sales of takeaway alcohol. First, Leedal, as a primarily Aboriginal organisation, bears responsibility. Although it was originally only half owned by Aboriginal interests, it was eventually fully Aboriginal owned. Leedal should have operated with more empathy and foresight. Rather than resisting (and in some cases undermining) those who expressed genuine concerns about the health and wellbeing of the community, and who had irrefutable evidence of alcohol-related harms, it could have collaborated with them. For the good of the community, it could have decided to cross-subsidise a reduction in its sales of alcohol by using income from its other enterprises. The deaths investigated by the coroner may not have occurred on the premises of the Crossing Inn; however, the alcohol sold there, its volume and manner of sale, was undoubtedly to blame. It is fortunate from Leedal's perspective that Australia does not treat liability for alcohol-related harms in the way that Canada does (Solomon & Payne 1996).

Second, the Indigenous development bureaucracies that funded and partnered with Leedal are responsible for prioritising commercial aspirations over social considerations. Without abandoning commercial aspirations, the ADC and other agencies should have been more alert to the (potentially adverse) social implications of their investments. Stephens rightly identified the ADC (followed by IBA and their joint partners) as being complicit in the perpetuation of aggressive off-premises sales at the Crossing Inn, which generated 'excessive profits and returns' for Leedal. Admittedly, the roles and policies of these agencies were complicated by a series of bureaucratic upheavals in Indigenous affairs that coincided with the planning phase for the Crossing Inn's purchase, as described in Chapter 2. The original loan for the Fitzroy Crossing businesses came from the ADC, and the original negotiations were conducted with the ADC. However, by the time the actual purchase of the businesses took place, the Audit Office had begun investigating the ADC, resulting in a tightening up of its governance and investment strategy. The minister wanted *more attention* paid to the commercial viability of the ADC's investments and demanded greater public accountability (Pratt & Bennett 2004). With the advent of ATSIC in 1990, local ADC staff—the people who had helped to broker early consultations over Leedal and the purchase of the enterprises—were redeployed. The creation of ATSIC's development arm, the CDC, continued the focus on investments along strictly commercial lines, as well as the promotion of joint ventures between Indigenous and non-Indigenous business people (WS Arthur 1996). However, these restructurings and political upheavals do not absolve these agencies from an ongoing duty of care. It is extraordinary that, only two years before the Crossing Inn was publicly excoriated for its role in alcohol-related dysfunction and mortality, IBA described it as one of its 'most successful strategic investments' (IBA 2005: 12). Within two years, IBA's position became so untenable that it *opted out* of its stake in the Crossing Inn, thus abdicating any further responsibility for it.

The third failure of responsibility lies with the state government's alcohol regulatory mechanisms, which were not mobilised until widespread and long-lasting social, cultural, physical and emotional harm had been done. The state's liquor licensing authority eventually swung into action to support the community mobilisation (once it gathered momentum) in

2007, but why was it left to the community to do this? It seems odd that the director of Liquor Licensing did not step in sooner, particularly in light of the extent of alcohol-related harm and suicide that was documented throughout the 1990s (Hunter 1993, Hall et al. 1993, Midford et al. 1994), not to mention the volatile and dangerous drinking practices near the Crossing Inn and the adjoining Billabong Park. Further, in view of irrefutable evidence of a specific licensed premises being directly associated with measurable harm, it is remarkable that, in 2005, the director of Liquor Licensing had apparently been so impressed with the 'strong', self-imposed restrictions adopted by the owners of the Crossing Inn that he used the hotel as a model for other remote hotels in Western Australia (IBA 2005: 12). Perhaps this was because the hotel had instituted *some*—albeit insufficient—adjustments to its sales practices in response to community requests?

The director of Liquor Licensing intervened only when compelled by strong community opinion and when faced with the prospect of a coronial inquest into numerous alcohol-related deaths that had occurred on his watch. Both he and the coroner were influenced by the political climate generated by the Australian government's tough new approach to alcohol consumption. The government's declaration of the Northern Territory Emergency Response (NTER) in June 2007 in response to reports of child sexual abuse, violence and neglect in remote Aboriginal communities demonstrated its willingness to override locally instigated regimes to tighten up alcohol controls.[58]

In addition to these three failures, there was also a failure to *keep track* of the health and wellbeing of the people of Fitzroy Valley. In retrospect, it seems anomalous that no external body was in a position to call attention to 'sentinel events' in the region much sooner: a spike in alcohol-related mortality, a spate of homicides, suicides and an increase in alcohol-related morbidity. ATSIC had shared responsibility for the oversight of Indigenous-specific health and alcohol program funding with federal and state health departments. All these bodies, in effect, ignored what turned

---

58   The NTER was initiated by the Australian Government in response to a Northern Territory inquiry into Aboriginal child sexual abuse that found it to be serious, widespread and often unreported (Altman & Hinkson 2007). The NTER included a number of measures, such as providing additional police officers in communities, and tightened existing alcohol-control measures. It declared Aboriginal communities, living areas and town camps to be 'prescribed areas', and banned the sale and consumption of alcohol in them (although there were already 107 restricted areas on Aboriginal land and only 15 allowed alcohol in one form or another); it also imposed restrictions on the sale of alcohol in the eight existing licensed clubs in remote communities.

out to be a deepening alcohol-related crisis in the Fitzroy Valley. Practical support, advice and ongoing evaluation of Indigenous governance was missing. An external review of Leedal's governance might have uncovered why board members felt powerless to change Leedal's direction.

Abandoning the ideals of a social enterprise

When preliminary discussions about the purchase of the Crossing Inn were taking place in 1988, people at Fitzroy Crossing were unaware of the rural communities in South Australia that owned their local pubs and had a say in how they were run; they were unaware that these cooperative efforts had a sound basis in alcohol-management and alcohol-control policies in Scandinavia and the United Kingdom. One of the founding principles of these community cooperatives, particularly those associated with the Gothenburg system, was that the hotel manager should not derive any personal profit from the sale of alcohol. 'Disinterested' management—the payment of a fixed salary to managers—was supposed to remove incentives for managers to encourage drunkenness. The coronial inquest in Fitzroy Crossing in 2007 disclosed that the managing partner of the Crossing Inn, Wayne Bowen of Mapigan Pty Ltd, had a remuneration package based on a formula in which he received 2 per cent of the hotel's sales and 10 per cent of its profit (Strutt 2007b).

Although Leedal's purchase of equity in the Crossing Inn was ostensibly motivated by harm reduction, which was supposed to be pursued by ending sales of packaged alcohol and relying on on-premises drinking, its policy was not modelled on the Gothenburg system, about which Leedal knew nothing.[59] Unhappily, packaged alcohol sales remained; the sale of alcohol contributed to widespread harm, and the profits derived from the hotel were not used for projects to reduce alcohol-related harm.[60] Without a community board specifically for the hotel, there was no focus on the hotel as a venue that required a special management style, aims, policies, serving practices, physical environment and facilities. As well, because the revenue from the hotel was not quarantined, its profits were Leedal's.

---

59   Bill Arthur (pers comm, 20 May 2015) observed that some useful lessons might have been learned from the 'Gothenburg' experiments in South Australian community-owned hotels had they known about them at the time.
60   This was the case up until 2010 and the establishment of the Yapawarnti Fund. However, this Fund is not explicitly oriented to reducing alcohol-related harm either.

By contrast, the profits generated by the South Australian community-owned hotels belonged to those hotels alone. With hotel boards made up of citizens from the local town, local people were able to decide on the allocation of a portion of these monies to local organisations, activities and facilities.

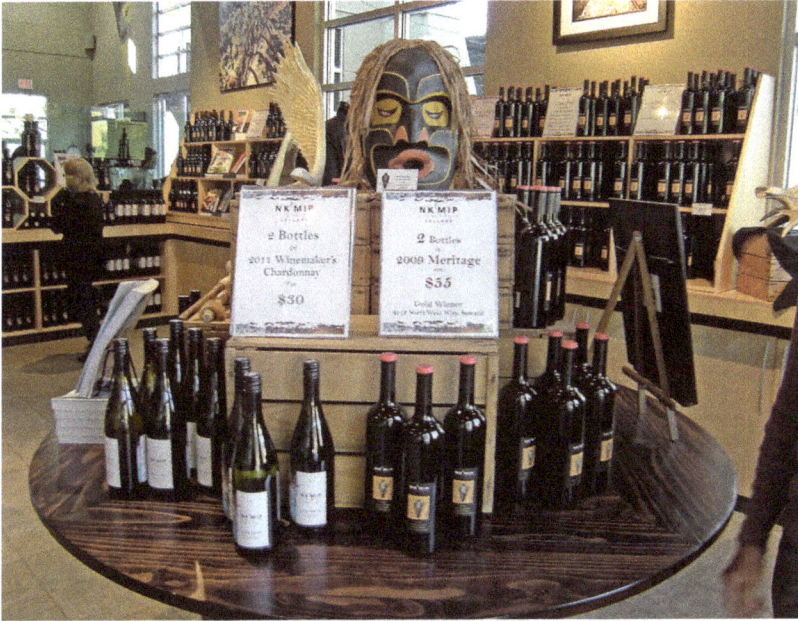

Fig. 33 Nk'Mip wine store, Osoyoos, British Columbia, 2013
Source: M Brady

Leedal's publicity material, although decorated with Aboriginal designs, does not market the Crossing Inn as 'community owned' or even 'Aboriginal owned'; instead, the hotel is described as 'The historic Crossing Inn'. The Fitzroy River Lodge does not mention that it is owned by Aboriginal communities either. This is in marked contrast to other, comparable Indigenous community projects associated with alcohol, such as the Aboriginal winegrowing venture at Murrin Bridge in New South Wales, which marketed its wine as coming from an Aboriginal-owned enterprise (McQuire 2011: 1). The Mt Ebenezer Roadhouse in northern South Australia openly states that it is owned by the Imanpa community. In Canada, the Nk'Mip Cellars and Resort in the Okanagan Valley of British Columbia makes a virtue out of the fact that it is 51 per cent owned by the Osoyoos Indian Band (Anderson et al. 2007).

The property is designed to attract tourists rather than members of the local First Nations band; nevertheless, Chief Clarence Louie's photograph is prominently displayed, holding a glass of red wine as if to demonstrate wine appreciation and moderate drinking. Like Leedal, Nk'Mip has many diversified investments; it owns and operates related enterprises catering to locals and tourists including a vineyard, winery, caravan park, golf course, cultural centre and museum, and a nature park. In the on-site shop, Nk'Mip sells its wine—with labels featuring indigenous rock art designs and artefacts—alongside First Nations masks, drums and other artefacts. In Australia and overseas, enterprises such as these have discovered that identifying and promoting themselves as being owned by the Indigenous community can be an effective marketing technique.

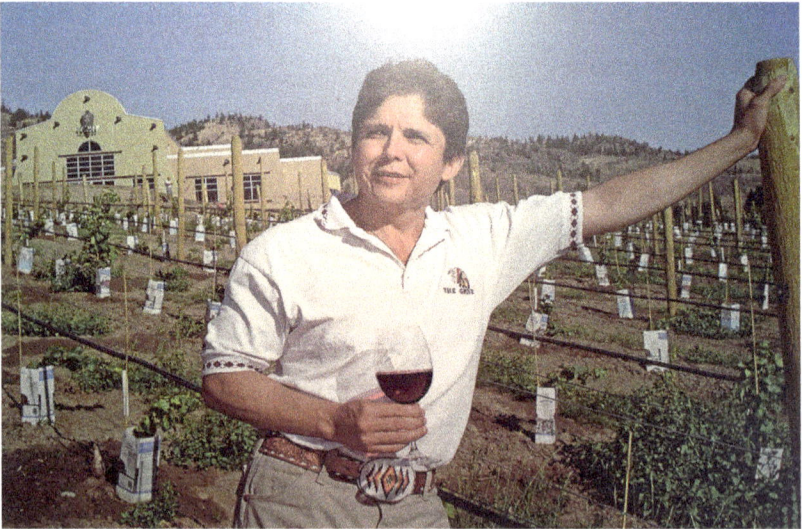

Fig. 34 Chief Clarence Louie, Nk'Mip, Osoyoos, British Columbia
Source: Nk'Mip promotional poster, 2013

The Crossing Inn is not a community-owned hotel in the 'classic' Gothenburg sense, nor is it a social enterprise of the kind discussed by researchers such as Defourny and Nyssens (2010). A social enterprise is generally understood as a market-oriented economic activity that serves a social goal. Commenting on the safeguards that protect the integrity of such enterprises, Defourny and Nyssens explain that, in Europe, governance structures for social enterprises aim for:

A democratic control and/or a participatory involvement of stakeholders [to] reflect the quest for more economic democracy, in the tradition of cooperatives. They therefore add to constraints on the distribution of profits with a view to protecting and strengthening *the primacy of the social mission, which is at the very heart of the organization.* (49, emphasis added)

Together with this kind of participatory cooperative governance, instituting strict constraints on who can benefit from the profits of such enterprises helps to avoid the risk that public subsidies will simply mean that more profits are distributed among owners or managers. Public support and subsidies are important, as they (usually) enable enterprises to avoid purely market-driven strategies. However, the Crossing Inn became part of the much larger business entity, Leedal, the Trustee for the Fitzroy Crossing Trust and, since profit is the bottom line of business, success in business is usually defined as monetary success (Foley 2003: 137).

During the planning process in 1988 and 1989, Arthur (1989b) drew attention to the fact that the project was set up as a Trust. 'It is the job of the Trustees', he observed:

> To be aware of the socio-economic realities of the valley, and the distribution of the benefits. The Trustees have the final say in the event that the project is not fulfilling its aims and objectives, else why bother to have a Trust in the first place?

As it turned out, this was a pertinent question, for the larger business entity and its members, together with the outside agencies charged with the financing, surveillance and governance of the enterprises, failed to fulfil the community's original aspirations for the hotel's purchase. Having a monopoly over alcohol sales in Fitzroy Crossing and the surrounding districts presented numerous opportunities, which the company squandered. Leedal should have been able to experiment with strategies designed to change the drinking habits of the Crossing Inn's customers, thereby diminishing alcohol-related harms in the region. This would have enabled the company to confront the moral hazard of profiting from the sale of alcohol. Instead, it suited Leedal's principals to subsume, and thus obscure, the complex issues surrounding the sale of alcohol by the Crossing Inn under their wider and pre-eminent remit to be a successful business enterprise.

8

Drinking, Indigenous policy and social enterprise

In this book, I set out to examine the centuries-long project to constrain and moderate—to 'civilise'—the drinking behaviour of Indigenous Australians; in doing so, I found that the story extended in several different directions. It led me into a socio-historical study of drinking and into the history of the idea that drinking is a *learned* behaviour. That led, inevitably perhaps, to a history of aspects of Australian Indigenous policy: assimilation, self-determination, and the influence of government advisory bodies and economic development agencies on alcohol management in Indigenous communities. Finally, the research moved into the area of social enterprise, focusing on the tensions and moral dilemmas that are inherent in both Indigenous and non-Indigenous social enterprises involved in the sale of alcohol.

The first part of this book presented a *socio-historical exploration of alcohol use*. It showed how Europeans have long tried either to suppress or improve the drinking behaviour of Aboriginal people—a process that began when Bennelong was taught to raise his glass of wine in a toast to the health of the king. Such overt efforts to introduce Aboriginal people to sociable drinking were soon abandoned, and the authorities resorted to prohibitions against Aboriginal drinking, which only disappeared around 50 years ago. Civil rights, including drinking rights, were achieved by Indigenous Australians during the post-prohibition era. This was when attention shifted from banning to 'improving' drinking behaviour. In Europe, there were parallel projects of suppression and improvement dating from the endeavours of the elite to create courtly manners and etiquette around food and drink, and to make these into accepted middle-class values. These European traditions of reform and improvement (rather than outright prohibition) in relation to alcohol gave rise to two developments that were relevant to my discussion. First, they prompted, or were accompanied by, theories of drinking as learned, and therefore malleable, behaviour. This novel idea had been hinted at in the eighteenth and nineteenth centuries, when colonised 'natives' (including Australian Aboriginal people) were thought to be natural imitators of their colonisers, learning what was expected of people who imbibed intoxicating drinks. In the twentieth century, theories of social learning emerged from clinical studies in the United States and Britain, which posited that, rather than being biologically determined and immovable, problematic drinking behaviours were learned and could be altered. This new way of thinking about alcohol problems counteracted the prevailing disease theory and raised questions about whether abstinence was the only viable treatment solution. Diffused to Australia, by the 1970s, ideas of social learning underpinned Australian government and mission experiments in providing rationed amounts of beer to Indigenous people in many remote communities.

European traditions of improvement in drinking behaviour also produced models for the reform of the drinking environment. The poor and underprivileged were thought to misuse alcohol because of their social and working conditions, their lack of 'rational' recreation and the unscrupulous behaviour of publicans who pushed sales of liquor. The most prominent and influential of the reformist models designed to deal with these factors was the Gothenburg system of local, social regulation. Its 'disinterested', salaried management of bars and liquor stores, quarantining of profits for the use and benefit of the municipality or local community and citizen participation, combined to reduce poor serving practices and intoxicated patrons. I described how politicians, government representatives and temperance thinkers from several countries, including Britain and Australia, became fascinated by this Scandinavian plan, and how its basic principles were taken up and put into practice by anti-prohibitionists and reformers of licensed public houses. In the late nineteenth and early twentieth centuries, Gothenburg-style ideas took hold in regional areas of South Australia, where residents bought shares in their local hotels, participated as board members in their management and decided on the distribution of profits. My account of this development, and how these community-owned hotels have fared over time, set the scene for the case studies presented later in the book as studies in Indigenous social enterprise.

Australian Indigenous policy formed the second major theme of this book, in particular, how Indigenous policy both affected and guided the approaches taken to alcohol availability and regulation. Unlike the United States, 'prohibition' for the general population in this country applied only to small and atypical districts, such as the 'temperance colony' along the Murray River, and a scattering of neighbourhoods that voted in local option polls to be 'dry'. However, for the Indigenous population (including Torres Strait and Pacific Islanders), prohibition applied to people according to their degree of 'assimilation'; it was lifted as part of a wider program of civil rights in which Indigenous people were supposed to be incorporated into Australian society as citizens, with all the accompanying rights and responsibilities of 'normal' (white) citizens.

The struggle for, and achievement of, the right to drink was really an assimilationist project: it was believed that 'they' should be able to drink like 'us'. However, as the old restrictions were repealed, jurisdiction by jurisdiction, and people began to act on their new freedoms, the question of how to *manage* these new rights arose. Once assimilation evolved into self-determination, merely having the same right to drink was not enough. Aboriginal people were expected—indeed, were obliged—to produce new forms of authority that could deal with the enactment of these rights. Previous traditional authority structures were repeatedly found to be inadequate; hence, the abandonment of some early experiments in alcohol rationing. As part of the transition from assimilation to self-determination, Aboriginal people were challenged to invent *new* modes of self-regulation through their local control and oversight of liquor sales from community-based clubs or via community purchases of public hotels. As illustrated in the case studies presented in this book, they did this by creating complex lists of rules that attempted to regulate the personal comportment of Aboriginal patrons and enforce their social and civic responsibilities; the lists also kept track of which patrons were excluded from the premises.

Aboriginal purchases of licensed hotels were facilitated by policy developments, such as the creation of development agencies and the promotion of Aboriginal entrepreneurship. As the case studies illustrated, the difficulties that followed were due, in large part, to the failure of these agencies—the ADC and its descendants, ATSIC and IBA—to foresee problems in underwriting projects that involved alcohol sales, and to create policies that would pre-empt these problems. A shift in policy, from an emphasis on social goals to primarily economic ones, further complicated matters, placing several Aboriginal enterprises at risk by impelling them to concentrate on alcohol sales, rather than the wellbeing of the community.

In the process of recounting the story of these Aboriginal enterprises, I showed the extent to which they had unwittingly resembled and replicated the strengths and weaknesses of the Gothenburg model of local control of liquor sales. I argued that Australian governments, and the agencies designed to promote Indigenous self-determination and economic independence—being ignorant of both the principles of the original Gothenburg model and its practical testing (through the experiences of community hotels in South Australia)—were apparently unable to devise an enterprise policy that was suited to *social* enterprise. This, in a sense, was what the Gothenburg system aimed to do; it sought create a viable liquor business that was socially responsible, avoided profiteering from alcohol sales and supported moderate consumption.

The licensed Indigenous entities discussed here, both the social clubs and hotels, needed a different policy framework—one that would have benefited by the experiences of Gothenburg-style premises. They also needed earlier intervention from external agencies to provide troubleshooting around governance matters, and to deflect problems of responsible service. In addition, they needed ongoing guidance and monitoring.

The third field of scholarship I explored in this book was *social enterprise*. I presented material from Europe and South Australia on the conscious diffusion of the Gothenburg system, and juxtaposed this with research from Aboriginal communities that revealed the *inadvertent*, unconscious mobilisation of this system. Remarkably, Indigenous and non-Indigenous community hotels existed in parallel, with each apparently unaware of the other. Indigenous hotels (and clubs) shared some goals in common with Gothenburg-style hotels: the expectation that ownership would enable greater local control over liquor sales, prevent sly grog sales, offer employment opportunities for Indigenous people and raise revenue for community causes. All the municipalities and communities involved experienced successes and failures, leading to the conclusion that while social enterprise of this kind is worth attempting, it requires considerable effort.

The business of establishing community-owned licensed premises is fraught with contradictions, hazards (moral and otherwise) and challenges. There is an inescapable tension within the definition of 'community benefit' that exists between the goal of moderating alcohol consumption and generating a surplus (which might be used to fund community projects) by selling it.

This tension is particularly severe in an Indigenous context, as Indigenous people experience a disproportionate physical and social cost from alcohol abuse. An Indigenous hotel or club that 'poisons its own people' is clearly an undesirable form of enterprise. The tension increases when an articulate temperance lobby (often led by women) draws attention to the inherent moral hazard of a social enterprise (often run by men) that sells alcohol. In this book, I documented the efforts of white Australian WCTU members and Aboriginal women in central and northern Australia who engaged in formal and informal acts of resistance against new and existing licences run by their menfolk; both groups, Aboriginal and non-Aboriginal, used similar arguments and rhetoric, pointing out the ethical dilemmas inherent in the use of 'grog money' for good works.

The research reported here revealed how the community governance of social enterprises is not purely a matter of good administration or compliance with the relevant liquor legislation. The administration of such enterprises is imbued with the additional challenges posed by political contestation, both within and beyond the communities involved. As Room (1982: 447) observed, all systems of local control, whether they are state licensing systems or systems of local option and decision-making around alcohol, share commonalities in that they:

> Create at least a partial monopoly for those inside them, whether they be state or private interests. They are thus usually very profitable for all concerned, and they create large and powerful vested interests in the continuance of the basic system, with gradual liberalisations of control for the benefit of those already inside.

This observation is borne out by what took place in numerous beer canteens and clubs in remote Aboriginal communities. If a club was already in place, and the majority of the community were drinkers, then, irrespective of the problems caused by the outlet, the popular vote would ensure that the desires of the drinkers (to oppose restrictions, to extend hours or to lobby for higher-alcohol content drinks) would be carried (Moran 2013: 199). The system comes with a built-in 'ratchet mechanism'—the community council (or Indigenous corporation or state) derives fiscal (and other) benefits from its franchise to sell alcohol; therefore, it is politically painful to extinguish that interest (Room 1982: 447).

It often takes a religious or popular uprising around alcohol before licences and revenues will be taken away (Room 1982). Examples of such uprisings were presented in this book: resistance to the Tyeweretye Club by Pitjantjatjara women; the wrecking of the Murrinh Patha Social Club at Wadeye; and the alarm raised by concerned women and men of the Kimberley over takeaway sales in Fitzroy Crossing. In each case, the systems of government needed a 'jolt' to force an appropriate level of response. It is to their credit that these Aboriginal protestors mobilised sufficient support to mount challenges that highlighted the moral contradictions inherent in these enterprises.

Bibliography

ABC News (2004). Hotels group rejects alcohol ban, 23 April 2004, www.abc.net.au/news/2004-04-23/hotels-group-rejects-alcohol-ban/174858.

ABC News (2007a). Industry body says alcohol warnings pointless, 25 June 2007, www.abc.net.au/news/2007-06-25/industry-body-says-alcohol-warnings-pointless/80230.

ABC News (2007b). Urgent action needed to stop Indigenous mothers drinking: doctor, 20 July 2007.

ABC News (2007c). Anger over inquiry into Kimberley alcohol sales, 26 July 2007.

ABIX (Australasian Business Intelligence) (2007). Frichot faces jail after judge upholds charges, 14 March.

Aborigines' Friends' Association (1888). *Thirtieth annual report,* Aborigines' Friends Association, Adelaide.

ADC (Aboriginal Development Commission) (1983). *Views of the commissioners on alcohol related problems and the advertising of alcoholic beverages,* ADC, Canberra.

ADC (Aboriginal Development Commission) (1989). *Annual report 1987–1988,* Australian Government Publishing Service, Canberra.

ADC (Aboriginal Development Commission) (1990). *Annual report, July 1989 – March 1990*, Australian Government Publishing Service, Canberra.

Adelaide Advertiser (1988). Outback town wants 'dry' future for its kids, 27 February 1988:4.

Adler M (1991). From symbolic exchange to commodity consumption: anthropological notes on drinking as a symbolic practice. In Barrows S & Room R (eds), *Drinking: behaviour and belief in modern history*, University of California Press, Berkeley:376–398.

Akesson G (2009). Fitzroy Crossing: the less obvious impact of take-away liquor restrictions. *ADCA News* 47(October):6–7.

Albrecht PGE (2002). *From mission to church 1877–2002, Finke River Mission*, Finke River Mission, Adelaide.

Alcorn G (1995). Spears, bullets, boomerangs fly in riot. *Sydney Morning Herald*, 29 December 1995.

Alexander K (1985). *Kava in the north: a study of kava in Arnhem Land Aboriginal communities*, North Australia Research Unit, Darwin.

Altman JC & Hinkson M (2007). *Coercive reconciliation: stabilise, normalise, exit Aboriginal Australia*, Arena Publications Association, Melbourne.

Altman JC & Smith DE (1994). *The economic impact of mining moneys: the Nabarlek case, Western Arnhem Land*, Discussion Paper 63/1994, Centre for Aboriginal Economic Policy Research, The Australian National University, Canberra.

Altman JC & Smith DE (1999). *The Ngurratjuta Aboriginal Corporation: a model for understanding Northern Territory royalty associations*, Discussion Paper 185/1999, Centre for Aboriginal Economic Policy Research, The Australian National University, Canberra.

Ambler C & Crush J (1992). Alcohol in southern African labor history. In Crush J & Ambler C (eds), *Liquor and labor in southern Africa*, Ohio University Press & University of Natal Press, Athens and Pietermaritzburg:1–55.

Anderson RB, Wingham DW, Giberson RJ & Gibson B (2007). Indigenous economic development: a tale of two wineries. In Campbell G and Guilbert N (eds), *The golden grape: wine, society and globalization: multidisciplinary perspectives on the wine industry*, Palgrave Macmillan, New York:201–20.

The Argus [Melbourne, Vic.: 1848–1954] (1922). Renmark Hotel: remarkable institution. How community benefits, 6 November 1922:14.

Armadale Public House Society (2001). *A celebration of 100 years of The Goth, 1901–2001*, Armadale, East Lothian (Scotland), www.armadale.org.uk/goth.htm.

Arthur JM (1996). *Aboriginal English: a cultural study,* Oxford University Press, Melbourne.

Arthur WS (1988). *Interim report: Fitzroy Project,* Aboriginal Economic Research Unit, Department of Education and Training, Perth.

Arthur WS (1989a). *Mid-term report: Fitzroy Project (January 1989),* Aboriginal Economic Research Unit, Department of Education and Training, Perth.

Arthur WS (1989b). *Fitzroy project: Briefing notes (February 1989),* Aboriginal Economic Research Unit, Department of Education and Training, Perth, mimeo.

Arthur WS (1996). *The Aboriginal and Torres Strait Islander Commercial Development Corporation: a new approach to enterprise?* Discussion Paper 113/1996, Centre for Aboriginal Economic Policy Research, Canberra.

Arthur WS (1999). *What's new? The 1997 Parliamentary Inquiry into Indigenous Business,* Discussion Paper 177/1999, Centre for Aboriginal Economic Policy Research, Canberra.

Australian Audit Office (1989). *Special audit report: the Aboriginal Development Commission and the Department of Aboriginal Affairs,* Australian Government Publishing Service, Canberra.

Australian Institute of Aboriginal Studies Uranium Impact Project Steering Committee (1984). *Aborigines and uranium: consolidated report on the social impact of uranium mining on the Aborigines of the Northern Territory,* Australian Government Publishing Service, Canberra.

Babor T, Caetano R, Casswell S, Edwards G, Giesbrecht N, Graham K, Grube J, Gruenewald P, Hill L, Holder H, Homel R, Österberg E, Rehm J, Room R & Rossow I (2003). *Alcohol: No ordinary commodity: research and public policy,* Oxford University Press, Oxford.

Backhouse J (1843). *A narrative of a visit to the Australian colonies,* Hamilton Adams, London.

Baker SJ (1978). *The Australian language,* Currawong Press, Milsons Point, NSW.

Bandler F (1989). *Turning the tide: a personal history of the Federal Council for the Advancement of Aborigines and Torres Strait Islanders,* Aboriginal Studies Press, Canberra.

Bane N (1996). Port Keats drinkers head to city: police. *Northern Territory News,* 7 March 1996:6.

Banks J (1963). *The endeavour journal of Joseph Banks 1768–1771,* ed Beaglehole JC, vols I & II, Trustees of the Public Library of New South Wales in association with Angus and Robertson, Sydney.

Barrass T (2007). Business arm told to quit grog sales. *The Australian,* 9 August 2007:6.

Barratt G (1981). *The Russians at Port Jackson 1814–1822,* Australian Institute of Aboriginal Studies, Canberra.

Bartlett B & Duncan P (2000). *Top End Aboriginal health planning study,* Plan Health Pty Ltd, NSW.

Baudin N (1974). *The journal of Post Captain Nicolas Baudin,* trans Cornell C, Libraries Board of South Australia, Adelaide.

Beckett J (1958). A study of a mixed blood aboriginal minority in the pastoral west of New South Wales, MA thesis, The Australian National University, Canberra.

Beckett J (1965). Aborigines, alcohol and assimilation. In Reay M (ed), *Aborigines now,* Angus and Robertson, Sydney:32–47.

Beeson MJ (1980). *Some Aboriginal women pathfinders, their difficulties and their achievements,* National Woman's Christian Temperance Union of Australia, Adelaide.

Berndt RM, Berndt CH & Stanton JE (1993). *A world that was: the Yaraldi of the Murray River and the lakes, South Australia,* Miegunya Press, Melbourne.

Berridge V (2005). *Temperance: its history and impact on current and future alcohol policy,* Joseph Rowntree Foundation, York.

Bertie CH (1924). Captain Cook and Botany Bay. *Royal Australian Historical Society Journal and Proceedings* 10(5):236–8.

Birch A & Macmillan DS (eds) (1962). *The Sydney scene 1788–1960,* Melbourne University Press, Melbourne.

Blocker JS, Fahey DM & Tyrrell IR (eds) (2003). *Alcohol and temperance in modern history: an international encyclopedia,* ABC/CLIO, Santa Barbara.

Blume AW, Lostutter TW, Schmaling KB & Marlatt GA (2003). Beliefs about drinking behaviour predict drinking consequences. *Journal of Psychoactive Drugs* 35(3):395–9. doi.org/10.1080/02791072.2003.10 400025

Bonner P (1989). Bathurst Is women want alcohol ban. *Northern Territory News,* 15 March 1989:3.

Botsman P (2015). *The sublime tragedy of kava in North East Arnhem Land,* Working Paper, www.workingpapers.com.au/papers/sublime-tragedy-kava-north-east-arnhem-land.

Bottral J (1990). Knockback curtails club plan. *Centralian Advocate,* 5 December 1990:3.

Bourbon D, Saggers S & Gray D (1999). *Indigenous Australians and liquor licensing legislation,* Curtin University of Technology, Perth.

Brady M (1988). *Where the beer truck stopped: drinking in a northern Australian town,* North Australia Research Unit, Darwin.

Brady M (1992). *Heavy metal: the social meaning of petrol sniffing in Australia,* Aboriginal Studies Press, Canberra.

Brady M (ed) (1995). *Giving away the grog: Aboriginal accounts of drinking and not drinking,* Department of Health and Ageing, Canberra.

Brady M (1999). The politics of space and mobility: controlling the Ooldea/Yalata Aborigines, 1952–1982. *Aboriginal History* 23:1–14.

Brady M (2002). *Indigenous residential treatment programs for drug and alcohol problems: current status and options for improvement*, Discussion Paper 236, Centre for Aboriginal Economic Policy Research, The Australian National University, Canberra.

Brady M (2004). *Indigenous Australia and alcohol policy: meeting difference with indifference*, University of New South Wales Press, Sydney.

Brady M (2005). *The grog book: strengthening Indigenous community action on alcohol,* revised edn, Department of Health and Ageing, Canberra.

Brady M (2008). *First taste: how Indigenous Australians learned about grog,* Foundation on Alcohol Research and Education, Canberra.

Brady M (2010). On- and off-premise drinking choices among Indigenous Australians: the influence of socio-spatial factors. *Drug and Alcohol Review* 29(4):446–51. doi.org/10.1111/j.1465-3362.2009.00144.x

Brady M (2014). *Lessons from a history of beer canteens and licensed clubs in Indigenous Australian communities*, Discussion Paper 290, Centre for Aboriginal Economic Research, The Australian National University, Canberra.

Brady M, Byrne J & Henderson G (2003). 'Which bloke would stand up for Yalata?' The struggle of an Aboriginal community to control the availability of alcohol, *Australian Aboriginal Studies* 2003/2:62–71.

Brady M, Nicholls R, Henderson G & Byrne J (2005). The role of a sobering-up centre in managing alcohol-related harm to Aboriginal people in South Australia. *Drug and Alcohol Review* 25:201–6. doi.org/10.1080/09595230600644657

Brady M & Palmer K (1984). *Alcohol in the Outback: two studies of drinking,* North Australia Research Unit, Darwin.

Broome R (2005). *Aboriginal Victorians. A history since 1800.* Allen and Unwin, Crows Nest, NSW.

Brown JB (1972). The temperance career of Joseph Chamberlain, 1870–1877: A study in political frustration. *Albion: A Quarterly Journal Concerned with British Studies* 4(1):29–44. doi.org/10.2307/4048365

Buckell J (1986). Contribution from the Tangentyere Liquor Committee, *Central Australian Rural Practitioners Association Newsletter*, 3 April 1986:8–10.

Burbank V (1994). *Fighting women: anger and aggression in Aboriginal Australia*, University of California Press, Berkeley.

Burnett J (1999). *Liquid pleasures: a social history of drinks in modern Britain*, Routledge, London and New York.

Burnham JC (1993). *Bad habits: drinking, smoking, taking drugs, gambling, sexual misbehaviour and swearing in American history*, New York University Press, New York.

Butler Rev W Corly (1899). Letter to the Editor, 'The Gothenburg System', *The West Australian* [Perth, WA: 1879–1954], 24 January 1899:3.

CAAC (Central Australian Aboriginal Congress) (1976). Submission to House of Representatives Standing Committee on Aboriginal Affairs, Hansard 5 July 1976:1196–7.

Cadbury D (2010). *Chocolate wars: the 150 year old rivalry between the world's greatest chocolate makers*, Public Affairs, New York.

Caddy GR & Lovibond SH (1976). Self-regulation and discriminated aversive conditioning in the modification of alcoholics' drinking behaviour. *Behavior Therapy* 7:223–30. doi.org/10.1016/S0005-7894(76)80279-1

Calley MJC (1957). Race relations on the north coast of New South Wales. *Oceania* 27:190–209. doi.org/10.1002/j.1834-4461.1957.tb00204.x

Calma T (2004). Address by the Aboriginal and Torres Strait Islander Social Justice Commissioner to the Australasian Liquor Licensing Authorities' Conference, Hobart, 26–29 October 2004.

Casson MR & Hirst WRC (1988). *Loxton district and town,* JC Irving & Co, Berri.

Cawte J (1988). Macabre effects of a 'cult' for kava. *Medical Journal of Australia* 148(11):545–6.

Centralian Advocate (1973). Liquor report slams Alice, 16 August 1973:1.

Centralian Advocate (1993a). Tough new drinking laws anger hoteliers, 9 March 1993:3.

Centralian Advocate (1993b). Chief Minister sacks Liquor Commissioner, 16 March 1993:3.

Centralian Advocate (1998a). Tyeweretye club must be allowed to survive: Hickey, 13 February 1998:2.

Centralian Advocate (1998b). Political war resumes over takeaway licence, 20 February 1998:5.

Centralian Advocate (1998c). Congress 'no' to takeaways, 27 February 1998:8.

Chafetz ME & Demone HW (1962). *Alcoholism and society,* Oxford University Press, New York.

Chenhall R (2007). *Benelong's haven: recovery from alcohol and drug abuse within an Aboriginal Australian residential treatment centre,* Melbourne University Press, Melbourne.

Chesterman J (2005). *Civil rights: how Indigenous Australians won formal equality,* University of Queensland Press, Brisbane.

Chlanda E (1998). Grog wars: Labor calls for 'zero tolerance'. *Alice Springs News,* 25 February 1998.

Chlanda E (2006). *Alice Springs News,* 14 September 2006.

Christie M & Young M (2011). The public problem of 'Aboriginal gambling': winning the struggle for an urban space. *Australian Journal of Social Issues* 46(3):253–72. doi.org/10.1002/j.1839-4655.2011. tb00218.x

Clough A, Burns CB & Mununggurr N (2000). Kava in Arnhem Land: a review of consumption and its social correlates. *Drug and Alcohol Review* 19:319–28. doi.org/10.1080/713659370

Clough A & Jones P (2004). Policy approaches to support local community control over the supply and distribution of kava in the Northern Territory (Australia). *Drug and Alcohol Review* 23:117–26. doi.org/10.1080/09595230410001645619

Cohen S (1972). *Folk devils and moral panics: The creation of the mods and rockers,* MacGibbon & Kee, London.

Collins D (1971). *An account of the English colony in New South Wales from its first settlement, in January 1788, to August 1801,* vols I & II, Australiana Facsimile editions no 76, Libraries Board of South Australia, Adelaide.

Collins RL & Marlatt GA (1981). Social modelling as a determinant of drinking behaviour: implications for prevention and treatment. *Addictive Behaviors* 6:233–9. doi.org/10.1016/0306-4603(81)90021-6

Collmann J (1979). Social order and the exchange of liquor: a theory of drinking among Australian Aborigines. *Journal of Anthropological Research* 35(2):208–24. doi.org/10.1086/jar.35.2.3629975

Collmann J (1988). *Fringe-dwellers and welfare: the Aboriginal response to bureaucracy,* University of Queensland Press, Brisbane.

Commonwealth of Australia (1977). *Alcohol problems of Aboriginals: final report,* House of Representatives Standing Committee on Aboriginal Affairs, Australian Government Publishing Service, Canberra.

Commonwealth of Australia (1989a). *Special audit report: the Aboriginal Development Commission and the Department of Aboriginal Affairs, March 1989,* Australian Government Publishing Service, Canberra.

Commonwealth of Australia (1989b). *Final report of special audit: the Aboriginal Development Commission and the Department of Aboriginal Affairs, October 1989,* Australian Audit Office, Australian Government Publishing Service, Canberra.

Cook PJ (2007). *Paying the tab: the economics of alcohol policy,* Princeton University Press, Princeton and Oxford.

Cooke JA (1978). *Yalata review report,* Department of Aboriginal Affairs, Adelaide, mimeo.

Cooke K (1988). Beer at centre of NT riot. *Sydney Morning Herald,* 5 December 1988:5.

Coppin BB (2006). Leedal Pty. Ltd.—A case study into an Aboriginal economic and social development initiative, in Fitzroy Crossing, BA(Hons) thesis, University of Notre Dame Australia, Western Australia.

Coroner's Court of South Australia (2011). Finding of inquest by Anthony Ernest Schapel, Deputy State Coroner, Inquest no 18/2011, Adelaide.

Coughlan F (1991). Aboriginal town camps and Tangentyere Council: the battle for self-determination in Alice Springs, MA thesis, LaTrobe University, Victoria.

Courier Mail (2013). Queensland police at odds with Premier Campbell Newman over lifting of alcohol ban in Aboriginal townships, 21 June 2013.

Critchett J (1998). *Untold stories: memories and lives of Victorian Kooris,* Melbourne University Press, Melbourne.

Cunningham P (1966). *Two years in New South Wales,* vol 2, Australian Facsimile edition no 31, Libraries Board of South Australia, Adelaide, original work published 1827.

Curthoys A (2002). *Freedom ride: a freedom rider remembers,* Allen & Unwin, Sydney.

DAA (Department of Aboriginal Affairs) (1974). *Report of activities for the period 19 December 1972 – 30 June 1974,* Australian Government Publishing Service, Canberra.

DAA (Department of Aboriginal Affairs) (1976). *Annual report 1974–75,* Australian Government Publishing Service, Canberra.

d'Abbs P (1987). *Dry areas, alcohol and Aboriginal communities: a review of the Northern Territory Restricted Areas legislation,* report for the Drug and Alcohol Bureau and Racing Gaming & Liquor Commission, Darwin.

d'Abbs P (1990). *Responding to Aboriginal substance misuse: a review of programs conducted by the Council for Aboriginal Alcohol Program Services (CAAPS), Northern Territory,* report for the Drug and Alcohol Bureau and ATSIC, Darwin.

d'Abbs P (1995). The power of kava or the power of ideas? Kava use and kava policy in the Northern Territory, Australia. *Canberra Anthropology* 18(1–2):166–83. doi.org/10.1080/03149099509508413

d'Abbs P (1998). Out of sight, out of mind? Licensed clubs in remote Aboriginal communities. *Australian and New Zealand Journal of Public Health* 22(6):679–84. doi.org/10.1111/j.1467-842X.1998.tb01469.x

d'Abbs P (2012). Problematizing alcohol through the eyes of the other: alcohol policy and Aboriginal drinking in the Northern Territory, Australia. *Contemporary Drug Problems* 39(Fall):371–96. doi.org/10.1177/009145091203900303

d'Abbs P (2014). Submission no 99 to the House of Representatives Standing Committee on Indigenous Affairs Inquiry into the Harmful Use of Alcohol in Aboriginal and Torres Strait Islander Communities, www.aph.gov.au/Parliamentary_Business/Committees/House/Indigenous_Affairs/Alcohol/Submissions.

d'Abbs P, Hunter E, Reser J & Martin D (1994). *Alcohol-related violence in Aboriginal and Torres Strait Islander communities: a literature review*, Report no 8, National Symposium on Alcohol Misuse and Violence, Australian Government Publishing Service, Canberra.

d'Abbs P & Jones T (1996). *Gunbang … or ceremonies? Combating alcohol misuse in the Kakadu/West Arnhem region*, Menzies School of Health Research Occasional Papers no 3/96, Darwin.

d'Abbs P, Togni S & Duquemin A (1999). *Evaluation of restrictions on the sale of alcohol from Curtin Springs Roadhouse Northern Territory*, Menzies School of Health Research, Darwin.

Daily Telegraph (1975). Blacks will buy the only pub in town, 3 May 1975.

Dalley C (2012). Social relations and layered identities in a remote Aboriginal town, Mornington Island, southern Gulf of Carpentaria, Australia, PhD thesis, Aboriginal Environments Research Centre, University of Queensland, Brisbane.

Defourny J & Nyssens M (2006). Defining social enterprise. In Nyssens M (ed), *Social enterprise at the crossroads of market, public policies and civil society*, Routledge, London and New York:3–25.

Defourny J & Nyssens M (2010). Conceptions of social enterprise and social entrepreneurship in Europe and the United States: convergences and divergences. *Journal of Social Entrepreneurship* 1:32–53. doi.org/10.1080/19420670903442053

Department of Indigenous Affairs (2008). *WA State Government response to the Hope Report, 7 April 2008*, Government of Western Australia, Perth.

Department of Justice (2010). *Annual report 2009/10 to the Minister for Racing, Gaming and Licensing*, Northern Territory Government, Darwin.

Department of Racing, Gaming and Liquor (2008). *Annual report 2007–2008.* Department of Racing, Gaming and Liquor, Perth.

Desmarchelier X (2001). A historical and cultural overview to the re-emergence of Thamarrurr: a traditional form of governance for the people of Wadeye, MA thesis, University of South Australia, Adelaide.

Dexter B (2015). *Pandora's box. The Council for Aboriginal Affairs 1967–1976*, ed Foley G & Howell E, Keeaira Press, Southport, Queensland.

Dingle AE (1980). 'The truly magnificent thirst': an historical survey of Australian drinking habits. *Historical Studies* 19(75):227–49. doi.org/10.1080/10314618008595636

Douglas M (1987). A distinctive anthropological perspective. In Douglas M (ed), *Constructive drinking: perspectives on drink from anthropology*, Cambridge University Press, Cambridge:3–15.

Downing J (1976). Submission to House of Representatives Standing Committee on Aboriginal Affairs, Hansard 5 July 1976.

Downing J (1988). *Ngurra Walytja, Country of my Spirit*, North Australia Research Unit, Darwin.

Drew LHR (1977). Changes in Australian drinking patterns: 1969–1976. *Australian Journal of Alcohol and Drug Dependence* 4(3):78–80.

East Arnhem Health Workers (1978). Our social environment: views from health workers. *Aboriginal Health Worker* 2(1):4–8.

Education and Health Standing Committee (2011). *Alcohol restrictions in the Kimberley: a window of opportunity for improved health, education, housing and employment*, Report no 8 in the 38th Parliament, Western Australia, www.parliament.wa.gov.au.

Edwards G, Anderson P, Babor TF, Casswell S, Ferrence R, Giesbrecht N, Godfrey C, Holder HD, Lemmens P, Mäkelä, K, Midanik LT, Norström T, Österberg E, Romeslsjö A, Room R, Simpura J & Skog O–J (1995). *Alcohol policy and the public good*, World Health Organisation Europe, Oxford University Press, Oxford.

Edwards RW, Jumper-Thurman P, Plested, BA, Oetting ER & Swanson, L (2000). Community readiness: research to practice. *Journal of Community Psychology* 28(3):291–307. doi.org/10.1002/(sici) 1520-6629(200005)28:3%3C291::aid-jcop5%3E3.3.co;2-0

Egan T (2008). *Due inheritance: reviving the cultural and economic wellbeing of First Australians: a model for consideration*, Niblock Publishing, Darwin.

Eggleston E (1976). *Fear, favour or affection: Aborigines and the criminal law in Victoria, South Australia and Western Australia*, Australian National University Press, Canberra.

Elias N (1978). *The Civilizing Process*, vol I, *The history of manners*, Pantheon Books, New York.

Elias N (1982). *The Civilizing Process*, vol II, *State formation and civilization*, Basil Blackwell, London.

Evans N (1992). Macassan loanwords in Top End languages. *Australian Journal of Linguistics* 12:45–91. doi.org/10.1080/07268609208599471

Falkenberg J (1962). *Kin and totem: group relations of Australian Aborigines in the Port Keats district*, Oslo University Press, Oslo.

FARE (Foundation for Alcohol Research and Education) (2016). *Annual poll 2016, Attitudes and behaviours*, FARE, Canberra, fare.org.au/2016/05/fare-annual-alcohol-poll-2016/.

Ferguson B (1986). Tangentyere Liquor Committee. *Central Australian Rural Practitioners Association Newsletter,* 3 April 1986:8–10.

Ferguson B (2003). Tyeweretye Clubs Inc., Submission no 96 to the Select Committee on Substance Abuse in the Community, Legislative Assembly of the Northern Territory, 22 September 2003.

Finnane K (1997). Wet canteens would 'open up the graves'. *Alice Springs News* 4(42):5.

Finnigan L (2015). Booze ban in Bournville ends after newsagent given permission to sell alcohol. *Daily Telegraph*, 30 September 2015.

Fitzgerald T (2001). *Cape York Justice Study*, Queensland Department of Premier and Cabinet, Brisbane.

Fitzpatrick JP, Latimer J, Carter M, Oscar J, Ferreira ML, Olson HC, Lucas BR, Doney R, Salter C, Try J, Hawkes G, Fitzpatrick E, Hand M, Watkins RE, Martiniuk ALC, Bower C, Boulton J & Elliott EJ (2015a). Prevalence of fetal alcohol syndrome in a population-based sample of children living in remote Australia: the Lililwan Project. *Journal of Paediatrics and Child Health* 51:450–7. doi.org/10.1111/jpc.12913_12

Fitzpatrick JP, Latimer J, Ferreira ML, Carter M, Oscar J, Martiniuk ALC, Watkins RE & Elliott EJ (2015b). Prevalence and patterns of alcohol use in pregnancy in remote Western Australian communities: the Lililwan Project. *Drug and Alcohol Review* 34:329–39. doi.org/10.1111/dar.12232

Fletcher C (1992). *Aboriginal politics,* Melbourne University Press, Melbourne.

Foley D (2003). An examination of Indigenous Australian entrepreneurs. *Journal of Developmental Entrepreneurship* 8(2):133–51.

Foote T & Hall A (1995). *More tales from Pormpuraaw: Kuthip Yirram Pormpuraawntam,* Thaayorre/English, Australian Institute of Aboriginal and Torres Strait Islander Studies, Canberra.

Ford C (1988). Alcohol warnings opposed. *Melbourne Herald*, 24 November 1988:5.

Foster G (1982). Community development and primary health care: their conceptual similarities. *Medical Anthropology* 6:183–95. doi.org/10.1080/01459740.1982.9987016

Frykman J & Löfgren O (1987). *Culture builders: a historical anthropology of middle-class life*, Rutgers University Press, New Brunswick and London.

Fua C & Lumsden L (1984). Aboriginal alcohol abuse and crime in Queensland. In Swanton B (ed), *Aborigines and criminal justice*, Australian Institute of Criminology Proceedings, Canberra:6–16.

Gaff B, Spink J & Price D (1997). *Alice Springs sobering-up shelter client profile*, Drug and Alcohol Services Association Alice Springs.

Gascoigne J (2002). *The Enlightenment and the origins of European Australia,* Cambridge University Press, Cambridge.

Gladman DJ, Hunter E, McDermott R, Merritt T & Tulip F (1997). *Study of injury in five Cape York communities,* Australian Institute of Health and Welfare and Tropical Public Health Unit, Cairns.

Goode E & Ben-Yehuda N (1994). Moral panics: culture, politics and social construction. *Annual Review of Sociology* 20:149–71. doi.org/10.1146/annurev.so.20.080194.001053

Gordon E (1911). *Breakdown of the Gothenburg system*, National Temperance Society and Publication House, New York.

Gould ERL (1893). *The Gothenburg system of liquor traffic: fifth special report of the Commissioner of Labor,* Government Printer, Washington.

Gray D (1996). Harm reduction and self-determination. *Drug and Alcohol Review* 15(4):409–10.

Gray D, Drandich M, Moore L, Wilkes T, Riley R & Davies S (1995). Aboriginal wellbeing and liquor licensing legislation in Western Australia. *Australian Journal of Public Health* 19(2):177–85. doi.org/10.1111/j.1753-6405.1995.tb00370.x

Greenaway J (1998). Policy learning and the drink question in Britain 1850–1950. *Political Studies* XLVI:903–18. doi.org/10.1111/1467-9248.00174

Greenaway J (2003). *Drink and British politics since 1830. A study in policy-making*, Palgrave Macmillan, London.

Gregory R & Cawte J (1988). The principle of alien poisons: contrasting psychopharmacology of kava in Oceania and Australia. In Prescott J & McCall G (eds), *Kava: use and abuse in Australia and the South Pacific,* National Drug and Alcohol Research Centre Monograph no 5, University of New South Wales, Sydney:29–39.

Grimshaw P (1999). Colonising motherhood: evangelical social reformers and Koorie women in Victoria, Australia, 1880s to the early 1900s. *Women's History Review* 8(2):329–46. doi.org/10.1080/09612029900200203

Guest S (1988). Aboriginal commission officers face sack. *Canberra Times,* 19 September 1988:1.

Gutzke DW (1989). *Protecting the pub: brewers and publicans against temperance,* Royal Historical Society, Boydell Press, Woodbridge, Suffolk.

Gutzke DW (1994). Gentrifying the British public house, 1896–1914. *International Labor and Working-Class History* 45(March):29–43. doi.org/10.1017/S0147547900012448

Gutzke DW (2007). Progressivism and the history of the public house, 1850–1950. *Cultural and Social History* 4(2):235–60. doi.org/10.2752/147800307X199065

Hall W, Hunter E & Spargo R (1993). Alcohol-related problems among Aboriginal drinkers in the Kimberley region of Western Australia. *Addiction* 88:1091–100. doi.org/10.1111/j.1360-0443.1993.tb02128.x

Hansen EE (1969). The Christian Church and Aboriginal welfare. In Warburton JW (ed), *The Aborigines of South Australia, their background and future prospects : proceedings of a conference held at the University of Adelaide June 13–16, 1969,* Department of Adult Education, University of Adelaide, Adelaide.

Hansen EE (1972). Aborigines and alcohol. *Forum 69* 4(2):5–9.

Harris J (1998). *We wish we'd done more: ninety years of CMS and Aboriginal issues in north Australia,* Openbook Publishers, Adelaide.

Hawke S (2014). *A town is born: the Fitzroy Crossing story*, Magabala Books, Broome.

Heath, DB (2000). *Drinking occasions: comparative perspectives on alcohol and culture*, Brunner/Mazel, Philadelphia.

Heather N & Robertson I (1989). *Problem drinking*, 2nd edn, Oxford University Press, Oxford.

Henderson-Yates L, Wagner S, Parker H & Yates D (2008). *Fitzroy Valley Liquor Restriction Report: an evaluation of the effects of a six month restriction on take-away alcohol relating to measurable health and social benefits and community perceptions and behaviours*, report to the Drug and Alcohol Office, University of Notre Dame Australia, Perth.

Hercus L & Sutton P (eds) (1986). *This is what happened: historical narratives by Aborigines*, Australian Institute of Aboriginal Studies, Canberra.

Hodge A & Emerson S (2002). Black councils to lose grog canteen licences. *The Australian*, 11 April 2002:3.

Hogan M (Director) (2009). *Yajilarra = to dream: Aboriginal women leading change in remote Australia* [Videorecoding]. Marinwarntikura Women's Resource Centre.

Holman CDJ & Quadros CF (1986). *Health and disease in the Aboriginal population of the Kimberley region of Western Australia 1980–1985*, Health Department of Western Australia, Perth.

Hope AN, State Coroner (2008). *Inquest into the deaths of EJ Riley, R Henry, C Atkins, T Beharral, M Brown, J Dick, L Dawson, B Dickens, IB Gepp, OGJ Hale, EJ Laurel, J Middleton, WR Miller, G Oscar, CA Shaw, S Surprise, DK Edwards, NM Cox, D Sampi, L Sampi, TJ O'Sullivan & Z Yamera*, Record of investigation into death ref 37/07, WA Coroner's Court, Western Australia, Perth.

Howard E (1902). *Garden cities of to-morrow*, 2nd edn, ebooks.adelaide. edu.au/h/howard/ebenezer/garden_cities_of_to-morrow/chapter7. html.

Hoy WE, Norman RJ, Hayhurst BG & Pugsley DJ (1997). A health profile of adults in a Northern Territory Aboriginal community, with an emphasis on preventable morbidities. *Australian and New Zealand Journal of Public Health* 21(2):121–6. doi.org/10.1111/j.1467-842x.1977.tb01356.x

HRSCAA (House of Representatives Standing Committee on Aboriginal Affairs) (1976). Alcohol problems of Aboriginals, Hansard, 4 July 1976.

Hungerfords KMG (1986). *Aboriginal controlled social clubs, Alice Springs: final report stage I for the Tyeweretye Clubs*, report for Tangentyere Council by KMG Club and Hotel Management Services, Sydney.

Hunter E (1993). *Aboriginal health and history: power and prejudice in remote Australia*, Cambridge University Press, Cambridge.

Hunter J (1968). *An historical journal of the transactions at Port Jackson and Norfolk Island by Captain John Hunter*, Australiana Facsimile editions no 148, Libraries Board of South Australia, Adelaide, original work published 1793.

Hunter W & Clarence C (1996). *Ideas for sports and social clubs: creating safer drinking environments*, Living with Alcohol Program, Darwin.

Hupkens CLH, Knibbe RA & Drop MJ (1993). Alcohol consumption in the European Community: uniformity and diversity in drinking patterns. *Addiction* 88:1391–404. doi.org/10.1111/j.1360-0443.1993.tb02026.x

Hutt M (1999). *Te Iwi Maori me to Inu Waipiro: He Tuhituhinga Hitori [Maori and alcohol: a history]*, Health Services Research Centre, Wellington, New Zealand.

IBA (Indigenous Business Australia) (2005). From little things big things grow, Submission no 104 to the Inquiry into Indigenous Employment, House of Representatives Standing Committee on Aboriginal and Torres Strait Islander Affairs, Canberra.

IBA (Indigenous Business Australia) (2007). *Annual report 2006–2007*, IBA, Canberra.

IBA (Indigenous Business Australia) (2008). *Annual report 2007–2008*, IBA, Canberra.

IBA (Indigenous Business Australia) (2009). *Annual report 2008–2009*, IBA, Canberra.

International Center for Alcohol Policies (2004). *Drinking patterns: from theory to practice,* ICAP Reports 15, Washington, DC.

International Order of Good Templars (1890). The bishop and the Scandinavian plan. *Temperance Tracts* XI(89).

Irving GM (2007). A report on an independent review of the Fitzroy Crossing IBA Joint Venture Businesses, for the Minister for Employment and Workplace Relations, John Toohey Chambers, Perth.

Ivory B (2009). Kunmanggur, legend and leadership: a study of Indigenous leadership and succession focussing on the northwest region of the Northern Territory of Australia, PhD thesis, Charles Darwin University, Darwin.

Jackson P (1988). Families flee riot. *Northern Territory News*, 5 December 1988:1.

Johnson YM (1997). *The Renmark Hotel 1897–1997. The first community hotel in the British Empire,* J. Irving & Co., Berri, South Australia.

Johnston E, Commissioner (1991). Report of the inquiry into the death of a man who died at Oodnadatta on 17 December 1983, SA6, 24 January 1991, websearch.aic.gov.au/firstaicPublic/fullRecord.jsp?recno=207877.

Jones A (1994). *Lyrup Village: a century of association 1894–1994,* Lyrup Village Centenary Committee, Lyrup, South Australia.

Jones R (2017). Pubs saved from last orders by local co-ops enjoy new lease of life. *The Guardian*, 8 July 2017:13.

Kamien, M (1975). Aborigines and alcohol: intake, effects and social implications in a rural community in western New South Wales. *Medical Journal of Australia* 8(March):291–7.

Kamien M (1978). *The dark people of Bourke*: a *study of planned social change,* Australian Institute of Aboriginal Studies and Humanities Press, Canberra and New Jersey.

Karskens G (1999). *Inside the Rocks: the archaeology of a neighbourhood,* Hale and Iremonger, Hong Kong.

Katz R (1993). *The straight path: a story of healing and transformation in Fiji,* Addison-Wesley Publishing, Reading, Massachusetts.

Keeffe K (2003). *Paddy's road: life stories of Patrick Dodson,* Aboriginal Studies Press, Canberra.

Kenny J (1973). *Bennelong: first notable aboriginal,* a report from original sources arranged by John Kenny, Councillor, Royal Australian Historical Society, Royal Australian Historical Society, Sydney.

Kesteven S (1984). The social impact of uranium, 3. Health, II, Alcohol and family life. In AIAS (Australian Institute of Aboriginal Studies) (ed), *Aborigines and uranium: consolidated report to the Minister for Aboriginal Affairs on the social impact of uranium mining on the Aborigines of the Northern Territory,* Australian Government Publishing Service, Canberra:192–203.

Kidd R (1997). *The way we civilise: Aboriginal affairs—the untold story,* University of Queensland Press, Brisbane.

King PG (1980). *The journal of Philip Gidley King, Lieutenant, R.N. 1787–1790,* eds Fidlon PG & Ryan RJ, Australian Documents Library, Sydney.

Kinnane S, Farringdon F, Henderson-Yates L & Parker H (2009). *Fitzroy Valley Alcohol Restriction Report: an evaluation of the effects of a restriction on take-away alcohol relating to measurable health and social outcomes, community perceptions and behaviours after a 12 month period,* A report by the University of Notre Dame Australia to the Drug and Alcohol Office, Perth.

Kirkby D (1997). *Barmaids: a history of women's work in pubs,* Cambridge University Press, Cambridge.

Kociumbas J (1995). *Possessions 1770–1860. The Oxford history of Australia,* Oxford University Press, Oxford.

Koeler H (2006). Some notes on the Aborigines on the East Coast of Gulf St. Vincent in South Australia 1837 and 1830, translated by Lois Zwek. In Muhlhausler P (ed), *Herman Koeler's Adelaide: Observations on the language and culture of South Australia by the first Australian visitor,* Australian Humanities Press, Adelaide:51–126.

Kolig E (1974). Kerygma and grog: elders revive 'tribal law' in the Kimberleys. *Department of Aboriginal Affairs Western Australia, Newsletter* 1(7):44–52.

Kolig E (2000). Social causality, human agency and mythology: some thoughts on history-consciousness and mythical sense among Australian Aborigines. *Anthropological Forum* 10(1):9–30. doi. org/10.1080/00664670050006730

Koori Mail (2013). Club has mix right on Cape, 28 August 2013:12.

Kuilboer T (1999). Club no closer in liquor fight. *Northern Territory News*, 21 February 1999:13.

Kunitz SJ & Levy JE (1974). Changing ideas of alcohol use among Navaho Indians. *Quarterly Journal of Studies on Alcohol* 35(1):243–59.

Kunitz SJ & Levy JE (1994). *Drinking careers: a twenty-five-year study of three Navajo populations*, Yale University Press, New Haven and London.

Kunitz SJ & Levy JE (2000). *Drinking, conduct disorder and social change: Navajo experiences*, Oxford University Press, Oxford.

Kunitz SJ, Levy JE, Odoroff CL & Bollinge J (1971). The epidemiology of alcoholic cirrhosis in two south-western tribes. *Quarterly Journal of Studies on Alcohol* 32:706–20.

La Housse P (1992). Drink and cultural innovation in Durban: the origins of the beerhall in South Africa, 1902–1916. In Crush J & Ambler C (eds), *Liquor and Labor in southern Africa*, Ohio University Press and University of Natal Press, Athens and Pietermaritzburg:78–114.

Lame Deer JF & Erdoes R (1972). *Lame Deer seeker of visions: the life of a Sioux medicine man*, Simon and Schuster, New York.

Lang E (1994). Community action regarding licensing issues. In Stockwell T (ed), *An examination of the appropriateness and efficacy of liquor licensing laws across Australia*, Department of Human Services and Health, Canberra:211–31.

Langton M, Ah Matt L, Moss B, Schaber E, Mackinolty C, Thomas M, Tilton E & Spencer L (1991). *Too much sorry business: the report of the Aboriginal Issues Unit of the Northern Territory*, Appendix D(I) in National Report, vol 5, Royal Commission into Aboriginal Deaths in Custody, Australian Government Publishing Service, Canberra.

Lapthorne AM (1947). *Mildura calling,* Bread and Cheese Club, Melbourne.

Larkins J & Howard B (1973). *Australian pubs,* Weldon Hardie and Rigby, Sydney.

Larkins KP & McDonald DN (1984). Recent Northern Territory liquor control initiatives. *Australian Alcohol/Drug Review* 3(1):50–64. doi.org/10.1080/09595238480000161

Leary Rev J, Dodson Rev P, Tipiloura B & Bunduk L (1975). *Alcoholism and Aborigines: a report*, Interdepartmental Committee on Alcoholism and Aborigines, Canberra.

Lebot V, Merlin M & Lindstrom L (1992). *Kava: the Pacific drug,* Yale University Press, New Haven and London.

Leedal Pty Ltd (2009). Submission to the Senate Select Committee on Remote Indigenous Communities, Senate Select Committee on Regional and Remote Communities.

Leedal Pty Ltd (2013). Submission to the Review of the Liquor Control Act 1988 [to John Atkins, Chair, Liquor Act Review Committee, Perth].

Leedal Pty Ltd (2014). Submission no 18 to the House of Representatives Standing Committee on Indigenous Affairs Inquiry into the Harmful Use of Alcohol in Aboriginal and Torres Strait Islander Communities, 11 April 2014.

Legislative Assembly of the Northern Territory (1991). *Measures for reducing alcohol use and abuse in the Northern Territory: interim report of the Sessional Committee on the Use and Abuse of Alcohol by the Community*, Report no 2, Government Printer of the Northern Territory, Darwin.

LHA (Laynhapuy Homelands Association Inc.) (2008). Submission to Senate Standing Committee on Legal and Constitutional Affairs Inquiry into the Appropriation (Northern Territory National Emergency Response) Bill (No.2) 2007–2008.

Lickiss JN (1971). Alcohol and Aborigines in cross-cultural situations. *Australian Journal of Social Studies* 6(3):210–16. doi.org/10.1002/j.1839-4655.1971.tb00476.x

Lincoln K & Slagle AL (1987). *The good red road: passages into Native America,* Harper & Row, New York.

Lisansky-Gomberg ES (1989). On terms used and abused: the concept of 'Codependency'. *Drugs and Society* 3(3–4):113–32. doi.org/10.1300/J023v03n03_05

Lloyd J (2014). Violent and tragic events: the nature of domestic violence-related homicide cases in Central Australia. *Australian Aboriginal Studies* 2014(1):99–110.

Long J (1992). *The go-betweens: patrol officers in Aboriginal affairs administration in the Northern Territory 1936–1974,* North Australia Research Unit, Darwin.

Lyon P (1990). *What everybody knows about Alice: a report on the impact of alcohol abuse on the town of Alice Springs,* Tangentyere Council, Alice Springs.

Lyon P (1991). Liquor licensing, Aborigines and take-away alcohol in Central Australia. *Aboriginal Law Bulletin* August:11–13.

MacAndrew C & Edgerton RB (1969). *Drunken comportment: a social explanation,* Aldine Publishing, Chicago.

Macknight CC (1976). *The voyage to Marege'. Macassan trepangers in northern Australia,* Melbourne University Press, Melbourne.

McBryde I (2000). 'Barter ... immediately commenced to the satisfaction of both parties'. Cross-cultural exchange at Port Jackson, 1788–1828. In Torrance R & Clarke A (eds), *The archaeology of difference: negotiating cross-cultural engagements in Oceania,* Routledge, London:238–77.

McCambridge J (2011). Fifty years of brief interventions effectiveness trials for heavy drinkers [Editorial]. *Drug and Alcohol Review* 30(November):567–8. doi.org/10.1111/j.1465-3362.2011.00379.x

McCorkindale I (1945). *The community hotel and the community centre* [Booklet], National WCTU of Australia, Adelaide.

McDonald H (2001). *Blood, bones and spirit: Aboriginal Christianity in an East Kimberley town,* Melbourne University Press, Melbourne.

McGrath A (1993). 'Beneath the skin'. Australian citizenship, rights and Aboriginal women. *Journal of Australian Studies* 37:99–114. doi.org/10.1080/14443059309387144

McIntyre J (2008). 'Bannelong sat down to dinner with Governor Phillip, and drank his wine and coffee as usual'. Aborigines and wine in early New South Wales. *History Australia* 5(2):39.1–39.14. doi.org/10.2104/ha080039

McIntyre J (2011). Adam Smith and faith in the transformative qualities of wine in Colonial New South Wales. *Australian Historical Studies* 42(2):194–211. doi.org/10.1080/1031461X.2011.560611

McIntyre J (2012). *First vintage: wine in colonial New South Wales,* University of New South Wales Press, Sydney.

McKenna M (2014). Pearson backs drinking for some dry townships. *Weekend Australian*, 15–16 February 2014:5.

McKnight D (2002). *From hunting to drinking: the devastating effects of alcohol on an Australian Aboriginal community,* Routledge, London and New York.

McLean NJ (1987). Implementing a controlled drinking program, *Australian Drug and Alcohol Review* 6:137–43. doi.org/10.1080/09595238780000251

McQuire A (2011). New beginning for the first Aboriginal winemakers, *Tracker: New South Wales LALC,* April.

Malins J (1899). The Gothenburg system, a lecture by Joseph Malins in the Collins Street Independent Church, Melbourne, 9 November 1899.

Mancall PC (1995). *Deadly medicine: Indians and alcohol in early America,* Cornell University Press, Ithaca and London.

Mansfield J (2013). The social organisation of Wadeye's heavy metal mobs. *The Australian Journal of Anthropology* 24(2):148–65. doi. org/10.1111/taja.12035

Mantziaris C & Martin D (2000). *Native title corporations: a legal and anthropological analysis,* Federation Press, Canberra.

Marks K (2007). Alcoholism in Australia: the wives who said time, gentlemen … *The Independent* [UK], 31 October 2007, www. independent.co.uk/news/world/australasia/alcoholism-in-australia-the-wives-who-said-time-gentlemen-398367.html.

Marsden Jacob Associates (2005). *Identifying a framework for regulation in packaged liquor retailing,* report for the National Competition Council as part of the NCC Occasional Series, Marsden Jacob Associates, Camberwell, Victoria.

Marshall M (1981). 'Four hundred rabbits': an anthropological view of ethanol as a disinhibitor. In Room R & Collins G (eds), *Alcohol and disinhibition: nature and meaning of the link*, Research Monograph no 12, US Department of Health and Human Services, Washington.

Marshall M (ed) (1982). *Through a glass darkly: beer and modernization in Papua New Guinea,* Monograph no 18, Institute of Applied Social and Economic Research, Boroko, Papua New Guinea.

Marshall P (ed) (1988). *Raparapa: stories from the Fitzroy River drovers,* Magabala Books, Broome.

Martin D (1993). Autonomy and relatedness: an ethnography of Wik people of Aurukun, Western Cape York Peninsula, PhD thesis, The Australian National University, Canberra.

Martin D (1995). *Money, business and culture: issues for Aboriginal economic policy,* Discussion Paper no 101, Centre for Aboriginal Economic Policy Research, The Australian National University, Canberra.

Martin D (1998). *The supply of alcohol in remote Aboriginal communities: potential policy directions from Cape York*, Discussion Paper no 162, Centre for Aboriginal Economic Policy Research, The Australian National University, Canberra.

Matthews J, Riley M, Fejo L, Munoz E, Milns NR, Gardner ID, Powers JR, Ganygulpa E & Gununuwawuy BJ (1988). Effects of heavy usage of kava on physical health: summary of a pilot survey in an Aboriginal community. *Medical Journal of Australia* 148(June):545–55.

Mattingly C (ed) (1988). *Survival in our own land: 'Aboriginal' experiences in 'South Australia' since 1836,* Wakefield Press, Adelaide.

May PA, Miller J & Wallerstein N (1993). Motivation and community prevention of substance abuse. *Experimental and Clinical Psychopharmacology* 1(1–4):68–79. doi.org/10.1037/1064-1297.1.1-4.68

Measham F (2006). The new policy mix: alcohol, harm minimisation, and determined drunkenness in contemporary society. *International Journal of Drug Policy* 17:258–68. doi.org/10.1016/j.drugpo.2006.02.013

Meggitt MJ (1975). *Desert people: a study of the Walbiri Aborigines of Central Australia,* Angus & Robertson, Sydney.

Meredith Mrs C (1973). *Notes and sketches of New South Wales during a residence in the Colony from 1839–1844,* Ure Smith, Sydney.

Midford R, Daly A & Holmes M (1994). The care of public drunks in Hall's Creek: a model for community involvement. *Health Promotion Journal of Australia* 4(1):5–8.

Mills KC, Sobell MB & Schaefer HH (1971). Training social drinking as an alternative to abstinence for alcoholics. *Behavior Therapy* 2:18–27. doi.org/10.1016/S0005-7894(71)80142-9

Moizo BR (1991). We all one mob but different: groups, grouping and identity in a Kimberley Aboriginal village, PhD thesis, The Australian National University, Canberra.

Moran M (2013). Mothers know best: managing grog in Kowanyama. *Griffith Review* 40(Winter):196–209.

Morphy F (2008). Whose governance, for whose good? The Laynhapuy Homelands Association and the neo-assimilationist turn in Indigenous policy. In Hunt J, Smith D, Garling S & Sanders W (eds), *Contested governance, culture power and institutions in Indigenous Australia,* Centre for Aboriginal Economic Policy Research, Research Monograph no 29, The Australian National University, Canberra.

Murdoch L & Skelton R (2011). Macklin could end grog ban. *The Age*, 23 May 2011.

Myers FD (1979). Emotions and the self: a theory of personhood and political order among Pintupi Aborigines. *Ethos: Journal of the Society for Psychological Anthropology* 7(4):343–69. doi.org/10.1525/eth.1979.7.4.02a00030

National Drug Research Institute (2007). *Restrictions on the sale and supply of alcohol: evidence and outcomes*, National Drug Research Institute, Curtin University of Technology, Perth.

National Drug Research Institute and the Lewin-Fordham Group (1999). *The public health, safety and economic benefits of the Northern Territory's Living with Alcohol program 1992/3 to 1995/6*, Curtin University of Technology, Perth.

New Dawn (1971). Walgett—then and now, August 1971:1–2.

Northern Territory Aboriginal News (1989). Kava education program, 5(2):9.

Northern Territory Department of Justice (2009). *Annual report 2008/9 to the Minister of Racing, Gaming and Licensing*, Darwin.

Northern Territory Licensing Commission (2009). *Reasons for decision: review of the declaration of Alice Springs Township as public restricted and review of alcohol supply measures introduced in Alice Springs*, 12 August 2009.

Northern Territory Liquor Commission (1997). *Reasons for decision: Tyeweretye Social Club variation of conditions hearing*, 11–15 March 1997.

Northern Territory Liquor Commission (2008). *Reasons for decision: complaint pursuant to S48 of the Liquor Act*, 13 October 2008.

Northern Territory Liquor Commission (2010a). *Reasons for decision: cancellation of liquor licence pursuant to s72(5)(a) of the Liquor Act*, 12 May and 7 September 2010.

Northern Territory Liquor Commission (2010b). *Reasons for decision: complaint pursuant to s48(2) of the Liquor Act*, 15 September 2010.

Northern Territory News (1988). Shots fired in Port Keats riot, 7 October 1988.

Northern Territory News (1993). 300 women in anti-grog rally, 24 April 1993:6.

Northern Territory News (1998). Grog Ban may go in new Port Keats plan, 1 April 1998.

O'Connor R (1983). A case of might-have-been: some reflections on the new 'Two Kilometre Law' in the Northern Territory. *Anthropological Forum* 5(2):201–7. doi.org/10.1080/00664677.1983.9967347

O'Connor R (1984). Alcohol and contingent drunkenness in Central Australia. *Australian Journal of Social Issues* 19(3):173–83. doi.org/10.1002/j.1839-4655.1984.tb00787.x

O'Loughlin G (1988). Bathurst to be almost grog free. *Northern Territory News*, 6 December 1988.

Ormerod P & Wiltshire G (2009). 'Binge' drinking in the UK: a social network phenomenon. *Mind and Society* 8:135–52. doi.org/10.1007/s11299-009-0058-1

Oscar J & Pedersen H (2011). Alcohol restrictions in the Fitzroy Valley: trauma and resilience. In Maddison S & Brigg M (eds), *Unsettling the settler state: creativity and resistance in Indigenous settler-state governance*, Federation Press, Sydney:83–97.

Ottosson Å (2014). To know one's place: belonging and differentiation in Alice Springs town. *Anthropological Forum* 24(2):115–35. doi.org/10.1080/00664677.2014.901212

Parsons M (1997). The tourist corroboree in South Australia to 1911. *Aboriginal History* 21:46–69.

Pedersen H & Woorunmurra B (2007). *Jandamarra and the Bunuba resistance*, Magabala Books, Broome.

Peele S (1993). The conflict between public health goals and the temperance mentality. *American Journal of Public Health* 83(6):805–10. doi.org/10.2105/AJPH.83.6.805

Pendery ML, Maltzman IM & West LJ (1982). Controlled drinking by alcoholics? New findings and a reevaluation of a major affirmative study. *Science* 217(9 July):169–74. doi.org/10.1126/science.7089552

Penny R (1979). *Aboriginal Drinking Project report*, Department of Psychology, University of Adelaide, Adelaide, mimeo.

Perkins C (1975). *A bastard like me*, Ure Smith, Sydney.

Petersen AR (1987). Alcohol policy and health promotion: rhetoric and reality. *Australian Journal of Social Issues* 22(1):333–44. doi.org/10.1002/j.1839-4655.1987.tb01210.x

Peterson N (2013). On the persistence of sharing: personhood, asymmetrical reciprocity, and demand sharing in the Indigenous Australian domestic moral economy. *The Australian Journal of Anthropology* 24:166–76. doi.org/10.1111/taja.12036

Petrie T (1904). *Tom Petrie's reminiscences of early Queensland (dating from 1837) recorded by his daughter*, Watson, Ferguson & Co., Brisbane.

Phelan B (2012). Trouble at Mount Ebenezer. *ABC Alice Springs*, 17 December 2012.

Pitjantjatjara Council Inc (1990). *Submission to the Sessional Committee on the Use and Abuse of Alcohol by the Community*, Legislative Assembly of the Northern Territory, Darwin.

Pitman RC (1877). *Alcohol and the state, a discussion: or the problem of law as applied to the liquor traffic*, National Temperance Society and Publication House, New York.

Plomley NJB (1983). *The Baudin expedition and the Tasmanian Aborigines 1802*, Blubber Head Press, Hobart.

Pratt A & Bennett S (2004). *The end of ATSIC and the future administration of Indigenous affairs*, Current Issues Brief no 4 2004–05, Information and Research Services, Parliamentary Library, Canberra.

Prestoungrange G (2004). The Prestoungrange Gothenburg. *East Lothian Life*, 28 November 2004:32–3.

Purtill T (2017). *The dystopia in the desert*, Australian Scholarly Publishing, North Melbourne.

Putt J (2011). *Review of the Substance Abuse Intelligence Desks and Dog Operation Units*, FaHCSIA, Canberra, www.dss.gov.au/sites/default/files/documents/05_2012/attachment-a-said-review-report-final-9-dec-11-clean.pdf.

Queensland Government (2002). *Meeting challenges, making choices*, the Queensland Government's response to the Cape York Justice Study, Brisbane, www.mcmc.qld.gov.au.

Race Discrimination Commissioner (1995). *Alcohol report: Racial Discrimination Act 1975. Race discrimination, human rights and the distribution of alcohol*, Australian Government Publishing Service, Canberra.

Racing, Gaming and Licensing Division (2003). *A review of Northern Territory wayside inns: still needed or a thing of the past?* Northern Territory Treasury, Darwin.

Rae KG (1989). *Application by Erldunda Motel Pty Ltd., Desert Oaks Motel before NT Racing, Gaming and Liquor Commission*, Alice Springs, 14–17 March 1989.

Raftery J (1987). God's gift or demon drink? Churches and alcohol in South Australia between the two World Wars. *Journal of the Historical Society of South Australia* (1987):16–41.

Read P (2001). *Charles Perkins: a biography*, Penguin Books, Melbourne.

Recorder (Port Pirie) (1939). Growing interest in community hotels, 5 January 1939:1.

Renmark Community Hotel (nd). *The Renmark Community Hotel: brief history*, Renmark, mimeo.

Renmark Pioneer (1895). Anti-prohibitionist [Correspondence], 20 July 1895:4.

Richards D (2009). Drinks club key to Alice drink problem. *Centralian Advocate*, 16 January 2009:5.

Rickard S (ed) (2001). *George Barrington's voyage to Botany Bay: retelling a convict's travel narrative of the 1790s*, Leicester University Press, London and New York.

Rifkin SB (1986). Lessons from community participation in health programmes. *Health Policy and Planning* 1(3):240–9. doi.org/10.1093/heapol/1.3.240

Room R (1976). Ambivalence as a sociological explanation: the case of cultural explanations of alcohol problems. *American Sociological Review* 41(December):1047–65. doi.org/10.2307/2094802

Room R (1982). A view from outside. In Marshall M (ed), *Through a glass darkly: beer and modernization in Papua New Guinea,* Monograph no 18, Institute of Applied Social and Economic Research, Boroko, Papua New Guinea:441–50.

Room R (1985). Dependence and society. *British Journal of Addiction* 80:133–9. doi.org/10.1111/j.1360-0443.1985.tb03263.x

Room R (1988). The dialectic of drinking in Australian life: from the Rum Corps to the wine column. *Australian Drug and Alcohol Review* 7:413–37. doi.org/10.1080/09595238880000741

Room R (1992). The impossible dream? Routes to reducing alcohol problems in a temperance culture. *Journal of Substance Abuse* 4:91–106. doi.org/10.1016/0899-3289(92)90030-2

Room R (1993). The evolution of alcohol monopolies and their relevance for public health. *Contemporary Drug Problems* 20(Summer):169–87.

Room R (2001). Intoxication and bad behaviour: understanding cultural differences in the link. *Social Science and Medicine* 53:189–98. doi.org/10.1016/S0277-9536(00)00330-0

Room R (2004). Alcohol and harm reduction, then and now. *Critical Public Health* 14:329–44. doi.org/10.1080/09581590400027536

Room R (2005). Stigma, social inequality and alcohol and drug use. *Drug and Alcohol Review* 24:143–55. doi.org/10.1080/09595230500102434

Room R (2011). Addiction and personal responsibility as solutions to the contradictions of neoliberal consumerism. *Critical Public Health* 21(2):141–51. doi.org/10.1080/09581596.2010.529424

Room R (2012). Individualised control of drinkers: back to the future? *Contemporary Drug Problems* 39(Summer):311–43. doi.org/10.1177/009145091203900207

Room R, Babor T & Rehm J (2005). Alcohol and public health. *The Lancet* 365(5 February):519–30. doi.org/10.1016/s0140-6736(05)70276-2

Room R & Mäkelä K (2000). Typologies of the cultural position of drinking. *Journal of Studies on Alcohol* 61(3):475–83. doi.org/10.15288/jsa.2000.61.475

Rowley C (1970). *The destruction of Aboriginal society: Aboriginal policy and practice*, vol I, Australian National University Press, Canberra.

Rowntree J & Sherwell A (1903). *British 'Gothenburg' experiments and public-house trusts*, 3rd edn, Hodder & Stoughton, London.

Rowse T (1996). *Traditions for health: studies in Aboriginal reconstruction*, North Australia Research Unit, Darwin.

Rowse T (1998). *White flour, white power: from rations to citizenship in Central Australia*, Cambridge University Press, Cambridge.

Rowse T (2015). Indigenous incorporation as a means to empowerment. In Brennan S, Davis M, Edgeworth B & Terrill L (eds), *Native title from Mabo to Akiba: a vehicle for change and empowerment?*, The Federation Press, Sydney.

Saggers S & Gray D (1998). *Dealing with alcohol: Indigenous usage in Australia, New Zealand and Canada*, Cambridge University Press, Cambridge.

Salmond A (2003). *The trial of the cannibal dog: Captain Cook in the South Seas*, Penguin, London.

Sansom B (1977). Aborigines and alcohol: a fringe camp example. *Australian Journal of Alcoholism and Drug Dependence* 4(2):59–62.

Sansom B (1980). *The camp at Wallaby Cross: Aboriginal fringe-dwellers in Darwin*, AIAS (Australian Institute of Aboriginal Studies), Canberra.

Schivelbusch W (1993). *Tastes of paradise: a social history of spices, stimulants, and intoxicants*, Vintage Books, New York.

Schulz D (1990). Walk against grog. *Territory Digest* 12(3):1–4.

Searcy, A (1984). *In Australian Tropics*, 2nd edn, Hesperion Press, Perth, original work published 1909.

Secker A (1993). The policy-research interface: an insider's view. *Addiction* 88(Suppl):115S–120S. doi.org/10.1111/j.1360-0443.1993. tb02169.x

Sellman D (2010). Ten things the alcohol industry won't tell you about alcohol. *Drug and Alcohol Review* 29:301–3. doi.org/10.1111/j.1465-3362.2009.00121.x

Sexton LD (1982). New beer in old bottles: an innovative community club and politics as usual in the Eastern Highlands. In Marshall M (ed), *Through a glass darkly: beer and modernization in Papua New Guinea,* Monograph no 18, Institute of Applied Social and Economic Research, Boroko, Papua New Guinea:105–18.

Shadwell A (1923). *Drink in 1914–1922: a lesson in control,* Longmans, Green & Co, London.

Sharma K (2005). *Indigenous governance,* KPS Publications, Canberra.

Shaw G, Brady M & d'Abbs P (2015). *Managing alcohol consumption. A review of licensed clubs in remote Indigenous communities in the Northern Territory,* report to the Northern Territory Department of Business, Bowchung Pty Ltd.

Shaw B & Gibson J (1988). *Invasion and succession: an Aboriginal history of the Oodnadatta region,* vol 1, report prepared for the Oodnadatta Housing Society and Aboriginal Heritage Branch, South Australia.

Shields B (1995). *This is a story for the beer rations in Umbakumba Community,* Living with Alcohol Program, Darwin.

Shore JA & Spicer P (2004). A model for alcohol-mediated violence in an Australian Aboriginal community. *Social Science and Medicine* 58:2509–21. doi.org/10.1016/j.socscimed.2003.09.022

Simmons L (1988). *Availability of alcohol in Alice Springs,* Discussion Paper for CAAC, Central Australian Aboriginal Congress, Alice Springs.

Simonsen R (2006). Joint ventures and Indigenous tourism enterprises. *Tourism, Culture and Communication* 6(2):107–19. doi.org/10.3727/109830406777410607

Simper E (1991). Pub with no beer offers hope. *The Australian,* 15 April 1991:4.

Smith KV (2001). *Bennelong: the coming in of the Eora, Sydney Cove 1799–1792*, Kangaroo Press, Sydney.

Smith M (2013). *The archaeology of Australia's deserts,* Cambridge University Press, Cambridge.

Smith T (2002). Indigenous accumulation in the Kimberley during the early years of 'self-determination': 1968–1975. *Australian Economic History Review* 42(1):1–33. doi.org/10.1111/1467-8446.t01-1-00020

Smith T (2006). Welfare, enterprise, and Aboriginal community: the case of the Western Australian Kimberley region, 1968–1996. *Australian Economic History Review* 46(3):242–67. doi.org/10.1111/j.1467-8446.2006.00180.x

Smyth AW (2013). *Physical deterioration: its causes and the cure,* Forgotten Books, London, original work published 1904.

Social Development Committee of the South Australian Parliament (2014). *Inquiry into the sale and consumption of alcohol*, 36th report of the Social Development Committee, Legislative Council of South Australia, Adelaide.

Solomon R & Payne J (1996). *Alcohol liability in Canada and Australia: sell, serve and be sued*, National Centre for Research into Prevention of Drug Abuse, Curtin University, Perth.

Sournia J-C (1990). *A history of alcoholism,* Basil Blackwell, Oxford.

Spicer P (1997). Toward a (dys)functional anthropology of drinking: ambivalence and the American Indian experience with alcohol. *Medical Anthropology Quarterly* 11(3):306–23. doi.org/10.1525/maq.1997.11.3.306

Stanley O (1985). *The mission and Peppimenarti: an economic study of two Daly River Aboriginal communities,* North Australia Research Unit, Darwin.

Stanner WEH (1979). *White man got no dreaming: essays 1938–1973,* Australian National University Press, Canberra.

Stark J (2008). Liquor advice too severe: industry. *The Age*, 22 January 2008:7.

Stead J (1980). Under the influence: a comparison of drinking in two Australian Aboriginal societies, BA(Hons) thesis, The Australian National University, Canberra.

Stockwell T & Crosbie D (2001). Supply and demand for alcohol in Australia: relationships between industry structures, regulation and the marketplace. *International Journal of Drug Policy*, 12:139–152.

Strickler DP, Bigelow G, Lawrence C & Liebson I (1976). Moderate drinking as an alternative to alcohol abuse: a non-aversive procedure. *Behavior Research and Therapy* 14:279–88. doi.org/10.1016/0005-7967(76)90003-6

Strickler DP, Bradlyn AS & Maxwell WA (1981). Teaching moderate drinking behaviors to young adult heavy drinkers: the effects of three training procedures, *Addictive Behaviors* 6:355–64. doi.org/10.1016/0306-4603(81)90051-4

Strutt J (2007a). ASIC must investigate profits from Fitzroy Crossing pub. *The West Australian*, 27 July 2007.

Strutt J (2007b). Fitzroy pub sales total $4m a year, coroner told. *ABC Friday West*, 23 November 2007.

Subcommittee of the Education and Health Standing Committee (2010). *Inquiry into the adequacy and appropriateness of prevention and treatment services for alcohol and illicit drug problems in Western Australia*, Transcript of evidence taken at Fitzroy Crossing, 29 July 2010, Parliament of Western Australia.

Sullivan P (1996). *All free man now: culture, community and politics in the Kimberley region, North Western Australia,* Aboriginal Studies Press, Canberra.

Sweatman J (1977). *The Journal of John Sweatman: a nineteenth century surveying voyage in North Australia and the Torres Strait,* eds Allen J & Corris P, University of Queensland Press, Brisbane.

Sydney Gazette (1813). Obituary, Bennelong, 9 January 1813.

Symons Rev GJ (1974). Submission by United Church in North Australia to the Inquiry into Sale and Consumption of Intoxicating Liquors, House of Representatives Standing Committee on Aboriginal Affairs, Transcript Nhulunbuy, 2 August 1974.

Symons GJ, Albrecht P & Long JPM (1963). *Report of 1961 Missions/ Administration Conference Sub-committee on Alcohol Problems*, Northern Territory Administration, Darwin.

Talbot P (2015). Disinterested management: an early example of corporate social responsibility (CSR). *International Journal of Social Science Studies* 3(5):26–32. doi.org/10.11114/ijsss.v3i5.960

Tangentyere Council (1991). Submission concerning the distribution of alcohol in Central Australia, Submission to the Human Rights and Equal Opportunity Commission, January 1991.

Tangentyere Council (1998). *Tyeweretye Club, 2 km law and public drinking*, August 1998, mimeo.

Taylor J (2004). *Social indicators for Aboriginal governance: insights from the Thamarrurr region, Northern Territory*, Centre for Aboriginal Economic Policy Monograph no 24, The Australian National University, Canberra.

Taylor J (2008). Counting the cost: Stanner and the Port Keats/Wadeye population. In Hinkson M & Beckett J (eds), *An appreciation of difference: WEH Stanner and Aboriginal Australia*, Aboriginal Studies Press, Canberra:217–30.

Taylor J (2010). *Demography as destiny: schooling, work and Aboriginal population change at Wadeye*, Centre for Aboriginal Economic Policy Research Working Paper no 64, The Australian National University, Canberra.

Taylor P (2007). Flood of beer in Fitzroy Crossing. *The Australian*, 29 September 2007.

Tench W (1996). *1788: comprising a narrative of the expedition to Botany Bay and a complete account of the settlement at Port Jackson*, ed Tim Flannery, Text Publishing Company, Melbourne.

Tennant Times (2000). Kava seized at Avon Downs, 30 June 2000:3.

Territory Health Services (nd). The Kava Management Act: what does it mean? [Pamphlet].

Thom B (1999). *Dealing with drink: alcohol and social policy from treatment to management*, Free Association Books, London and New York.

Thorburn K (2011). 'Indigenous governance' and Aboriginal political practice: the gulf between two organisations in the Fitzroy Valley, West Kimberley, PhD thesis, The Australian National University, Canberra.

Tilmouth W (2001). Reference: needs of urban dwelling Aboriginal and Torres Strait Islander people, House of Representatives Standing Committee on Aboriginal Affairs, Hansard 1 May 2001.

Tondorf C (1993a). Tyweretye licence to help grog fight: Maley. *Centralian Advocate*, 2 April 1993:2.

Tondorf C (1993b). Aboriginal women call on CM to reduce liquor outlets. *Centralian Advocate*, 27 April 1993:3.

Trewartha S (1999). *The Ceduna Foreshore Hotel: '… the view across the bay'*, Ceduna Community Hotel, Ceduna.

Troy J (1994). *The Sydney language,* Australian Institute of Aboriginal and Torres Strait Islander Studies, Canberra.

Tyeweretye Clubs Inc. (1999). *Tyeweretye constitution* [Pamphlet], Alice Springs.

UNCA (United Church in North Australia) (1974). *Free to decide: the United Church in North Australia Commission of Enquiry, Arnhem Land*, United Church in North Australia, Darwin.

Vangopoulos K (2014). NT Licensing Commission to be replaced in favour of new licensing authority. *Northern Territory News*, 18 June 2014.

von Hugel C (1994). *New Holland Journal, November 1833 – October 1834,* Melbourne University Press, Melbourne.

Walker J (1995). Dreamtime. *The Australian Magazine*, 6–7 May 1995:12–17.

Wallace AR (1989). *The Malay Archipelago*, Oxford University Press, Singapore.

Walsh N (2005). *Review of Centacare NT Alcohol and other Drug Services provided to the Tiwi Islands and Wadeye*, mimeo.

Warner J (2006). Are you a closet Fabian? Licensing schemes then and now [Editorial]. *Addiction* 101:909–10. doi.org/10.1111/j.1360-0443.2006.01499.x

Warner WL (1957). *A black civilization: a social study of an Australian tribe,* Harper and Brothers.

Watson C, Fleming J & Alexander K (1988). *A survey of drug use patterns in Northern Territory Aboriginal communities: 1986–1987,* Northern Territory Department of Health and Community Services, Drug and Alcohol Bureau, Darwin.

Watson DW & Sobell MB (1982). Social influence on alcohol consumption by black and white males. *Addictive Behaviors* 7:87–91. doi.org/10.1016/0306-4603(82)90031-4

Wauchope L (1975). *40 gallons a head: alcohol in Alice,* a report for the Regional Council for Social Development, Alice Springs.

Wearne B (2001). An evaluation of the Miwatj Health Aboriginal Corporation outreach program, BMedSci thesis, Monash University, Victoria.

Weekend Australian (2000). Light justice in outback community, 4–5 November 2000:1–2.

Welborn S (1987). *Swan. The history of a brewery,* University of Western Australia Press, Perth.

Wells S, Graham K, Purcell J (2009). The widespread practice of 'predrinking' or 'pregaming' before going on to public establishments. *Addiction* 104:4–9. doi.org/10.1111/j.1360-0443.2008.02393.x

The West Australian (2014). Venturex settles sale of Whim Creek pub, 3 July 2014.

Western Australian Department of Health (2009). *From death we learn,* Office of Safety and Quality in Healthcare, Department of Health, East Perth.

Westman D (1989). High hopes for Liquor Commission. *Katherine Weekend Advertiser,* 8 July 1989.

Whimpress B (nd). *Corroboree: Adelaide Oval 1885,* Adelaide Oval Museum, Kent Town, Adelaide.

Whitaker A (1933). *Bacchus behave! The lost art of polite drinking,* Frederick A. Stokes Company, New York.

Whitelock D (1985). *Adelaide: from colony to Jubilee: a sense of difference*, Savvas Publishing, Adelaide.

Williams M (1990). A dream turned nightmare for Australia's Aborigines—Group here for convention laments the loss of spiritualism to alcoholism. *The Seattle Times*, 2 July 1990.

Willis J (2002). *Potent brews: a social history of alcohol in East Africa 1850–1999*, James Currey, Oxford.

Wilson F (1946). Community hotels: an address on Station 2CH (24 March) by Francis Wilson for the N.S.W. Temperance Alliance. *The Methodist*, 30 March 1946:1–2.

Wilson JM (1894). The Scandinavian plan [of regulating the liquor trade]: a sermon preached on Temperance Sunday, 18 November 1894 [LSE selected pamphlets], www.jstor.org/stable/60222451.

Worgan GB (1978). *Journal of a First Fleet surgeon,* Library Council of New South Wales, Sydney.

Wright A (1997). *Grog war,* Magabala Books, Broome.

Young PF & Secker AJ (1984). *Review of South Australian liquor licensing laws,* South Australia, Adelaide.

Zagar C (2000). *Goodbye riverbank: the Barwon-Namoi people tell their story,* Magabala Books, Broome.

Zinberg NE (1984). *Drug, set and setting: the basis for controlled intoxicant use,* Yale University Press, New Haven and London.

Index

Note: page numbers in *italics* indicate tables, figures or other illustrative material. Footnotes are indicated by page numbers in the form '3n5', this example meaning footnote 5 on page 3.

supports Aboriginal hotel
purchases, 59, 147, 181,
184n16, 185, 187, 189, *202*
Woden Town Club, 190–1
permit systems, 24n39, 39, 113
see also drinking rights
philanthropy, 5
Phillip, Arthur, 8, 9, 10
Pitjantjatjara Council, 161n40, 193,
205n44, 206
Pitjantjatjara lands *see* Anangu
Pitjantjatjara Yankunytjatjara
lands
Pitjantjatjara people, 18, 137, 144,
148, 160–1, 163, 168, 169, 191
poker machines, 54, 146, 151–2,
167, 189, 190, 197
politeness *see* etiquette
politics
of alcohol availability through
clubs, 99–100
local political struggles, 101–2
Port Keats *see* Wadeye (Port Keats),
NT
Port Sunlight, 5
port (wine) *see* fortified wine
Presbyterian missions, 78, 80–1 *see
also* United Church in Northern
Australia
Prime Minister's Department Office
of Aboriginal Affairs, 73
problem drinking *see* alcohol
problems; alcohol-related harm;
alcoholism treatment
profits from alcohol
beer canteens, 88–9, 98–9
community hotels, 48, 49, 50, 51,
54–6, 64
debates over, 50
distribution to community, 65
elimination of, 36–7 *see also*
Gothenburg system
Renmark Community Hotel, 48,
50, 51

prohibition in Australia
for Indigenous Australians, xvii,
24, 29, 259, 261
Indigenous Australians' exemption
certificates, 24n39, 68,
179–80
for Indigenous Australians, repeal
of, 5–6, 25, 29–30, 69–70
Leedal's use of term, 247
local prohibition, xvii–xviii, 5, 29,
43–6, 163n45, 261
spatial constraints, 141–2,
163n45
see also abstinence; drinking rights
prohibition in US, xvii, 1
Protestant missions, 77–81, *82–3*
public houses *see* hotels
Pukatja (Ernabella), SA, 69, 74, 81

Quakers, 5, 77
capitalists, 5, 8n13, 19, 40–1
Queensland
beer canteens, 70, 82–3, 88–9,
93, 95n53, 99

random breath testing, 25n40
rationing
of alcohol, xviii, 6, 30, 39, 86, 91,
93–4, 95, 97, 112, 128, 194,
195, 197
of food, 86
recreational time, notion of, 4
Renmark Community Hotel, 44–8,
50, 51, 53n21, 54
Renmark, SA, 29, 43–8, 53, 203
rights *see* civil rights; drinking rights
rituals of drinking *see* toasting rituals
Riverland region, SA, 29, 43–9, 53,
203–4
Room, Robin, 20, 30, 169, 263
Rowley, Charles, 68, 96
Rowntree, Joseph, 5, 40–1, 47

Wadeye (Port Keats), NT, xix, 74n16, 81, 107, 108, *108*, 110, 129–31, 136 *see also* Murrinh Patha Social Club

Walgett, NSW, 180–1
Oasis Hotel, 175, 180, 181, 185–6, 190, *202*, 204, 209

Walkabout Hotel, Nhulunbuy, 73n12, 182

Walker, Kath, 29

Warlpiri people, 144, 161, 163, 168, 169

Wayside Inn, Timber Creek, NT, 175, 196–201, *202*, 208

wayside inns, 199–200, 212

Welfare Branch (NT), 72, 74, 78

wet canteens *see* beer clubs/canteens in Aboriginal communities

Whim Creek Hotel, Pilbara, WA, 175, *202*

Whitaker, Alma, 1–2, 29, 31

Whitlam government, 73, 183

wine
choices of Aboriginal people, 32
'civilised' status of, 4, 12
civilising influence of, 7–13
cultivation of, 12–13
fortified, 24n39, 32, 54, 109, 188, *202*, 225
offered to Indigenous people, 6–9
sales of, 25
toasting with, 9–12

Woden Town Club, Canberra, ACT, xix, 175, 189–91, *202*

Woman's Christian Temperance Union (WCTU), xvii, 189, 263
on alcohol education for Aboriginal people, 70
on effect of drinking on women and children, 162
offices, Adelaide, *52*
opposition to community licences, 50–3, 263
pamphlet, *71*

Women against Alcohol movement, 160–2, 217–18, 229
march, Alice Springs, 137, 161–2, *162*
see also Aboriginal women

women and children
adverse effects of alcohol and drinking, 105, 118n27, 119, 132, 137, 157, 162n43

women's activism, xx, 29, 52, 136–8, 160–2, 217, 229, 263, 264

Yalata, SA, *79*, 80, 83, 92–3, 97n54, 98n56, 104, 185

Yapawarnti Fund Inc., 240, 254n60

Yirrkala, NT, 17, 34, 62–3, 73n12, 182

Yolngu people, 17, 23, 34, 61

Zinberg, Norman, 90–1

CAEPR Research
Monograph Series

1. *Aborigines in the economy: a select annotated bibliography of policy relevant research 1985–90*, LM Allen, JC Altman and E Owen (with assistance from WS Arthur), 1991.

2. *Aboriginal employment equity by the year 2000*, JC Altman (ed.), published for the Academy of Social Sciences in Australia, 1991.

3. *A national survey of Indigenous Australians: options and implications*, JC Altman (ed.), 1992.

4. *Indigenous Australians in the economy: abstracts of research, 1991–92*, LM Roach and KA Probst, 1993.

5. *The relative economic status of Indigenous Australians, 1986–91*, J Taylor, 1993.

6. *Regional change in the economic status of Indigenous Australians, 1986–91*, J Taylor, 1993.

7. *Mabo and native title: origins and institutional implications*, W Sanders (ed.), 1994.

8. *The housing need of Indigenous Australians, 1991*, R Jones, 1994.

9. *Indigenous Australians in the economy: abstracts of research, 1993–94*, LM Roach and HJ Bek, 1995.

10. *The native title era: emerging issues for research, policy, and practice*, J Finlayson and DE Smith (eds), 1995.

11. *The 1994 National Aboriginal and Torres Strait Islander Survey: findings and future prospects*, JC Altman and J Taylor (eds), 1996.

12. *Fighting over country: anthropological perspectives*, DE Smith and J Finlayson (eds), 1997.

13. *Connections in native title: genealogies, kinship, and groups*, JD Finlayson, B Rigsby and HJ Bek (eds), 1999.

14. *Land rights at risk? Evaluations of the Reeves Report*, JC Altman, F Morphy and T Rowse (eds), 1999.

15. *Unemployment payments, the activity test, and Indigenous Australians: understanding breach rates*, W Sanders, 1999.

16. *Why only one in three? The complex reasons for low Indigenous school retention*, RG Schwab, 1999.

17. *Indigenous families and the welfare system: two community case studies*, DE Smith (ed.), 2000.

18. *Ngukurr at the millennium: a baseline profile for social impact planning in south-east Arnhem Land*, J Taylor, J Bern and KA Senior, 2000.

19. *Aboriginal nutrition and the Nyirranggulung Health Strategy in Jawoyn country*, J Taylor and N Westbury, 2000.

20. *The Indigenous welfare economy and the CDEP scheme*, F Morphy and W Sanders (eds), 2001.

21. *Health expenditure, income and health status among Indigenous and other Australians*, MC Gray, BH Hunter and J Taylor, 2002.

22. *Making sense of the census: observations of the 2001 enumeration in remote Aboriginal Australia*, DF Martin, F Morphy, WG Sanders and J Taylor, 2002.

23. *Aboriginal population profiles for development planning in the northern East Kimberley*, J Taylor, 2003.

24. *Social indicators for Aboriginal governance: insights from the Thamarrurr region, Northern Territory*, J Taylor, 2004.

25. *Indigenous people and the Pilbara mining boom: a baseline for regional participation*, J Taylor and B Scambary, 2005.

26. *Assessing the evidence on Indigenous socioeconomic outcomes: a focus on the 2002 NATSISS*, BH Hunter (ed.), 2006.

27. *The social effects of native title: recognition, translation, coexistence*, BR Smith and F Morphy (eds), 2007.

28. *Agency, contingency and census process: observations of the 2006 Indigenous Enumeration Strategy in remote Aboriginal Australia*, F Morphy (ed.), 2008.

29. *Contested governance: culture, power and institutions in Indigenous Australia*, J Hunt, D Smith, S Garling and W Sanders (eds), 2008.

30. *Power, culture, economy: Indigenous Australians and mining*, J Altman and D Martin (eds), 2009.

31. *Demographic and socioeconomic outcomes across the Indigenous Australian lifecourse*, N Biddle and M Yap, 2010.

32. *Survey analysis for Indigenous policy in Australia: social science perspectives*, B Hunter and N Biddle (eds), 2012.

33. *My Country, mine country: Indigenous people, mining and development contestation in remote Australia*, B Scambary, 2013.

34. *Indigenous Australians and the National Disability Insurance Scheme*, N Biddle, F Al-Yaman, M Gourley, M Gray, JR Bray, B Brady, LA Pham, E Williams and M Montaigne, 2014.

35. *Engaging Indigenous economy: debating diverse approaches*, W Sanders (ed.), 2016.

36. *Better than welfare? Work and livelihoods for Indigenous Australians after CDEP*, K Jordan (ed.), 2016.

37. *Reluctant representatives: blackfella bureaucrats speak in Australia's north*, E Ganter, 2016.

38. *Indigenous data sovereignty: toward an agenda*, T Kukutai and J Taylor (eds), 2016.

Centre for Aboriginal Economic Policy Research,
College of Arts and Social Sciences,
The Australian National University, Canberra, ACT, 2601

Information on CAEPR Discussion Papers, Working Papers and Research Monographs (Nos 1–19) and abstracts and summaries of all CAEPR print publications and those published electronically can be found at the following website: caepr.anu.edu.au.

www.ingramcontent.com/pod-product-compliance
Lightning Source LLC
Chambersburg PA
CBHW050806270326
41926CB00026B/4585